~~FIONA. E. SINCLAIR~~

J. Totten

13–38

85 – 91

17th June – Exam.

Pages

74 – 85

139 – 140

173 – 193

Figures	page 133	64	78
	140	65	80
	180	69	83
	185	75	
	189	76+77	

OXFORD MEDICAL PUBLICATIONS

CUNNINGHAM'S MANUAL OF PRACTICAL ANATOMY

CUNNINGHAM'S MANUAL OF PRACTICAL ANATOMY

THIRTEENTH EDITION

REVISED BY

G. J. ROMANES, *C.B.E.*

B.A., PH.D., M.B., CH.B., F.R.C.S.ED., F.R.S.E.

Professor of Anatomy in the University of Edinburgh

VOLUME II

THORAX AND ABDOMEN

LONDON

OXFORD UNIVERSITY PRESS

NEW YORK BOMBAY

Oxford University Press, Ely House, London W. 1

GLASGOW NEW YORK TORONTO MELBOURNE WELLINGTON
CAPE TOWN IBADAN NAIROBI DAR ES SALAAM LUSAKA ADDIS ABABA
DELHI BOMBAY CALCUTTA MADRAS KARACHI LAHORE DACCA
KUALA LUMPUR SINGAPORE HONG KONG TOKYO

ISBN 0 19 263122 5

Dissector's Guide 1879
Manual of Practical Anatomy 1889
Present Series
First Edition 1893
Thirteenth Edition 1968
Reprinted 1969, 1972 and 1973

Printed in Great Britain by R. & R. Clark, Ltd., Edinburgh

CONTENTS

PREFACE
TO THE THIRTEENTH EDITION

This volume has been rewritten in keeping with the principles set out in the Preface to Volume I. The over-all length has been reduced considerably to meet the needs of the shortened curricula which have been or are about to be introduced in many medical schools. This has been done without the sacrifice of any material which is essential to a proper understanding of the gross anatomy of the thorax and abdomen; indeed several new subjects have been introduced, including some elementary notes on the embryology and histology of those organs and systems in which the structure or function are made more readily intelligible by their inclusion.

The total number of changes is considerable, but only the major alterations are mentioned here.

It has long been felt that the usual method of dissection of the heart tends to distort the relations of its parts to each other and increases the difficulty of visualizing the heart and great vessels as they lie within the thorax in the living. A new dissection has been devised which demonstrates all parts of the heart *in situ* and permits the student to see the position of these parts in relation to each other and to the anterior thoracic wall throughout the dissection. It also gives a clearer demonstration of the course taken by the blood through the right and left sides of the heart and of the relative position of the atria to each other and to the structures posterior to them.

The dissection of the pelvis and perineum raises a number of difficulties for the student. It is not possible to obtain an ideal exposure of all parts of these important structures in a single specimen, so it has been decided to base the dissection of the pelvis on a median section. Inevitably this sacrifices the complete exposure of the levator ani muscles as a unit, but it gives the student a clearer picture of the structures in the pelvis which may be examined by rectal or vaginal examination, and leaves intact the structures on the lateral walls of the pelvis and in the proximal parts of the lower limbs.

The descriptions of the male and female pelvis are treated together. This method highlights the similarities and differences in the two sexes, and lessens the tendency of the student to concentrate on the arrangement in his own specimen to the exclusion of that in the opposite sex.

More than forty entirely new illustrations and explanatory diagrams have been added. These and the remaining illustrations, which have all been redrawn and modified where necessary, are the work of Miss M. Benstead, Mrs. C. Clarke, and Mr. R. N. Lane to whose skilful assistance the new edition owes so much. The radiographs have been replaced by a new series which, it is hoped, will prove more useful to the student.

It is a pleasure to acknowledge the indebtedness of this edition to Dr. H. S. Barrett for her continuing help with the reading of the manuscript and proofs, and to the Medical Department of the Oxford University Press for their tolerance in dealing with editorial foibles and for their careful attention to every detail throughout the preparation of all three volumes.

EDINBURGH
October 1967

G. J. Romanes

THE THORAX

INTRODUCTION

The thorax is that part of the trunk which extends from the root of the neck to the abdomen. It contains the lungs, separated by a thick but movable median septum (the **mediastinum**). The heart, and the great vessels connecting it with the body and lungs, lie in the mediastinum which transmits the oesophagus (gullet), the sympathetic trunks, and the vagus nerves from the neck to the abdomen, the trachea (windpipe) to the lungs, and the phrenic nerves to the diaphragm.

Movements of the thorax are primarily concerned with increasing and decreasing intrathoracic pressure so that air is alternately expelled from the lungs (expiration) through trachea, larynx (voice box), pharynx (throat) and nasal cavities, and drawn into the lungs through the same passages (inspiration). The walls of the thorax are strengthened to allow these movements and to resist the tendency of the atmospheric pressure to compress them when the internal pressure is lowered during inspiration. The strengthening is achieved by the presence of the sternum (breast bone) and of the ribs with their anterior extensions, the costal cartilages. Each rib and its costal cartilage is joined to the adjacent members by sheets of muscle which not only move the ribs and costal cartilages, but also make the spaces between them rigid so that these spaces do not move out and in with changes in intrathoracic pressure.

Shape and Framework of Thorax

The thorax is the shape of a truncated cone which tapers superiorly to the root of the neck and expands inferiorly to surround the superior part of the abdominal cavity from which the cavity of the thorax is separated by the dome-shaped diaphragm. The thorax is flattened anteroposteriorly to accommodate the scapulae on its posterolateral aspects and to give attachment to the powerful muscles of the upper limb which overlap the thorax.

Each **rib** articulates with the vertebral column posteriorly, and sweeps round the trunk from this articulation, passing obliquely downwards to its anterior extremity, to which a costal cartilage is fused.

The **costal cartilages** are flexible extensions of the ribs. The upper cartilages continue the sweep of the ribs to the sternum. The lower members become progressively more angulated, the anterior part passing superiorly either to reach and articulate with the sternum (the upper seven or true ribs), or to articulate with the upturned part of the cartilage above (eighth to tenth or false ribs), or to end blindly (eleventh and twelfth or floating ribs). These articulations of the costal cartilages and of the ribs with the vertebral column are synovial joints, and together with the flexible costal cartilages constitute the sites at which respiratory movements take place. The first costal cartilage differs from the others in being fused to the upper part (**manubrium**) of the sternum, and is frequently calcified or even ossified. Thus the manubrium of the sternum and first ribs tend to move as one piece around the articulation of these ribs with the vertebral column, while there is more independent movement of the other ribs, especially the false and floating ribs.

The ribs inferior to the seventh become progressively shorter, and fail to reach as far anteriorly, their upturned cartilages forming the diverging **costal margins** which sweep downwards, laterally and backwards from the sternum [FIG. 2]. Because of this, the

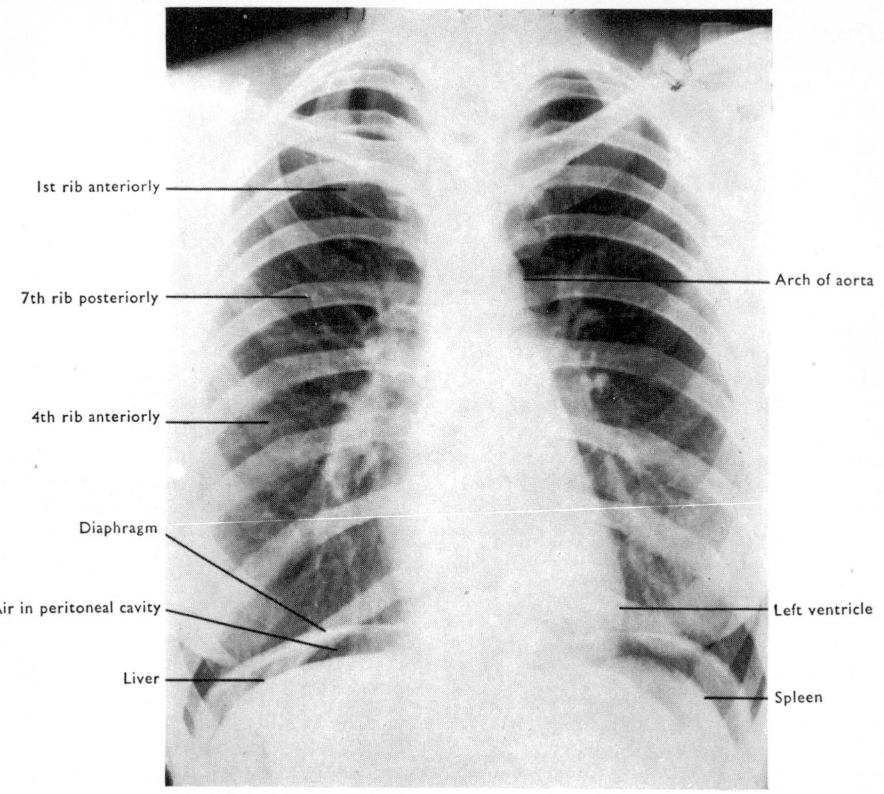

FIG. 1 An anteroposterior radiograph of the thorax in a patient with air in the peritoneal cavity. The air outlines the inferior surface of the diaphragm.

anterior wall of the thorax is much shorter than the lateral or posterior walls. Thus the inferior end of the sternum lies approximately opposite the ninth thoracic vertebra, while the lowest part of the costal margin (eleventh costal cartilage in the mid-axillary line) lies at the level of the third lumbar vertebra close to the iliac crest [FIG. 2], and may even touch the iliac crest in elderly individuals.

In transverse section, the thorax is kidney-shaped because the vertebral bodies project anteriorly into it, leaving a deep **paravertebral groove** on each side formed by the backward sweep of the posterior parts of the ribs. The posterior parts of the lungs lie in the paravertebral grooves, while the mediastinum lies for the most part anterior to the vertebral bodies [FIG. 3].

SURFACE ANATOMY

All the structures which lie in the thorax are mobile to a greater or lesser degree and undergo changes in position during respiratory movements, but these changes are relatively slight compared with movements which can take place in certain pathological conditions the diagnosis of which depends partly on the demonstration of an abnormal displacement of the thoracic contents. Thus, if one lung collapses, the mediastinum is shifted to that side carrying the heart with it. This may be demonstrated readily, provided the normal relationship between the thoracic contents and the thoracic wall is known. It is important therefore to know and be able to demonstrate the surface features of the thorax both from in front and from behind, so that later when the contents are dissected their position relative to these features may be understood.

The superior margin of the sternum (**jugular notch**) is easily felt between the medial ends of the clavicles in the midline. A finger drawn downwards from the notch in the midline passes downwards and slightly forwards for about 5 cm. over the superior part (**manubrium**) of the sternum, and then over a marked angulation (the sternal angle) on to the more vertical **body of the sternum**. The body ends inferiorly in the angle between the costal margins by becoming continuous with the flexible **xiphoid process** which extends into the upper part of the anterior abdominal wall in the midline.

The **sternal angle** is an important landmark. The **second costal cartilage** joins the lateral margin of the sternum at this level, and can be felt through the pectoralis major muscle lateral to the angle. Even in obese individuals it is possible to identify the sternal angle and to find the second costal cartilage from it; the lower ribs may then be identified by counting downwards from the second costal cartilage. The sternal angle lies opposite the disc between the fourth and fifth thoracic vertebrae, while the jugular notch lies opposite the disc between the second and third. These and other levels which are mentioned in the text are approximate only, and apply to the young adult. In old age the sternum tends to sag to a lower level, and the relative positions of sternum and vertebral column are greatly

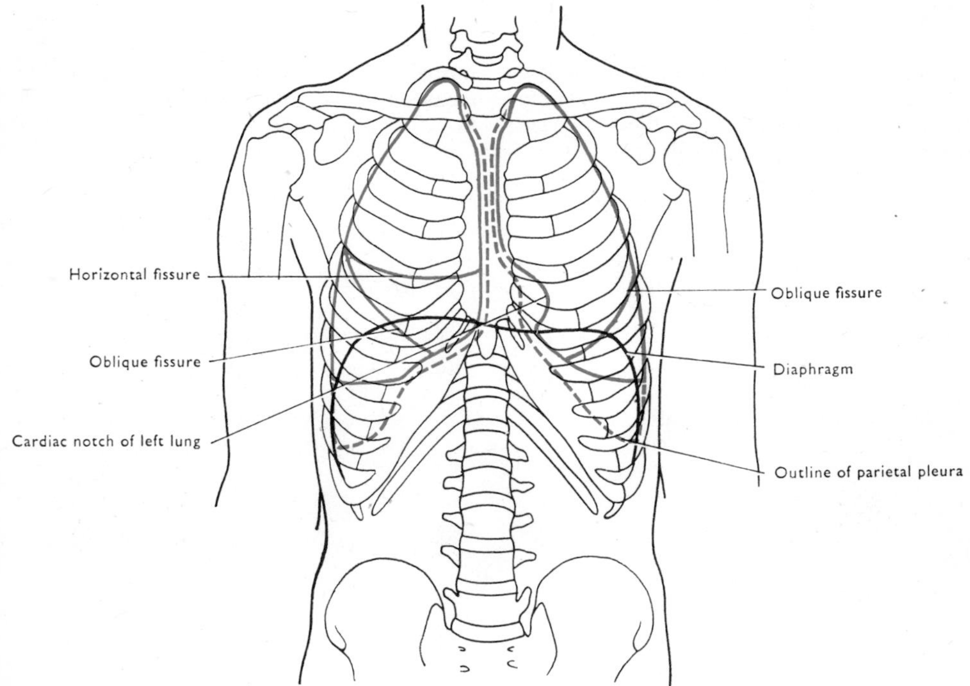

FIG. 2 The anterior aspect of the trunk to show the position of the lungs (blue stipple) and their fissures (solid blue lines), the pleural sacs (broken blue lines), and the diaphragm.

disturbed by pathological curvatures of the vertebral column, by disease of the lungs, and by dilatation of the heart.

The **first rib** is hidden from view by the clavicle, but may be felt as a deep resistance if a finger is pressed inferiorly in the supraclavicular fossa posterior to the medial one third of the clavicle.

The lateral surfaces of the ribs may be palpated; the superior ribs by pressing the fingers upwards into the axilla with the arm by the side to relax the fascia of the axillary floor. The posterior surfaces of the ribs are partly covered by the scapulae, and medially are hidden by the long muscles of the back (**erector spinae**). The **twelfth rib** may be so short that it scarcely appears lateral to the erector spinae, or it may almost reach the iliac crest.

All the thoracic **vertebral spines** are palpable; the first is the lower of two knobs at the root of the back of the neck (the upper is the **vertebra prominens**, the spine of the seventh cervical vertebra); the **third** lies midway between the roots of the spines of the scapulae; the **seventh** is midway between the inferior angles of the scapulae with the arms by the sides. All the thoracic spines slope obliquely downwards so that their palpable tips lie below the bodies from which they arise, those of the middle of the series are the most oblique.

The **nipple** is very inconstant in position, especially in the female, but often overlies the fourth intercostal space approximately 10 cm. from the median plane in the adult male.

LUNGS

The lungs (pulmones) are a pair of sponge-like, elastic organs which fill the greater part of the cavity of the chest. They consist of a myriad (approximately 300×10^6) of minute, air filled cavities (**alveoli**) which are connected by a branching tubular system (**bronchi** and **bronchioles**) to the windpipe. The interalveolar walls are very thin, and are formed of a layer of blood capillaries interspersed with **elastic fibres** and some connective tissue cells, sandwiched between two layers of flattened epithelium continuous with the lining of the bronchial tree. In many places this flattened epithelium is only separated from the capillary endothelium by a thin layer of structureless material (basement membrane) and the whole thickness of tissue separating blood from air is often as little as 0·002 mm. The over-all surface area of the alveolar walls is approximately seventy square metres, and through this enormous surface gaseous exchange occurs between blood circulating through the pulmonary capillaries and the air in the alveoli which is changed as a result of respiratory movements.

The lungs are separated by a broad, median septum (the **mediastinum**) which extends from the posterior aspect of the sternum to the anterior surface of the vertebral column. The medial surface of each lung is attached to the mediastinum by a narrow root through which bronchi, blood and lymphatic vessels, and

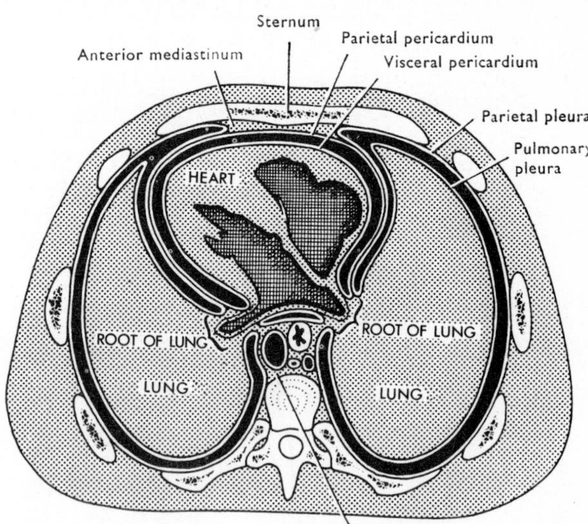

FIG. 3 A diagrammatic horizontal section through the thorax to show the positions of the major structures in it. The pleural and pericardial cavities are shown in black.

nerves enter and leave the lung. Elsewhere the lung lies free in the thoracic cavity, surrounded by a narrow space (the **pleural cavity**) which separates the lung from the internal surface of the thoracic wall **(parietes)** and from the parts of the mediastinum to which the root is not attached. This space is surrounded by a smooth, glistening membrane (the **pleura**) which lines the internal surface of the thoracic wall and covers the lateral surface of the mediastinum (**parietal pleura**) except at the lung root around which it is continuous with the pleura that covers the surfaces of the lung **(pulmonary pleura)**.

The pleural cavity contains a small quantity of thin serous fluid. This lubricates the apposed pleural surfaces and allows the lung and pulmonary pleura to slide freely over the parietal pleura during respiratory movements, thus equalizing the pressure changes throughout the cavity whichever part of the thoracic wall is moving.

The lungs, and the mediastinum between them, rest inferiorly on the **diaphragm.** This musculotendinous sheet separates the thoracic and abdominal cavities, and arches superiorly into the thorax from its attachments to the internal surfaces of the vertebral column, costal margins, and xiphoid process to reach as high as the eighth thoracic vertebra. It thus greatly decreases the vertical extent of the thoracic cavity, particularly in the midline anteriorly, and allows the upper abdominal contents to extend under cover of the ribs so that they are overlapped by the thoracic cage and lungs, especially on the posterior and lateral aspects. The diaphragmatic surface of each lung is deeply concave to fit the corresponding **dome of the diaphragm,** and the inferior margins are sharp where they extend downwards into the acute angle formed by the diaphragm passing to its attachment to the internal surface of the lower margin of the thoracic wall [FIG. 48]. Thus the thorax is fitted over the upper part of the abdominal cavity, and penetrating wounds of the lower thorax frequently involve the abdomen, the upper part of which is most easily approached by the surgeon through the pleural cavity and diaphragm.

APERTURES OF THORAX

Superiorly the thorax tapers to its **superior aperture** at the root of the neck. This is a

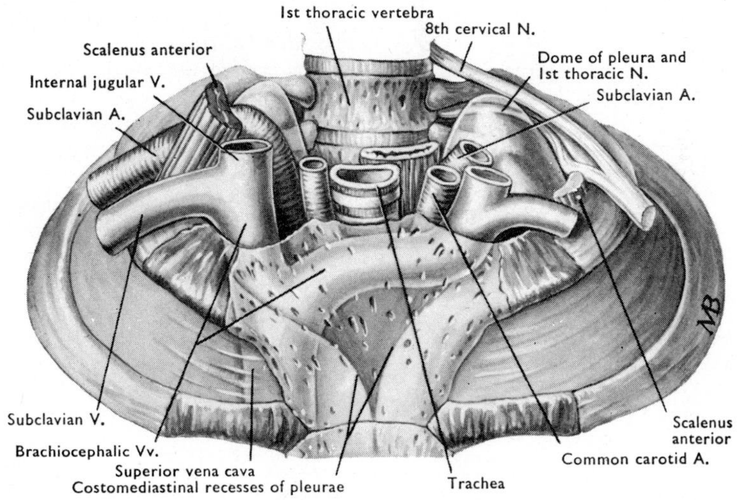

FIG. 4 The superior aperture of the thorax. The anterior margins (costomediastinal recesses) of the pleural sacs and the great veins are shown through the sternum. Cf. FIG. 16.

narrow opening (5 cm. anteroposteriorly) which is bounded by the body of the first thoracic vertebra, the first ribs and the superior border of the sternum. The margin of the aperture slopes steeply downwards and forwards, and thus the apex of each lung, which reaches superiorly to the neck of the first rib, projects above its costal cartilage [FIG. 4]. The superior aperture transmits the structures which pass between the thorax and the upper limbs and neck.

The **inferior aperture** is much larger, and slopes downwards and backwards following the curved costal margins from the xiphisternal joint to the tip of the twelfth rib, and then passes upwards along that rib to the twelfth thoracic vertebra. It is closed by the diaphragm which is pierced by the structures that pass between the mediastinum and the abdomen.

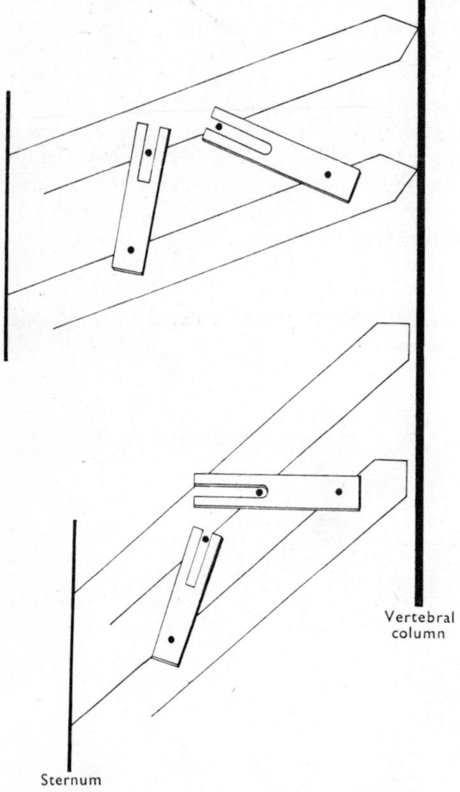

FIG. 5 A diagram to demonstrate that depression of the ribs decreases the anteroposterior diameter of the thorax. Note also that the internal intercostal muscle fibres are elongated in elevation of the ribs, while muscle fibres of the external intercostal muscle are shortened. The opposite occurs in depression of the ribs, *i.e.*, on expiration.

RESPIRATORY MOVEMENTS

These are dealt with more fully at a later stage, but it is important to have a general idea of the mechanism of respiration and to keep this in mind while dissecting the thoracic wall. Some of the features are shown diagrammatically in FIGURES 5 and 78. **Inspiration** is achieved by elevating the anterior parts of the ribs around the axis of their joints with the vertebral column. This increases the anteroposterior, transverse, and vertical diameters of the thorax, and thus reduces the intrathoracic pressure so that the tendency of the elastic lung to shrink down on to its root is overcome, and air flows into the lung, allowing it to expand. These movements are assisted by: (1) the contraction of the diaphragm which depresses the abdominal contents and increases the vertical extent of the thorax, and (2) by muscles of the posterior abdominal wall which hold down the lower ribs and thus make the elevation of the upper ribs more effective in increasing the vertical diameter of the thorax.

Expiration is mainly due to the elastic recoil of the lungs, but this is assisted by the weight of the thoracic cage, and in forced expiration can be facilitated by any muscles which depress the anterior parts of the ribs or increase the intra-abdominal pressure so as to force the relaxed diaphragm upwards into the thoracic cavity. In certain pathological conditions the elasticity of the lungs is lost and the thorax tends to remain permanently in a position of inspiration, thus causing great respiratory difficulty, particularly in expiration. The considerable **elasticity of the normal lung** is well shown by the fact that if a hollow needle is introduced into the pleural cavity through the thoracic wall, air will flow through it into the cavity even during expiration, and the lung

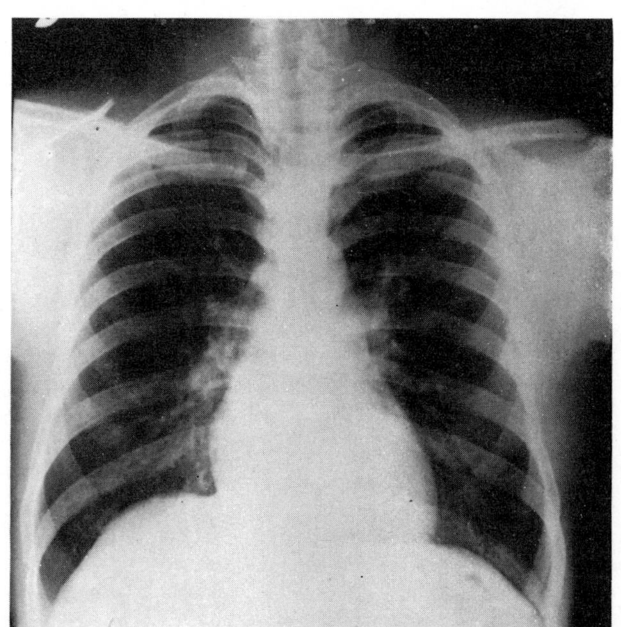

FIG. 6 An anteroposterior radiograph of the thorax in inspiration. Note that the right dome of the diaphragm lies below the level of the tenth rib posteriorly, and the outline of the diaphragm and the costodiaphragmatic recesses are clear owing to the air content in the lungs.

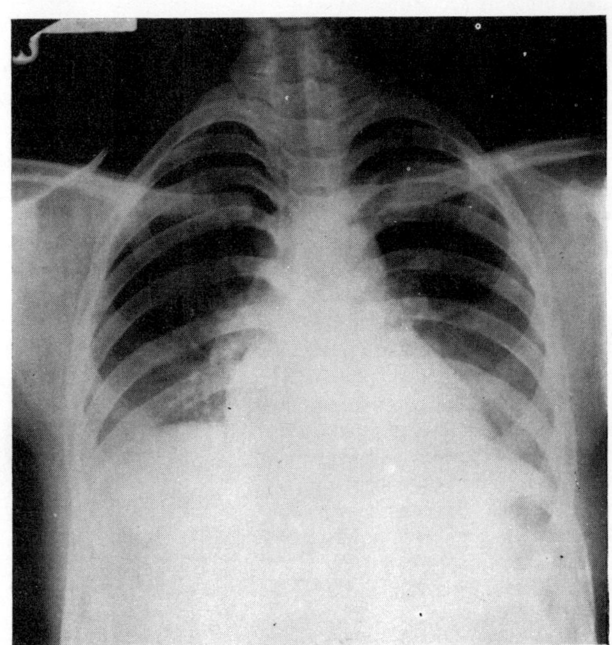

FIG. 7 An anteroposterior radiograph of the same individual as FIG. 6 but in expiration. Note that the right dome of the diaphragm reaches the level of the eighth rib posteriorly, and that the shadow of the diaphragm and costodiaphragmatic recesses are poorly defined because of the increased density of the basal parts of the lungs due to loss of air. Note also that the heart is shorter and broader in association with the raised diaphragm.

shrinks down on to its root until it is a mere fraction of its normal size. This shrinkage is caused by contraction of the elastic tissue in the lung unopposed by the normal negative pressure in the pleural cavity which is maintained by the rigidity of the thoracic wall.

THE WALLS OF THE THORAX

SUPERFICIAL STRUCTURES

The upper limbs having been dissected before the thorax, only remnants of muscles, nerves, and blood vessels will be found, but these should be identified as far as possible.

Anteriorly. (1) The **pectoralis major** is attached to the sternum and the cartilages of the upper six ribs. It is pierced at the sternal ends of the intercostal spaces by the anterior cutaneous branches of the ventral rami (**intercostal nerves;** FIG. 10) of the corresponding thoracic nerves (except the first which has no such branch) accompanied by the perforating branches of the internal thoracic artery. (2) The **rectus abdominis** is attached to the xiphoid process and the cartilages of the seventh to fifth ribs. (3) The **pectoralis minor** is attached to the third to fifth ribs near their cartilages.

Laterally. (1) The **serratus anterior** is attached to the upper eight ribs along a curved line on the side of the thorax. Its lower four attachments interdigitate with the upper four attachments of the **obliquus externus abdominis.** (2) The lateral cutaneous branches of the ventral rami of the thoracic nerves (except the first) emerge between the digitations of the serratus anterior and of obliquus externus a little anterior to the mid-axillary line [FIG. 89].

Posteriorly. The cutaneous branches of the dorsal rami will have been removed by the dissectors of the upper limb. The remnants of trapezius, the rhomboids, and latissimus dorsi may be seen, and the cut ends of the nerves may be visible as they pass through the thoracolumbar fascia.

DISSECTION. Remove the remains of serratus anterior and the pectoral muscles from the upper ribs, but retain the cutaneous branches of the intercostal

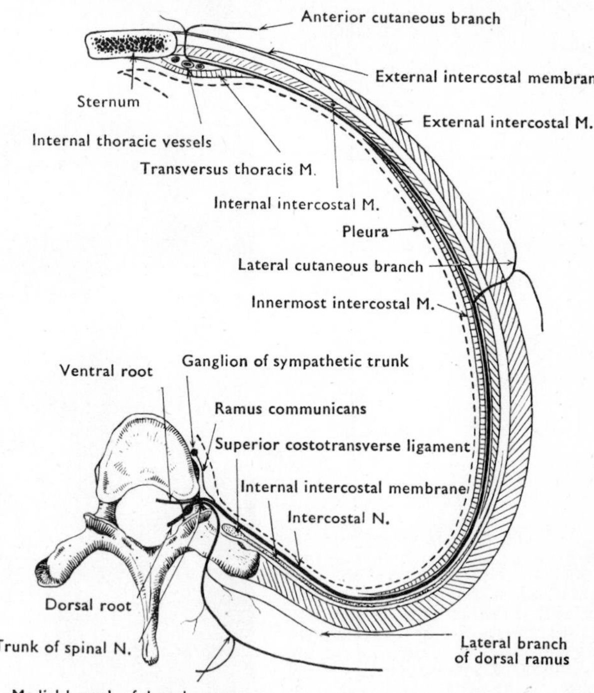

FIG. 8 A diagram of an upper thoracic spinal nerve in an intercostal space.

nerves. Clean the external intercostal muscle in one or two of the spaces between the ribs, and follow it anteriorly to the external intercostal membrane which replaces it between the costal cartilages.

INTERCOSTAL MUSCLES AND MEMBRANES

Each intercostal space contains two layers of muscle (the external and internal intercostal muscles) and an incomplete third layer, internal to both, which consists of three muscles: transversus thoracis, subcostals, and the innermost intercostals.

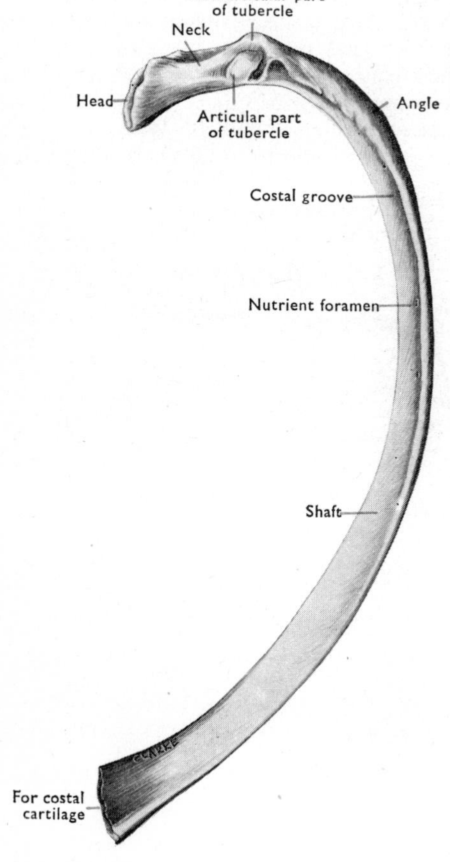

FIG. 9 The inferior aspect of a rib from the middle of the series.

External Intercostal Muscles

These muscles run obliquely downwards and forwards between the adjacent borders of two ribs. They extend from the tubercles of the ribs posteriorly, to the beginning of the costal cartilages anteriorly. Anterior to this (in the upper spaces) each is replaced by an **external intercostal membrane** which reaches the anterior extremity of the intercostal space. Nerve supply: the intercostal nerves. Action: they are inspiratory muscles [p. 6].

DISSECTION. Divide the external intercosta muscles and membranes along the lower borders of two spaces, and turn them upwards. Avoid injury to the branches of the intercostal vessels and nerve. This exposes the internal intercostal muscle.

Internal Intercostal Muscles

These are similar to the external intercostal muscles, but their fibres run postero-inferiorly from the floor of the costal groove of one rib to the upper margin of the rib below. The muscle extends from the anterior extremity of its intercostal space to the angle of the rib [FIG. 9] where it is replaced by the **internal intercostal membrane.** This membrane is continuous anteriorly with the fascia between the intercostal muscles, and thickens posteriorly to fuse with the superior costotransverse ligament. In the lowest two intercostal spaces, the internal intercostal muscle is continuous with the internal oblique muscle of the abdomen where it is attached to the costal margin. Nerve supply: intercostal nerves. Action: this is an expiratory muscle [p. 6].

Innermost Intercostal Muscle

This deeper muscle has all the appearances of the internal intercostal muscle, but is separated from it by the intercostal vessels and nerve. It arises from the inner surface of the rib immediately superior to the costal groove and is inserted into the upper margin of the rib below. Its extent is variable, but it usually passes further posteriorly than the internal intercostal and not so far anteriorly as the external [FIG. 8]. Nerve supply and action: as internal intercostal.

DISSECTION. Dissect out the intercostal nerve and vessels in two or three spaces by picking up the lateral cutaneous branch and following it under cover of the lower margin of the rib, cutting away as much of the rib as is necessary to expose the trunk of the nerve. Follow the trunk anteriorly and posteriorly, displaying the artery and vein as far as possible. Note the branches of the nerve to the intercostal muscles.

INTERCOSTAL NERVES

These are the ventral rami of the upper eleven thoracic nerves. The twelfth lies in the abdominal wall inferior to the twelfth rib (the **subcostal nerve**) and the first (and sometimes the second) sends its greater part into the brachial plexus.

Course. Each intercostal nerve emerges from the intervertebral foramen inferior to the corresponding vertebra, and is immediately connected to a ganglion of the **sympathetic trunk** [FIGS. 27, 28] by a **white** and a **grey ramus communicans**; the former passing to the sympathetic trunk from the nerve, the other in the opposite direction. The nerve then enters an intercostal space between the parietal pleura and the internal intercostal membrane, and runs anteriorly between the internal and innermost intercostal muscles in the costal groove of the corresponding rib. It then crosses anterior to the transversus thoracis and the internal thoracic vessels [FIG. 11], and turning forwards as the **anterior cutaneous branch,** 1 cm. from the margin of the sternum, pierces the internal intercostal muscle, the external intercostal membrane, and pectoralis major. The above description applies only to the third to sixth intercostal nerves, for the first and second run the early part of their course on the pleural surfaces of the corresponding ribs, and the first has no anterior cutaneous branch. When they reach the end of their intercostal spaces the seventh

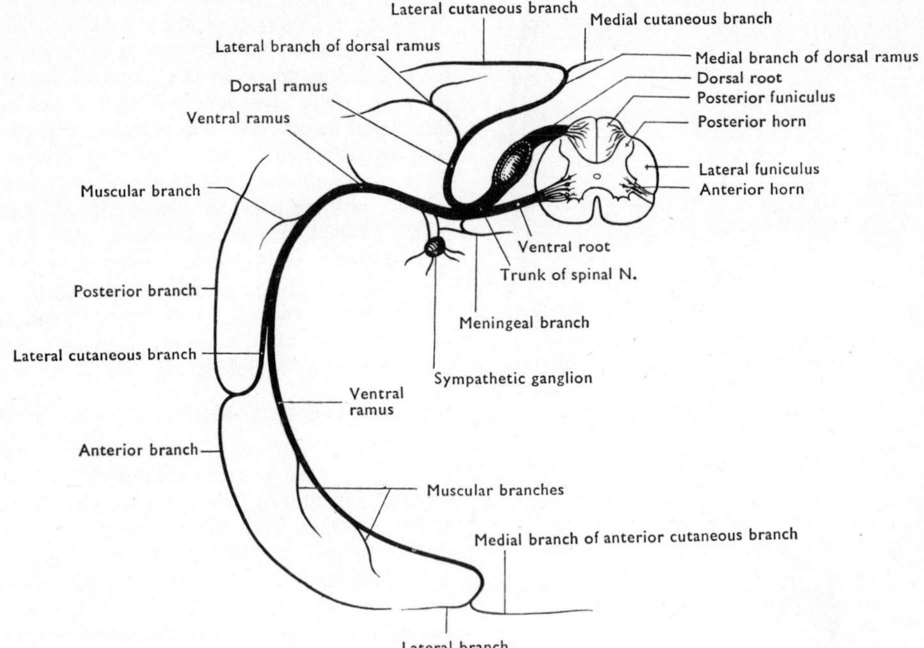

FIG. 10 A diagram of a typical upper thoracic spinal nerve. In the lower half of the trunk the lateral branch of the dorsal ramus gives the cutaneous branch. Both branches of the dorsal ramus supply the erector spinae throughout the trunk.

to eleventh intercostal nerves enter the anterior abdominal wall either directly (10th and 11th) or deep to the upturned end of the next costal cartilage, and supply the structures of the anterior abdominal wall.

Branches. 1. **Rami communicantes** [pp. 10, 30].

2. A **collateral branch** arises near the angle of the rib and runs along the upper margin of the rib below to supply the intercostal muscles. It may rejoin the parent stem, or be absent.

3. **Anterior cutaneous branch,** see above.

4. **Lateral cutaneous branch.** This arises at a variable point beyond the angle of the rib, and is thicker than the continuation of the nerve. About half way round the chest it pierces the internal and external intercostal muscles and divides into anterior and posterior branches. It is frequently absent from the first intercostal nerve; the second forms the large **intercostobrachial nerve** to the floor of the axilla and medial side of the arm; the lower five supply the muscles and skin of the abdominal wall.

5. **Muscular branches** also supply the subcostal, transversus thoracis, levator costae, and the serratus posterior muscles. *It should be noted however that they take no part in the supply of the muscles of the upper limbs which arise from the thorax*, *i.e.*, pectoral muscles, serratus anterior, latissimus dorsi, rhomboids, and trapezius.

INTERCOSTAL ARTERIES AND VEINS

Each intercostal space receives three arteries. The largest is the single **posterior intercostal artery** which accompanies the intercostal nerve and, like it, gives a collateral branch along the superior margin of the rib below. Both arteries end by anastomosing with the two small **anterior intercostal arteries.** These enter the space either from the internal thoracic artery beside the sternum (upper six spaces) or from its musculophrenic branch [FIG. 11] which runs along the costal margin also deep to the cartilages (seventh to ninth spaces). The corresponding **anterior intercostal veins** drain into the musculophrenic and internal thoracic veins. In the last two spaces the posterior intercostal artery and its collateral branch continue into the anterior abdominal wall, and there is no anterior intercostal artery. The arteries and veins which lie subjacent to the mammary gland become greatly enlarged during lactation.

The origin of the posterior intercostal arteries and the termination of the corresponding veins will be seen when the posterior thoracic wall is exposed from within.

DISSECTION. Remove the intercostal muscles and membranes from the anterior part of the first and second intercostal spaces, and expose a part of the internal thoracic artery and veins about 1 cm. from the side of the sternum.

Cut transversely through the manubrium of the sternum immediately inferior to its junction with the first costal cartilage, taking care not to carry the saw deeper than the bone. Cut through the parietal pleura of the first intercostal space on both sides as far back as the mid-axillary line. Then with bone forceps and knife cut inferiorly through the ribs (from the second) and intercostal spaces to the level of the xiphisternal joint. Divide the internal thoracic vessels in the first intercostal space, and gently elevate the inferior part of the sternum with the costal cartilages and the anterior parts of the ribs. Close to the midline, the pleura will be seen turning posteriorly (reflected) from the back of the sternum on to the mediastinum on both sides. Divide this where it leaves the sternum, and as the anterior wall of the thorax is lifted away and hinged on the superior part of the anterior abdominal wall, continue to cut the pleura along the line of its reflexion from the sternum on to the mediastinum, to the level of the lower border of the heart. Note the position of this reflexion and its differences on the two sides [Fig. 2].

When the anterior thoracic wall has been hinged downwards, note the smooth pleura on the posterior aspect, its cut margin, and the manner in which the cut margin on the mediastinum is continuous with the pleura forming the lateral surface of the mediastinum.

Strip the pleura from the back of the sternum and costal cartilages and expose the transversus thoracis muscle and the internal thoracic vessels [Fig. 11].

Transversus Thoracis

This muscle consists of four or five slips which arise from the xiphoid process and the lower part of the body of the sternum, and pass superolaterally to the second to sixth costal cartilages close to their junctions with

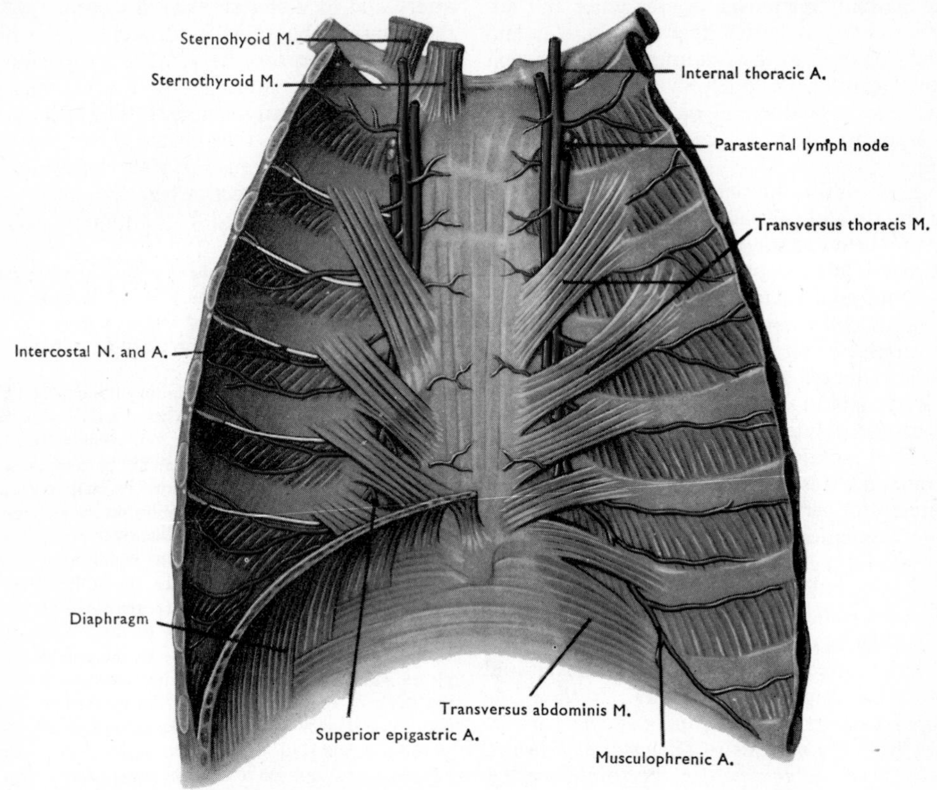

FIG. 11 A dissection of the posterior surface of the anterior thoracic wall.

the ribs. Note that it becomes directly continuous with a transversely placed muscle on the posterior surface of the anterior abdominal wall, the **transversus abdominis.** Nerve supply: the corresponding intercostal nerves. Action: a weak expiratory muscle.

INTERNAL THORACIC ARTERY

This artery arises in the root of the neck from the first part of the subclavian artery, and enters the thorax posterior to the clavicle and the first costal cartilage. This part of its course can easily be exposed by a little dissection upwards from the cut end of the artery posterior to the first costal cartilage, and downwards from the root of the neck. Note the small **pericardiacophrenic artery** passing to the phrenic nerve from this part of the artery. The internal thoracic artery then descends about 1 cm. from the edge of the sternum, at first anterior to the pleura and then to transversus thoracis. It is posterior to the upper six costal cartilages, the intercostal spaces between them, and the terminal parts of the intercostal nerves. It ends at the sixth intercostal space by dividing into the **superior epigastric** and **musculophrenic arteries** [FIG. 11].

Branches

In addition to the terminal branches, it gives off many small branches to the mediastinum, the **anterior intercostal arteries** to the upper six spaces, and the **perforating branches** which accompany the anterior cutaneous branches of the intercostal nerves. The latter are particularly large in the second, third, and fourth spaces in the female, for they play an important part in the supply to the **mammary gland.** Running with these perforating vessels are the corresponding veins and a number of invisible lymphatics. The latter drain from the anterior thoracic wall and the medial part of the mammary gland into the small **parasternal lymph nodes** which lie along the internal thoracic artery.

Superior Epigastric Artery. This branch passes into the sheath of the rectus muscle in the anterior abdominal wall by running between the sternal and costal origins of the diaphragm. In that sheath it anastomoses with a similar branch of the external iliac artery, the **inferior epigastric artery.**

Musculophrenic Artery. This branch runs inferolaterally along the superior surface of the costal origin of the diaphragm deep to the costal cartilages. At the eighth costal cartilage it pierces the diaphragm and runs on its abdominal surface, supplying it.

Internal Thoracic Veins

These vessels are venae comitantes of the internal thoracic artery and drain the territory each supplies. On each side they usually join to form a single vessel opposite the third costal cartilage, and this drains into the corresponding brachiocephalic vein [Fig. 41].

DISSECTION. Clean out the intercostal spaces on the reflected flap of anterior thoracic wall, but leave it attached inferiorly. It may then be replaced in its original position, and the relation of the ribs to the subjacent organs established as these are dissected.

THE CAVITY OF THE THORAX

MEDIASTINUM

The general division of the thoracic contents into a more or less median mediastinum and the laterally placed pleural cavities has already been described [p. 1]. The student should realize that the mediastinum, though thick, is movable, and that it extends supero-inferiorly from the root of the neck to the diaphragm, and anteroposteriorly from the sternum to the vertebral column [Fig. 3]. For the purpose of description, the mediastinum is subdivided by an imaginary plane which passes anteroposteriorly from the sternal angle to the lower border of the fourth thoracic vertebral body. The part superior to this is the **superior mediastinum;** the part inferior to the plane is further subdivided into: (1) the **middle mediastinum** which consists of the pericardial sac and its contents with a phrenic nerve on each side; (2) the **anterior mediastinum** between the middle mediastinum and the sternum; and (3) the **posterior mediastinum** between the pericardium and diaphragm anteriorly and the vertebral column posteriorly [Fig. 12]. Because of the anterior concavity of the thoracic vertebral column, the superior mediastinum has a smaller anteroposterior depth than the remainder. Also, because of the curve of the diaphragm [Fig. 12], the posterior mediastinum extends furthest inferiorly for it passes into the angle between the diaphragm and the vertebral column to reach the level of the twelfth thoracic vertebra.

LATERAL PARTS OF THORACIC CAVITY AND PLEURA

These consist of the **pleural cavities,** each almost completely filled by a lung which gives the impression of having invaginated this cavity from the mediastinum. Each lung is everywhere covered with a smooth glistening layer of **pulmonary pleura** except where its root is attached to the mediastinum. Here the pleura ensheathes the root [Fig. 13] to become continuous with the **parietal pleura** which (1) covers the lateral aspect of the mediastinum, (2) lines the thoracic wall, (3) covers the superior surface of the diaphragm lateral to

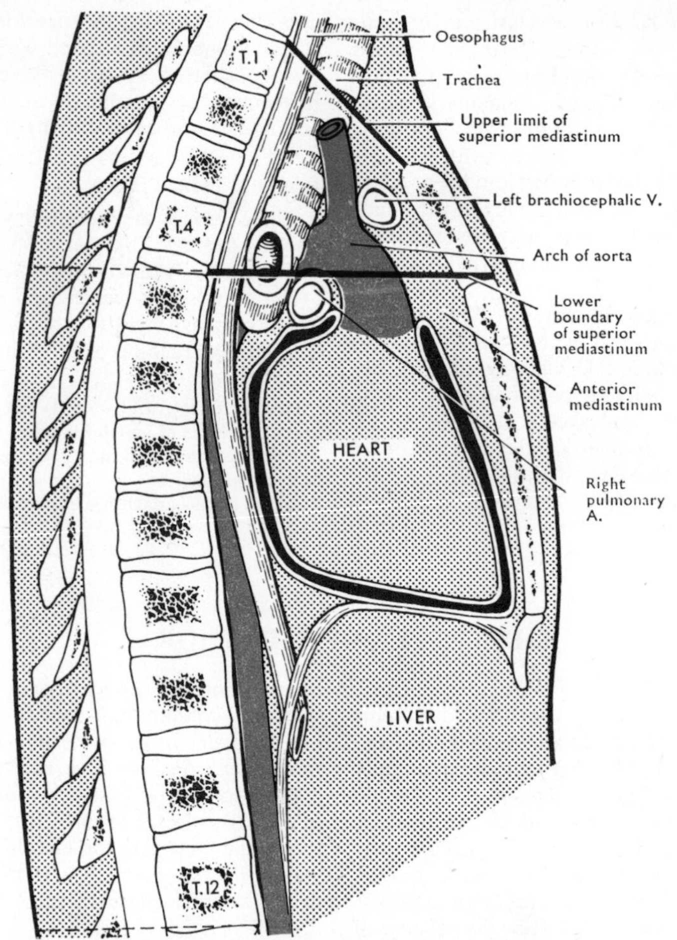

FIG. 12 A diagram of a median section through the thorax to show the general disposition of the structures in the mediastinum. The heart in the pericardium forms the middle mediastinum, while the anterior and posterior mediastina lie between it and the sternum and vertebral column respectively; the posterior mediastinum also extends downwards behind the diaphragm.

the mediastinum, and (4) extends through the superior aperture of the thorax into the lower part of the root of the neck, the **dome of the pleura.** The parietal pleura is applied to the pulmonary pleura, but is separated from it by a narrow interval, the **pleural cavity**, which contains a little fluid. In effect the lung bears the same relation to the pleural cavity as an object which pushes in one wall of a hollow sphere and then expands to fill the cavity, stretching the wall which is carried with it till that wall is applied to the internal surface of the sphere, the original cavity of the sphere being reduced to a mere slit. Neither the object nor the lung are inside the cavity, but are separated from it by the layer which immediately covers them [FIG. 14]. This arrangement is also found in the peri-

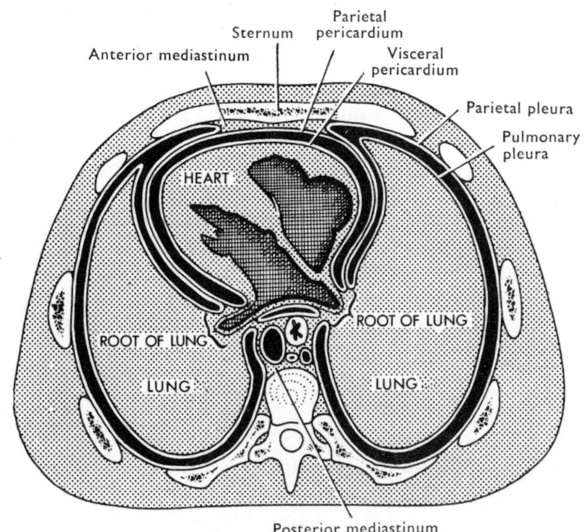

FIG. 13 A diagrammatic horizontal section through the thorax to show the positions of the major structures in it. The pleural and pericardial cavities are shown in black.

cardial and peritoneal (abdominal) cavities which have the same embryological origin as the pleural cavity, and it permits free movement of organs within the body, in much the same manner as a tendon sheath allows a tendon to slide on the surrounding tissues.

The **parietal pleura** differs from the pulmonary pleura in having a thick outer fibrous layer. The various parts are named according to the structures on which they lie: *i.e.*, mediastinal pleura, costal pleura, diaphragmatic pleura, and dome of the pleura.

From what has been said it should be clear that once the pleural cavity has been opened in a completely healthy individual, it is possible to lift the lung and pulmonary pleura away from the parietal pleura except on the mediastinal surface. Here the two parts of the pleura become continuous around the lung root, with a fold of pleura extending inferiorly, the **pulmonary ligament.** In aged individuals it is common to find that the pulmonary and parietal layers of the pleura are adherent at various points owing to the spread of inflammatory or cancerous processes from the lung. Such adhesions interfere with respiration to a greater or lesser degree, and make it difficult to confirm the extent of the pleural cavity by dissection. Nevertheless the cavity should be carefully explored and its extent noted. More especially the anterior part of the lung should be drawn laterally and the root of the lung identified together with the pulmonary ligament [FIGS. 32, 33].

DISSECTION. Having identified the roots of the lungs and the pulmonary ligaments, divide them from above downwards, close to the medial surface of each

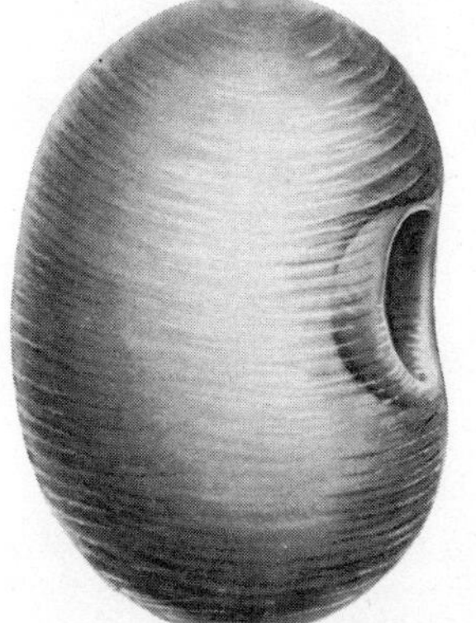

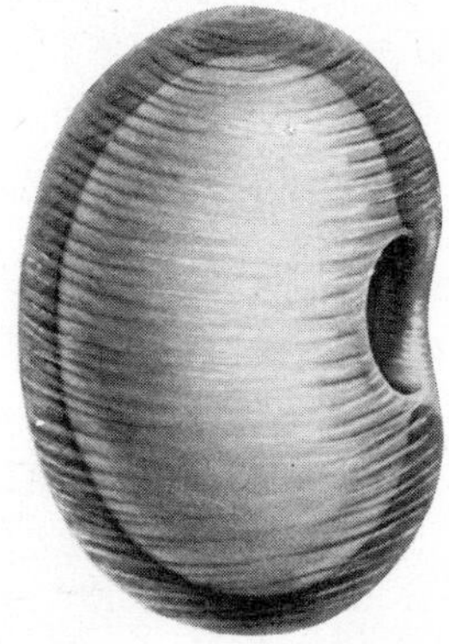

FIG. 14 A diagram to show how a structure may grow into a cavity carrying part of the wall in front of it as a covering. By expanding within the cavity the structure reduces it to a mere slit between the outer shell (parietal layer) and the layer intimately covering the structure (visceral layer). A thin film of fluid separates these two layers and allows free movement of the structure and the visceral layer within the parietal layer. This is the arrangement of the lung within the pleural cavity. The heart in the pericardial cavity and the gut in the peritoneal cavity are similarly placed, though the method of development is not exactly the same.

lung. Remove the lungs and store them damped in a plastic bag or other container to prevent drying.

Dome of Pleura

This rounded extension of the parietal pleura passes through the superior aperture of the thorax into the **root of the neck.** The highest point on the dome lies opposite the neck of the first rib, but is 3–5 cm. above the anterior end of the rib which slopes antero-inferiorly [FIGS. 4, 16, 18]. The dome has a number of important structures in contact with it [FIGS. 15, 16] and many of these are easily identified if the neck has been dissected already. If not, then feel the **subclavian artery** as it arches across the front of the dome a little below its highest point by placing a finger in the dome. If full of blood clot, the **subclavian vein** may also be felt antero-inferior to the artery. The internal thoracic artery may also be felt running inferomedially across the anterior surface of the dome, and its direction can be confirmed from the cut end of this vessel. If the inner margin of the first rib is palpated, the edge of **scalenus anterior** may be felt anterior to

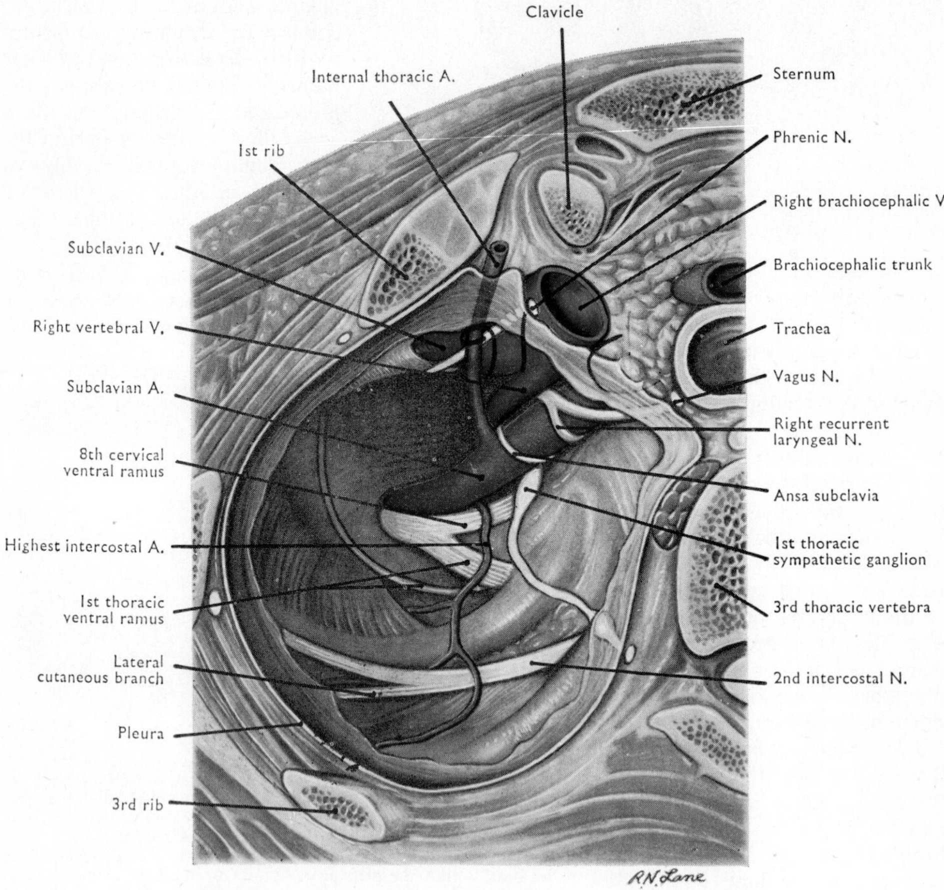

FIG. 15 A dissection of the dome of the pleura seen from below.

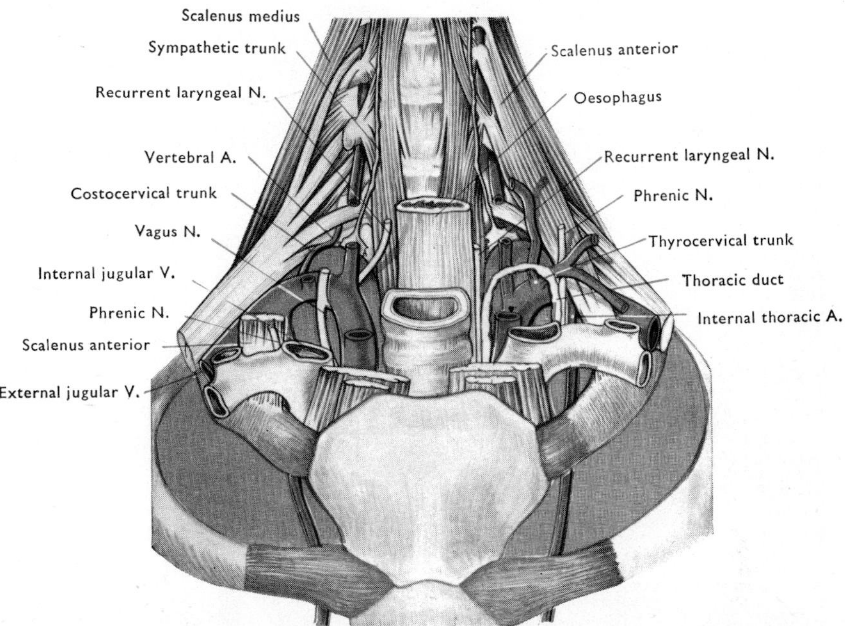

FIG. 16 A dissection of the root of the neck to show the structures adjacent to the dome of the pleura (blue).

the subclavian artery, but both are often obscured by a layer of fascia (**suprapleural membrane**) which spreads from the transverse process of the seventh cervical vertebra to the medial margin of the first rib. This fascia supports the dome of the pleura and minimizes its movement during changes in intrathoracic pressure. It may be tightened by some muscle fibres, **scalenus minimus.** These structures will be seen when the dome of the pleura is dissected.

Pleural Recesses

These recesses are the parts of the pleural cavity which are not occupied by the lung except in full inspiration, and they lie where the different parts of the parietal pleura meet at an acute angle. The **costomediastinal** recess lies along the anterior margin of the pleura, while the **costodiaphragmatic** recess lies inferiorly where the costal pleura extends into the angle between the thoracic wall and the diaphragm. Here the pleura is attached to the diaphragm and the adjoining costal cartilages by a narrow ribbon of fascia (**phrenico-pleural fascia**) which holds this part of the pleura in place during respiratory movements.

Margins of Pleural Cavity

Place a finger in the dome of the pleura and note that its highest point rises 1–2 cm. superior to the medial third of the clavicle, and that it is widely separated from its fellow by the structures which occupy the median part of the neck, *i.e.*, the trachea and oesophagus, and the vessels passing to and from the neck.

Traced from the domes, the **anterior margins** of the two pleurae converge as they descend posterior to the sternoclavicular joints, to meet at the sternal angle [FIGS. 18, 19]. Inferior to this the margins remain in apposition to the level of the fourth costal cartilage. Here the anterior margin of the left pleura deviates to the left and descends posterior to

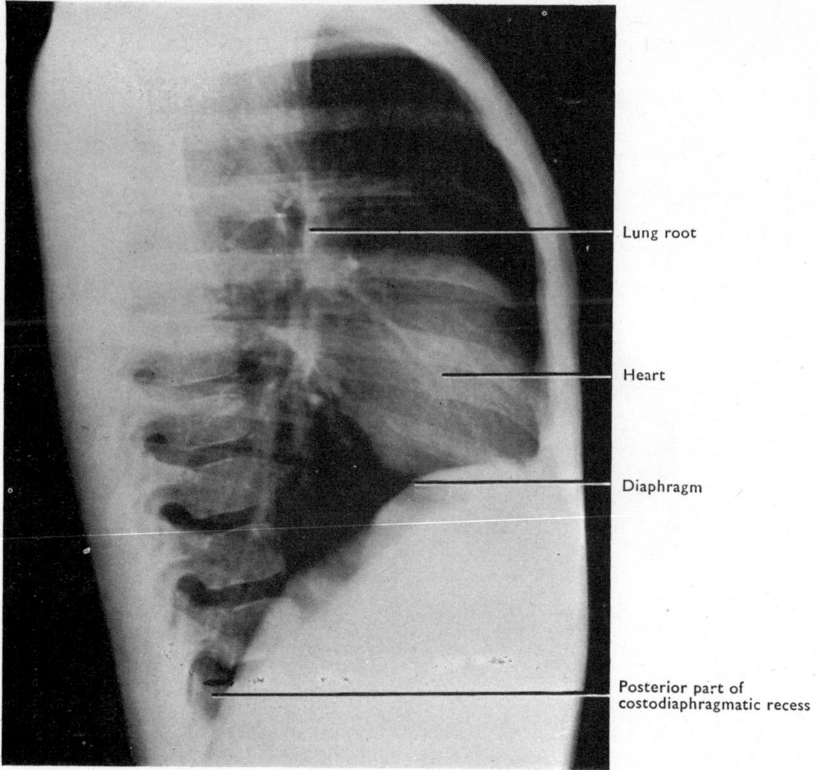

FIG. 17 A lateral radiograph of the thorax. Note the extension of the lung into the costodiaphragmatic recess posterior to the diaphragm and the upper abdominal contents.

the fifth and sixth costal cartilages close to the margin of the sternum, while the right descends vertically. Each anterior margin becomes continuous with the corresponding inferior margin at the level of the xiphisternal joint.

With a finger in the **costodiaphragmatic recess** trace the **inferior margin** of the pleural cavity. It passes posterior to the cartilage of the seventh rib, and running postero-inferiorly in a curve which is convex downwards, crosses the tenth rib in the mid-axillary line, about 5 cm. superior to the costal margin. It then crosses the eleventh and twelfth ribs to reach the side of the vertebral column inferior to the medial part of the twelfth rib, approximately opposite the twelfth thoracic spine. The fact that the pleural cavity reaches so far inferiorly should always be remembered, otherwise it may be damaged in clinical procedures involving the upper abdomen. It should also be appreciated that the costodiaphragmatic recess does not quite reach the level of attachment of the diaphragm to the thoracic wall.

The **posterior margin** of the pleural cavity extends along the vertebral column from the dome to the termination of the inferior margin.

The **inferior margin of the lung** does not extend into the costodiaphragmatic recess in quiet respiration, but follows a course from a point lateral to the xiphisternal joint through the eighth rib in the mid-axillary line (*i.e.*, 10 cm. above the costal margin) to meet the vertebral column opposite the tenth thoracic vertebral spine.

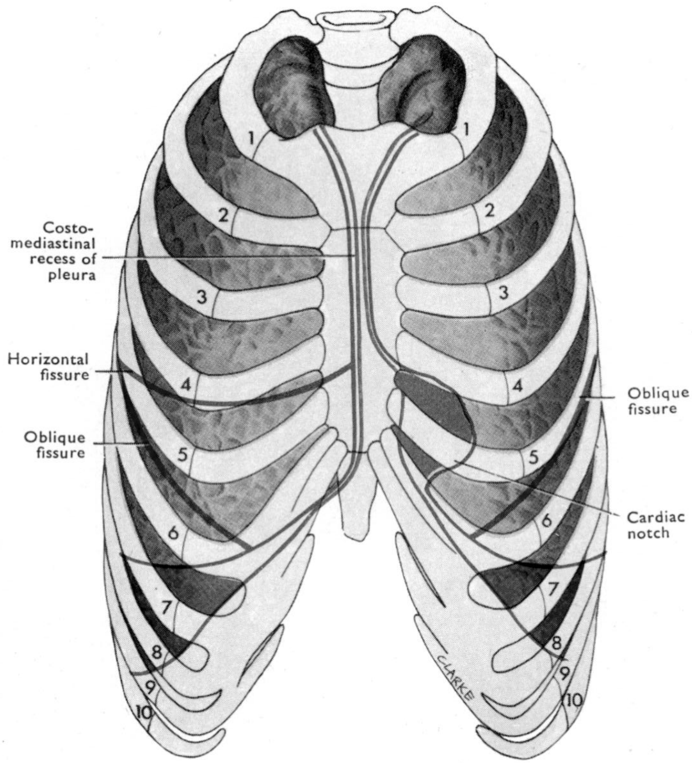

FIG. 18 A diagram to show the relation of the lungs (red) and pleurae (blue) to the anterior thoracic wall.

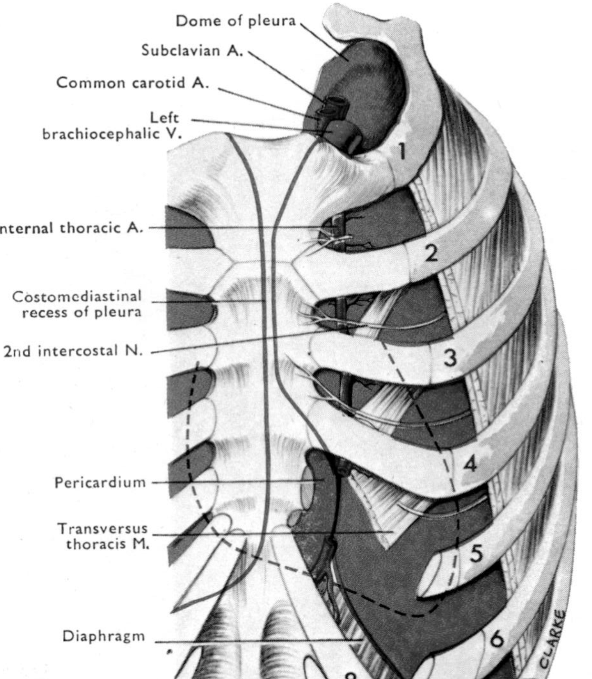

FIG. 19 A diagram to show the structures anterior to the pericardium and heart. Outline of the heart, broken red line; pleura, blue. 1-8, ribs and costal cartilages.

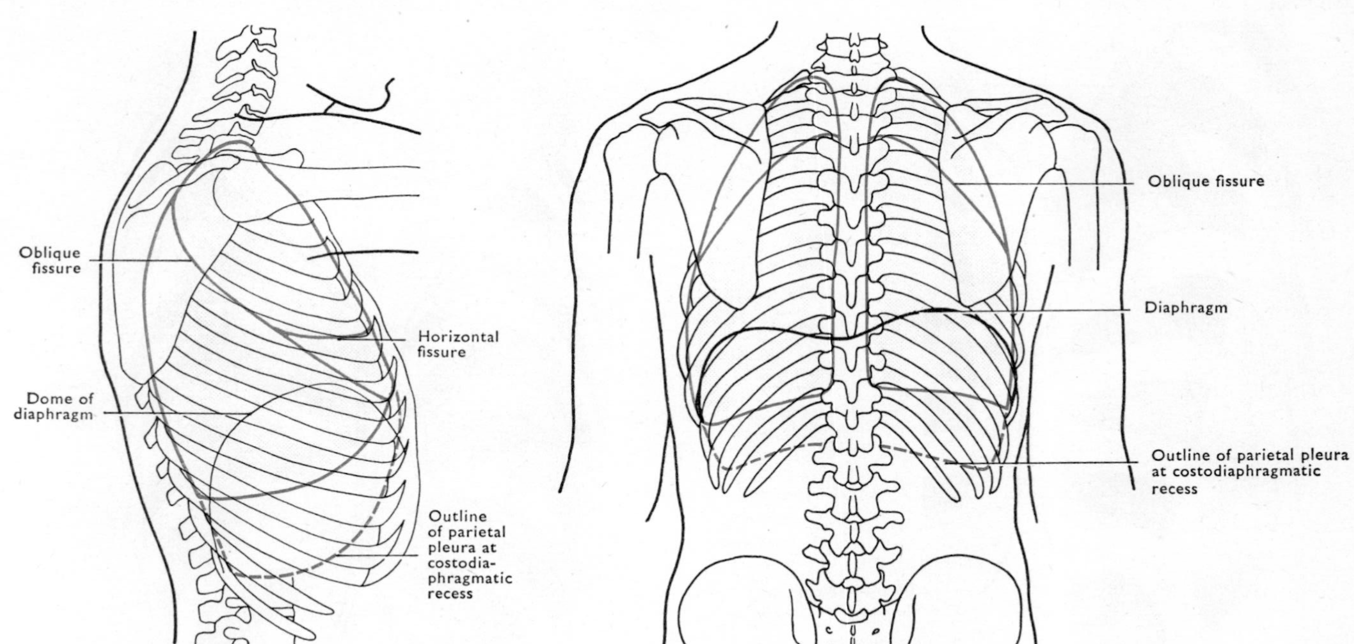

Fig. 20 The right lateral aspect of the trunk to show the position of the right lung (blue stipple) and its fissures (solid blue lines), the pleural sac (broken blue line), and the diaphragm.

Fig. 21 The posterior aspect of the trunk to show the position of the lungs (blue stipple) and their fissures (solid blue lines), the pleural sacs (broken blue lines), and the diaphragm.

GENERAL STRUCTURE AND POSITION OF HEART

The human heart and the great arteries which arise from it form a U-shaped tube which lies obliquely across the thorax more or less in the sagittal plane [FIGS. 25, 52]. The bend of the U lies antero-inferiorly (close to the sternum), while the ends of the two limbs are in a posterosuperior position (close to the vertebral column), one anterosuperior to the other. The tube is divided longitudinally by a continuous septum into right and left channels, the walls of which are mainly fused. Each channel is further subdivided by two transversely placed valves one of which lies approximately at the middle of each limb of the U. These valves are so placed as to direct the flow of blood from the inferior limb through the bend to the superior limb, and respectively they separate the right and left ventricles, which lie at the bend of the U, (1) from the right and left atria in the inferior limb (**atrioventricular valves**), and (2) from the pulmonary trunk and aorta (the great arteries) in the superior limb (**valves of the pulmonary trunk and aorta**).

The atria and ventricles are distended to form chambers, and each atrium is separated from the corresponding ventricle by a narrower portion at which the atrioventricular valve lies. The great arteries are parallel-sided tubes without the muscle which is found in the atria and ventricles. The arteries are the only parts of the right and left channels in which the walls are completely separate from each other [FIG. 55].

In the same manner as the lungs are invaginated into the pleural cavities, the U-shaped heart tube is 'invaginated' into the pericardial cavity. The two ends of the U (atria and great arteries) corresponding to the root of the lung, are the site at which the **parietal pericardium** (the outer wall of the pericardial cavity) becomes continuous with the layer which surrounds the heart (the **visceral pericardium**) and are therefore relatively fixed. The ventricles on the other hand are fully invaginated into the pericardium and have the greatest freedom of movement.

The thin-walled atria receive the veins at their vertebral extremities. The left is filled with oxygenated blood from the lungs through two pairs of pulmonary veins, while the right receives the deoxygenated blood from the rest of the body through the superior and inferior venae cavae. At the entry of these veins the parietal and visceral parts of the pericardium become continuous, so that the walls of the atria are almost completely covered by pericardium.

The atria discharge into the corresponding thick-walled ventricles (through the atrioventricular valves) and these in turn pump the

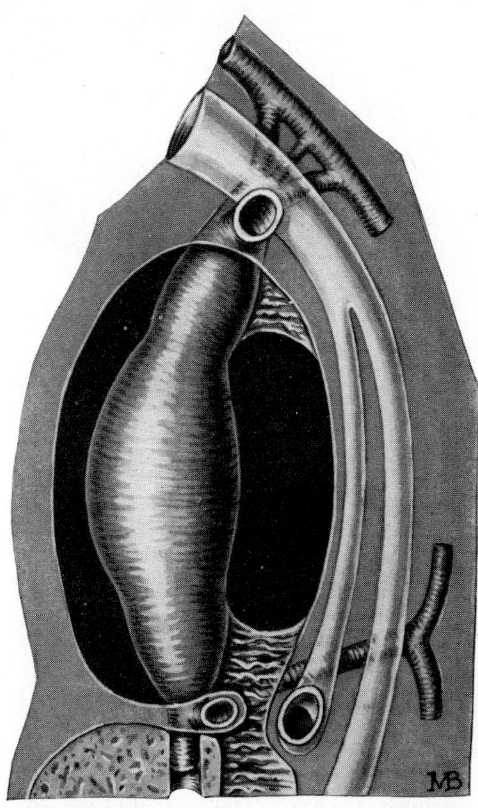

FIG. 22 A diagram of the early embryonic heart in the pericardial cavity. Cf. FIG. 23.

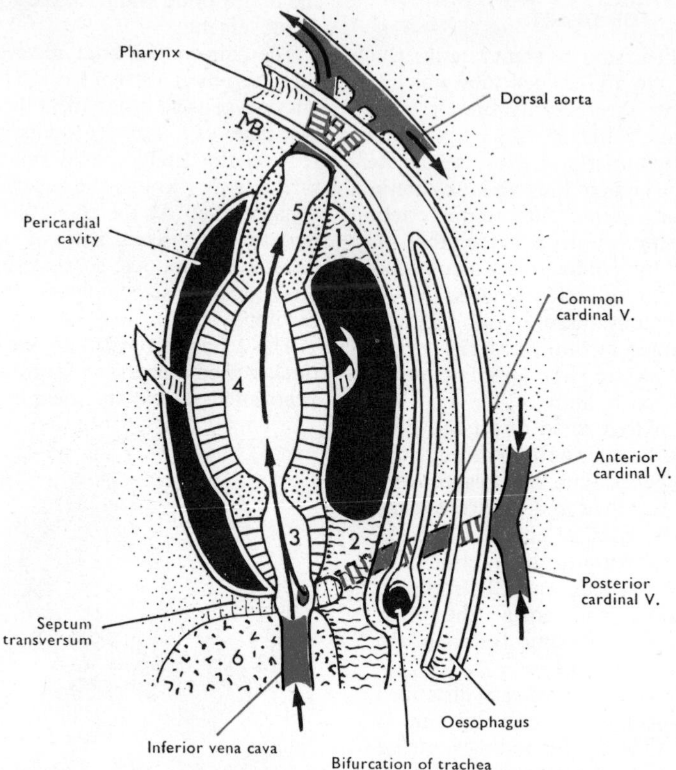

FIG. 23 A diagrammatic sagittal section through the heart shown in FIG. 22. The arrow passes through the transverse sinus of the pericardium.

1.} 2.} Remnants of the dorsal mesocardium.
3. Atrial chamber.
4. Ventricular chamber.
5 Bulbus cordis, outflow part of the heart.
6. Liver in the septum transversum.

blood either through the pulmonary trunk to the lungs (right ventricle), or through the aorta to the rest of the body (left ventricle).

In many quadrupeds, where the dorsoventral diameter of the thorax is much greater than its transverse diameter, the heart retains the simple sagittal position described above, but in Man, where the thorax is flattened antero-posteriorly, the heart is (*a*) rotated to the left around the long axis of the U and (*b*) the bend of the U (apex of the heart) is displaced to the left. The results of the rotation are: (1) The longitudinal septum lies obliquely, the right chambers lying anterior and to the right of the corresponding left chambers which lie posterior and to the left. (2) The left atrium lies in a posterior position against the vertebral column, and all but disappears from the left (pulmonary) surface of the heart, leaving the left ventricle to form the greater part of this

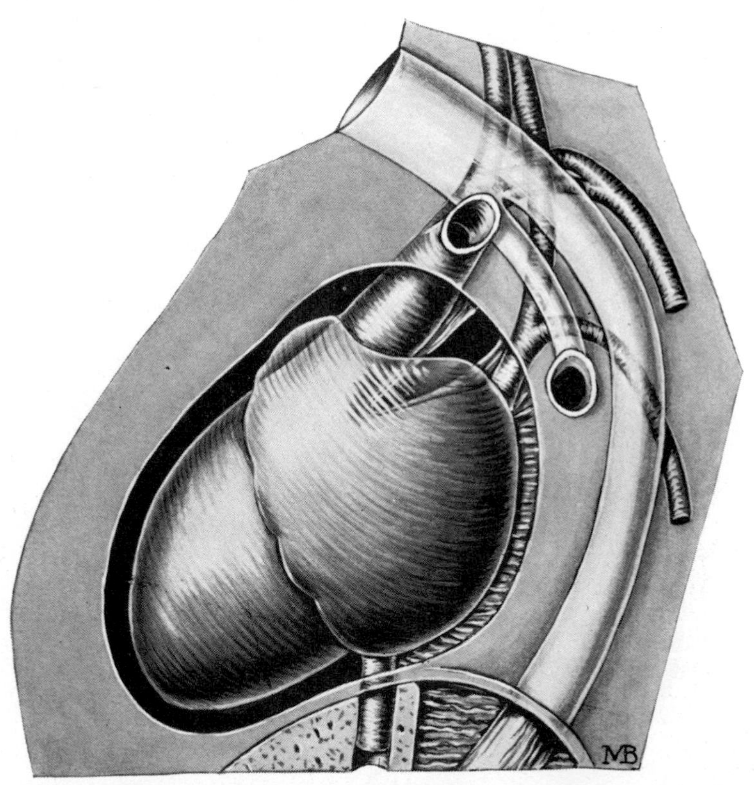

FIG. 24 A diagram of the embryonic heart in the pericardial cavity at a later stage of development than that shown in FIG. 22. To show the folding of the heart tube. Cf. FIG. 25.

surface [FIG. 40]. Since the left atrium lies at the opposite end of the heart from the apex, it forms the **base of the heart** close to the vertebral column [FIG. 63].

The results of the displacement of the apex to the left are: (1) The **apex** points antero-inferiorly and to the left, and lies in the fifth left intercostal space just medial to a vertical line dropped from the mid-point of the clavicle (the mid-clavicular line). (2) The right ventricle is displaced to an inferior position, leaving the right atrium to form the entire right margin of the heart. Thus the heart in its pericardial cavity bulges the left wall of the middle mediastinum far to the left, and deeply indents the pleural cavity and lung on that side. The right border of the heart, formed by the gently convex surface of the right atrium, indents the right pleural cavity and lung to a slight extent.

ROOTS OF LUNGS

[FIGS. 26, 28, 32, 33]

With the help of the above figures check the positions of the main structures in the sectioned roots of the lungs. Note the difference in the arrangement of the bronchi in the two lung roots due to the earlier division of the right principal bronchus. In addition it may be possible to see branches of the right bronchial artery and the two left bronchial arteries on the posterior surfaces of the corresponding bronchi, and a number of bronchial lymph nodes, which are easily distinguished by the black carbon deposits in them.

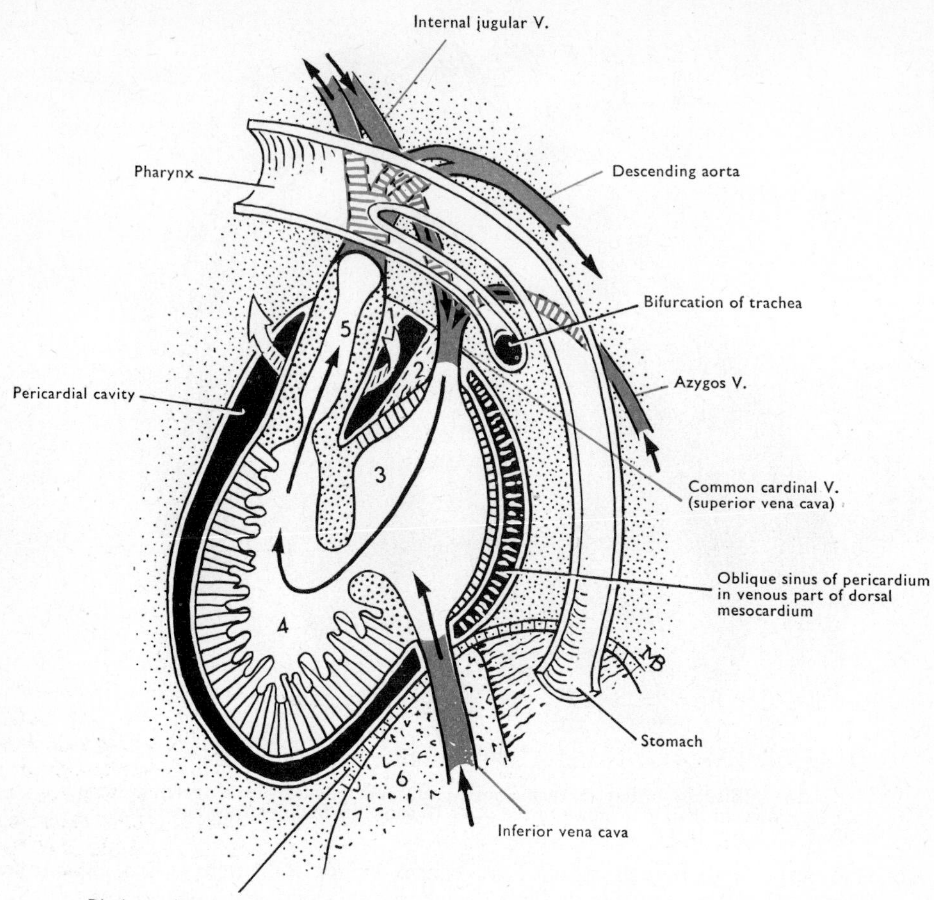

FIG. 25 A diagrammatic sagittal section through the heart shown in FIG. 24. The arrow passes through the transverse sinus of the pericardium.

1.
2. } Remnants of the dorsal mesocardium.
3. Atrium.
4. Ventricle.
5. Bulbus cordis.
6. Liver.

STRUCTURES VISIBLE THROUGH PLEURA

Unless the pleura is greatly thickened by disease it is possible to identify a number of structures through it, and this should be done before removing the pleura to avoid damage to them.

On the *right side* [FIG. 26], identify the bulge of the heart antero-inferior to the lung root, and note two longitudinal ridges extending from the superior and inferior extremities of the bulge. The superior is due to the **right brachiocephalic vein** above the inferior border of the first costal cartilage, and to the **superior vena cava** below this. The inferior ridge is very short and is formed by the thoracic part of the **inferior vena cava.** The **phrenic nerve** and its accompanying vessels form a vertical ridge along the posterolateral surface of the right brachiocephalic vein and the superior vena cava. They then cross a little anterior to the lung root, and descend over the posterior part of the bulge of the heart and the anterior border of the inferior vena caval ridge. The **vena azygos** can be seen arching over the superior surface of the lung root to join the superior vena cava, and above this the **trachea** can be seen or felt with the **right vagus nerve** descending postero-inferiorly across it. The **oesophagus** may be felt posterior to the trachea and lung root, and posterior to the oesophagus, the bodies of the thoracic vertebrae and the posterior parts of the ribs. The **sympathetic trunk** may be seen or felt as it descends over the heads of the upper ribs and the sides of the lower vertebral bodies, with the roots of the greater splanchnic nerve passing antero-inferiorly from it.

On the *left side* [FIG. 28], the large bulge of

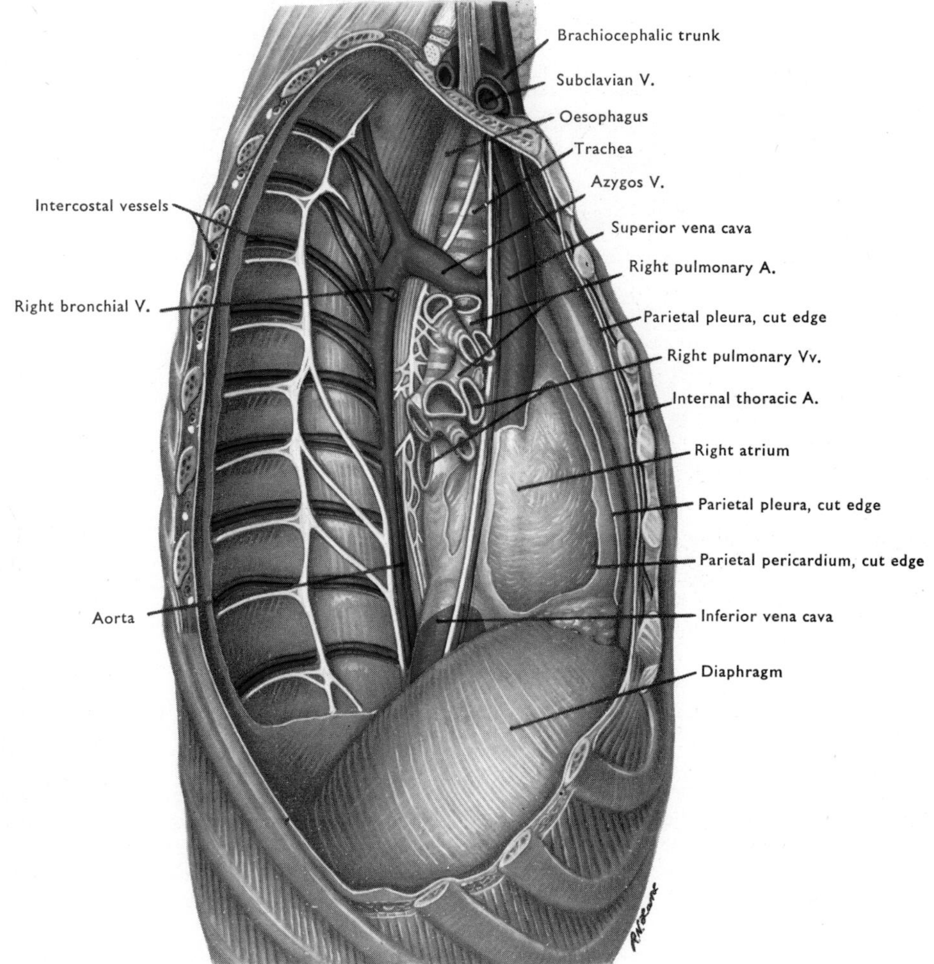

FIG. 26 The right side of the mediastinum and thoracic vertebral column. The pleura has been removed together with part of the pericardium.

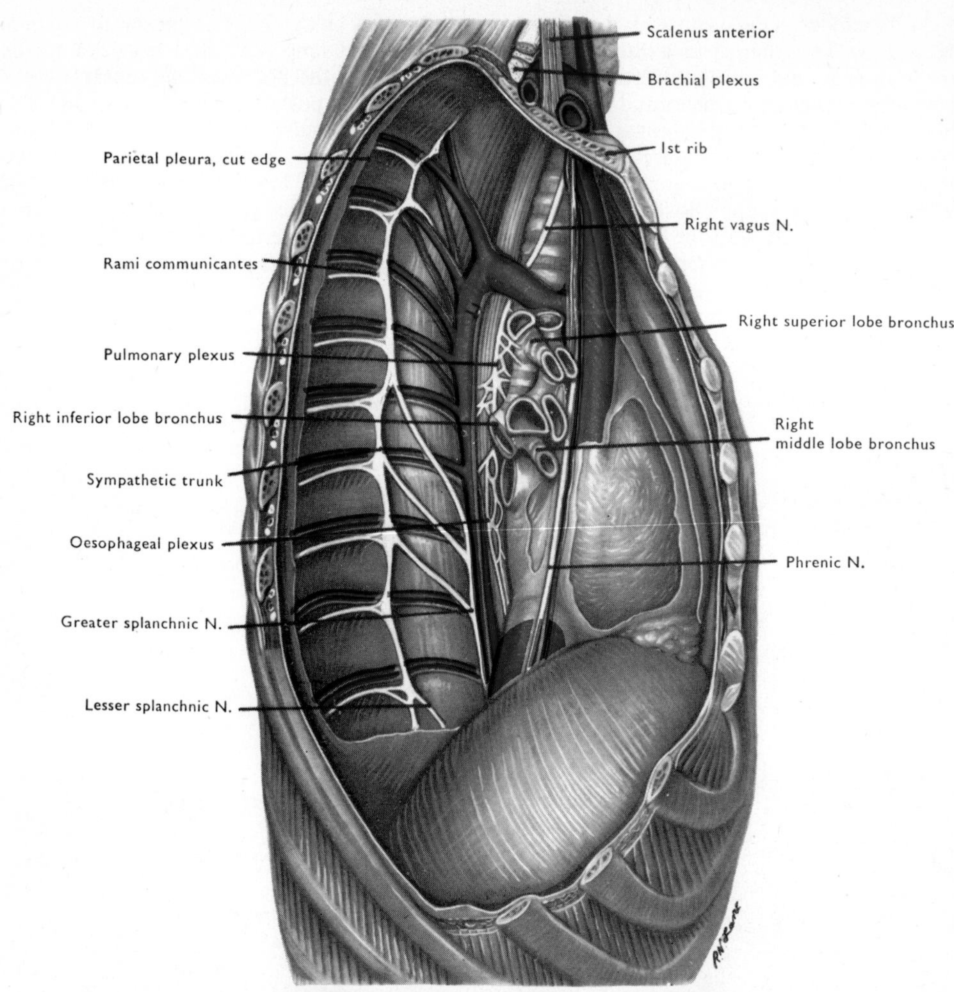

FIG. 27 The right side of the mediastinum and thoracic vertebral column. The pleura has been removed together with part of the pericardium.

the heart in the pericardium is antero-inferior to the lung root, and both are separated from the vertebral column by the **descending aorta,** with the **oesophagus**, deviating to the left inferiorly, appearing between pericardium and aorta. The **arch of the aorta** curves over the superior surface of the lung root and has the left common carotid and subclavian arteries passing superiorly from its convex surface anterior to the oesophagus. The phrenic nerve and vessels descend on the common carotid artery with the vagus nerve posterior to them. Both nerves cross the arch of the aorta, the vagus passing posteriorly to reach the posterior surface of the root of the lung, while the phrenic nerve descends vertically over the bulge of the heart to the diaphragm. The **thoracic duct** may be seen on the lateral

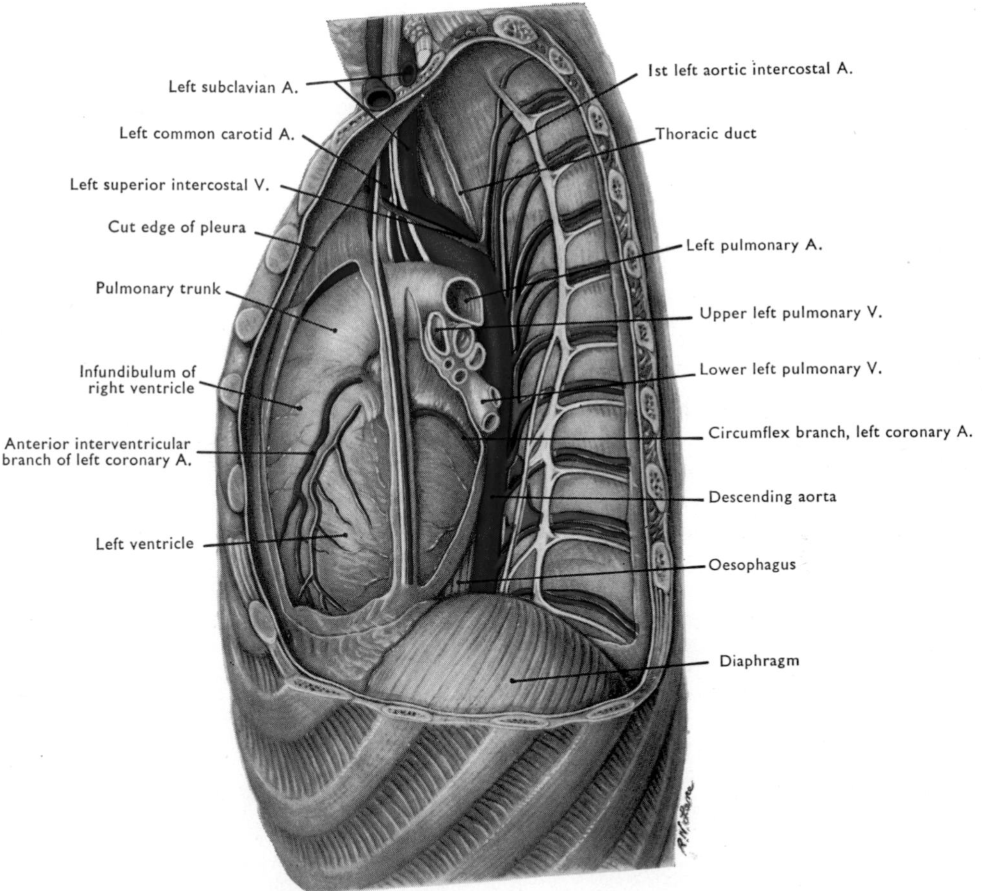

FIG. 28 The left side of the mediastinum and thoracic vertebral column. The pleura and part of the pericardium have been removed.

surface of the oesophagus posterior to the subclavian artery. The **sympathetic trunk** and the roots of the greater splanchnic nerve occupy the same position as on the right side, lying on the intercostal vessels as they cross the vertebral column.

DISSECTION. Make two vertical incisions through the mediastinal pleura, one anterior and one posterior to the phrenic nerve. Strip the posterior sheet of pleura completely (removing it from the lung root) from the mediastinum and ribs, but avoiding injury to the underlying structures. Turn the anterior flap forwards to uncover the anterior surface of the pericardium and the superior vena cava on the right, and the arch of the aorta on the left. Remove the pleural flaps, but leave a narrow strip of mediastinal pleura close to the costomediastinal recess.

Clean the whole sympathetic trunk and its branches which run anteriorly towards the pulmonary plexus on the lung root, and antero-inferiorly to form the splanchnic nerves. Slender branches may also be traced towards the cardiac plexus on the bifurcation of the trachea. Select two or three of the ganglia on the trunk and trace the rami communicantes which connect each with the corresponding intercostal nerve. In most cases there are two such rami (grey and white) to each

intercostal nerve, but they may be combined, and one ganglion may send rami to two intercostal nerves [Figs. 10, 27, 29].

Clean the intercostal vessels on the vertebral column and in the posterior parts of the intercostal spaces. Trace the highest intercostal artery (first two spaces) and the vein (first space) to the neck of the first rib, and follow the other intercostal veins towards the azygos vein on the right and to the left superior intercostal and hemiazygos veins on the left. Clean the azygos and hemiazygos veins as far as possible.

Find the vagus nerve on each side [Figs. 27, 29] and trace it to the posterior surface of the corresponding lung root. Note the recurrent laryngeal branch of the left vagus curving medially round the concavity of the aortic arch, and the fine branches which each vagus gives to the anterior surface of the lung root. Clean the pulmonary plexus and the branches of the bronchial arteries on the posterior surfaces of the bronchi. Trace the branches of the vagi to the plexus on the oesophagus.

On the right side, clean the surface of the trachea and the oesophagus as far inferiorly as the lung root, and clean the superior and inferior venae cavae and the pericardium, leaving the phrenic nerve in situ.

On the left side [Fig. 28], follow the superior intercostal vein obliquely across the arch of the aorta (superficial to the vagus and deep to the phrenic nerve) to the left brachiocephalic vein posterior to the manubrium of the sternum. Between the phrenic and vagus

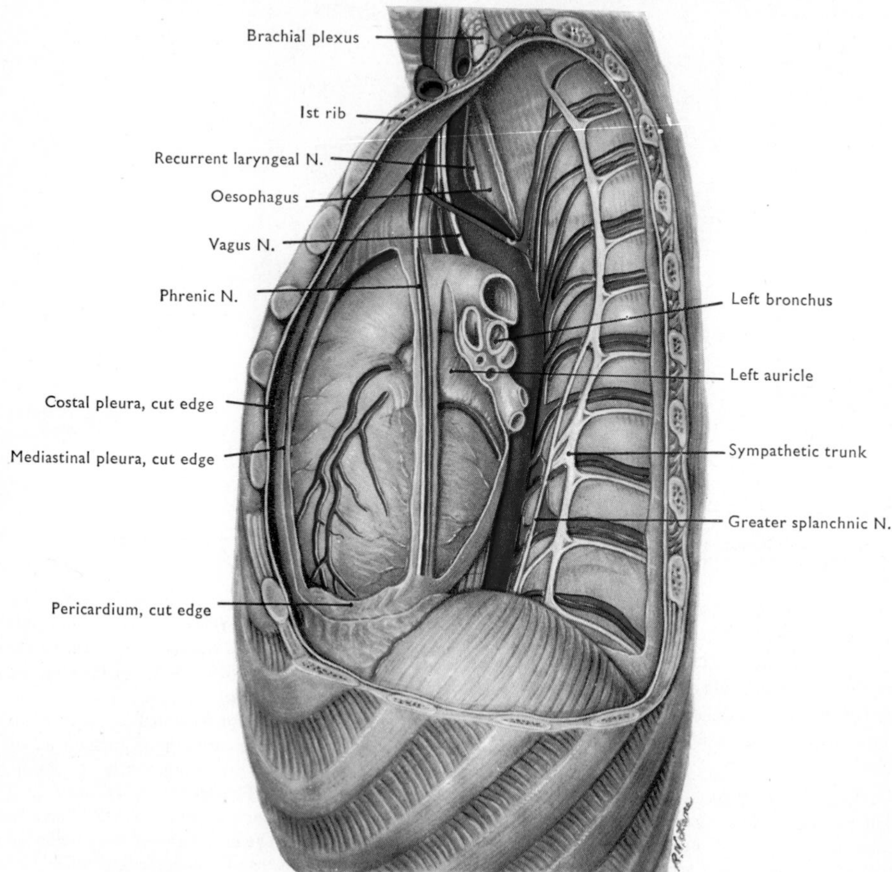

FIG. 29 The left side of the mediastinum and thoracic vertebral column. The pleura and part of the pericardium have been removed.

nerves on the arch of the aorta, find the superior cervical cardiac branch of the left sympathetic trunk and the inferior cervical cardiac branch of the left vagus. Trace them superiorly as far as possible, and inferiorly to the concavity of the aortic arch. Clean the left subclavian artery and the left surface of the oesophagus. Avoid damage to the recurrent laryngeal nerve, which lies anterior to the oesophagus, and to the thoracic duct on its left surface.

AUTONOMIC NERVOUS SYSTEM

The **sympathetic trunks** form an important element in the sympathetic part of the autonomic nervous system. This system consists essentially of peripherally situated groups (ganglia) of motor nerve cells concerned with the innervation of involuntary structures, such as smooth muscle and glands, through nerve fibres (postganglionic) which arise in the cells of the ganglia. It is connected to the central nervous system by nerve fibres (preganglionic) which carry impulses to the cells in the autonomic ganglia. The system also transmits the processes of sensory neurons which are distributed in the visceral territory, but have no immediate functional connexion with the motor cells in the autonomic ganglia, though they pass through them. The system as a whole has two divisions.

PARASYMPATHETIC PART

This part receives preganglionic nerve fibres through certain cranial nerves and the second and third, or third and fourth, sacral spinal nerves. It is concerned with the innervation of the gut tube and the structures developed in its wall. Its ganglia lie in or near the structures which it innervates, and thus its preganglionic fibres end close to these organs. The parasympathetic nerves of the thorax are the vagus nerves, and they are principally concerned with the innervation of the heart, lungs, trachea, and oesophagus.

SYMPATHETIC PART

This part receives preganglionic fibres (**white rami communicantes**) from all the thoracic and the upper two or three lumbar nerves, and its ganglia are concerned not only with the innervation of the gut tube and the structures which develop in its walls, but they also supply blood vessels throughout the body and the other involuntary structures in the body wall such as sweat glands, arrectores pilorum, etc. The sympathetic ganglia usually lie at some distance from the organs which they innervate, and their postganglionic nerve fibres are often distributed along blood vessels. The sympathetic part is composed of two readily distinguishable elements. (1) The **sympathetic trunks.** These extend from the upper cervical region to the coccyx on the front of the vertebral column, and their ganglia send postganglionic nerve fibres to most of the cranial and all of the spinal nerves (**grey rami communicantes**) through which the postganglionic fibres are distributed mainly to the body wall. The sympathetic trunks also transmit preganglionic fibres and send some postganglionic fibres through the **splanchnic nerves** to the sympathetic plexuses. (2) The **sympathetic plexuses** are networks of fine nerve fibres containing scattered ganglia, and they are associated with the viscera and the blood vessels which supply them. The chief plexuses are found in the thorax (cardiac and pulmonary), the abdomen (coeliac, superior mesenteric, and aortic), and the pelvis (hypogastric). These plexuses frequently transmit some parasympathetic fibres.

Sympathetic Trunk

In the thorax this trunk consists of approximately eleven ganglia joined by longitudinal bundles of preganglionic and postganglionic fibres in which are scattered a variable number of ganglion cells. In the superior part of the thorax it lies on the necks or heads of the ribs, but inferiorly it passes on to the bodies of the vertebrae as these increase in width. The **first thoracic ganglion** is frequently fused with the inferior cervical ganglion to form the **cervicothoracic ganglion** on the neck of the first rib. This ganglion may also include the second thoracic ganglion, and is commonly called the **stellate ganglion** because of its star-like shape.

Branches. 1. **Grey and white rami communicantes** join each ganglion to one or more intercostal nerves. The white rami (preganglionic fibres) passing from the nerve to the trunk, while the grey rami (postganglionic fibres) pass to the nerve from ganglion cells in the trunk, and are distributed through the branches of the spinal nerve, including its dorsal ramus.

2. **Aortic** and **oesophageal** branches pass to these organs in the thorax from the upper five ganglia and from the greater splanchnic nerve.

3. **Cardiac** and **pulmonary** nerves run antero-inferiorly on the vertebral bodies from the third and fourth ganglia to the side of the oesophagus, and thence to the cardiac and pulmonary plexuses.

4. The **greater splanchnic nerve** is formed by branches of the fifth to ninth ganglia which run antero-inferiorly over the vertebral bodies, unite, and enter the abdomen by piercing the crus of the diaphragm. In the thorax, branches pass to the oesophagus and aorta (from the greater splanchnic nerve and from the small **splanchnic ganglion** which lies on it opposite the twelfth thoracic vertebra) and traverse the diaphragm with these structures.

5. The **lesser splanchnic nerve** is formed by branches from the ninth and tenth ganglia of the sympathetic trunk. It passes to the abdomen through the crus of the diaphragm.

6. When present, the **lowest splanchnic nerve** arises from the last thoracic ganglion, and passes to the abdomen with the lesser splanchnic nerve.

DISSECTION. Clean the posterior parts of the ntercostal spaces as far as the angles of the ribs, where the internal intercostal muscles end.

Subcostal Muscles

These are thin muscular slips which run in the same direction as the internal intercostal muscles, but lie internal to them. The subcostal muscles cross two or three intercostal spaces, and may either form a complete sheet on the posterior part of the thoracic wall, or be represented by a few slips, or be totally absent. They form part of the incomplete internal muscular layer of the thorax with transversus thoracis and the innermost intercostals.

Internal Intercostal Membranes. These membranes are a medial continuation of the fascia between the internal and external intercostal muscles. They lie posterior to the corresponding intercostal vessels and nerves [FIG. 8] and are continuous medially with the superior costotransverse ligament, which passes from the neck of the rib to the transverse process of the vertebra above. If the membranes are removed, the posterior fibres of the external intercostal muscles are exposed.

Vena Azygos [FIGS. 26, 33, 48, 75]

This vein usually arises in the abdomen from the posterior surface of the inferior vena cava, and enters the thorax either immediately to the right of the aorta and thoracic duct, or through the right crus of the diaphragm. In the thorax it ascends to the right of the thoracic duct and aorta, at first posterior to the diaphragm and later to the right border of the oesophagus. It arches anteriorly over the root of the right lung to enter the superior vena cava immediately superior to the pericardium at the level of the fourth thoracic vertebra. The arch of the vein separates the pleura from the oesophagus, trachea and vagus nerve, and it grooves the medial aspect of the lung superior to the root. Occasionally a part of the lung (**azygos lobe**) surrounded by pleural cavity, extends upwards between the arch of the vein and the structures medial to it.

Tributaries. The azygos vein receives the second to eleventh right posterior intercostal veins, the subcostal vein, and blood from the posterior abdominal wall through the **ascending lumbar vein.** It also drains a similar territory on the left side from the fourth intercostal space inferiorly via the **hemiazygos** and **accessory hemiazygos veins.** Two or more **bronchial veins** from the right lung and some **oesophageal veins** also enter the azygos vein. The latter veins communicate with the gastric veins through the oesophageal orifice of the diaphragm, forming one route of communication between the systemic system of veins and the portal system in the abdomen. Through its communication with the inferior vena cava and that of the hemiazygos vein with the left renal vein, it forms an anastomosis between the superior and inferior venae cavae. This is enhanced by the communication of the inferior vena cava and the azygos and hemiazygos veins through the valveless **internal vertebral venous plexus** [FIG. 180].

Left Superior Intercostal Vein

This vein is formed by the union of the posterior intercostal veins of the second and third left intercostal spaces, with communications from the adjacent spaces. It descends to the vertebral end of the aortic arch, runs anterosuperiorly across the left side of the aortic arch, lateral to the vagus and medial to the phrenic nerve [FIG. 28], and enters the left brachiocephalic vein, often uniting with the left **pericardiacophrenic vein.**

DISSECTION. Remove the strip of pleura covering the phrenic nerve on both sides. Trace the nerve and the pericardiacophrenic vessels which accompany it, superiorly and inferiorly as far as possible.

Phrenic Nerves

These important nerves are the sole motor supply to the diaphragm, and transmit sensory fibres from other structures developed in or from the septum transversum (*i.e.*, pericardium, liver and biliary apparatus, and inferior vena cava). They arise in the neck from the **fourth cervical ventral rami,** with additional fibres from the third and fifth. Each descends to the thorax posterolateral to the corresponding internal jugular vein, and is joined by the pericardiacophrenic branch of the internal thoracic artery at the root of the neck. They pass inferiorly on the side of the mediastinum a short distance anterior to the root of the lung, immediately medial to the mediastinal pleura.

The **right phrenic nerve** traverses the thorax lateral to the right brachiocephalic vein and the superior vena cava, crosses the pericardium (which separates it from the right atrium) and runs on the inferior vena cava to the diaphragm [FIG. 27].

The **left phrenic nerve** descends between the left common carotid and subclavian arteries, crosses the left surface of the arch of the aorta, and courses along the side of the pericardium superficial to the left auricle and left ventricle of the heart.

Both nerves pierce the diaphragm and are distributed on its inferior surface together with sympathetic filaments from the plexus on the inferior phrenic arteries.

LUNGS

[p. 4]

Each of these two organs has the shape of half a cone, and is comparatively light because of its large content of air. The right lung of a healthy adult weighs approximately 620 g., while the left weighs 570 g., and they float freely in water unless consolidated by disease.

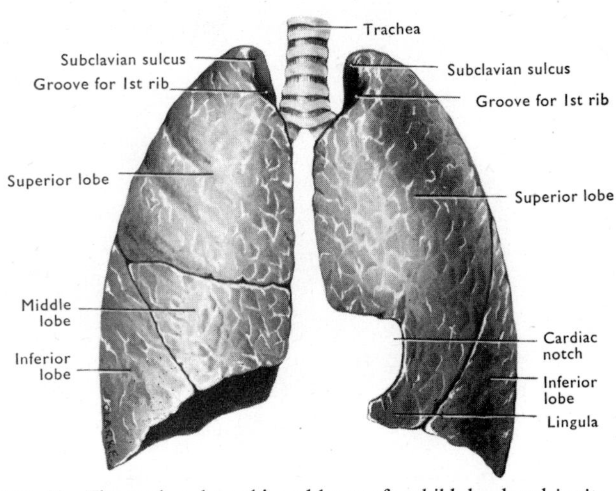

FIG. 30 The trachea, bronchi, and lungs of a child, hardened *in situ*.

The lungs contain a high proportion of elastic tissue, and if distended with air in the fresh state, will contract down and expel most of the air. It is this elasticity which is responsible for most of the expiratory force in quiet respiration, and the loss of this elasticity in disease (*e.g.*, emphysema) leads to permanent distension of the lungs and grave embarrassment of respiration.

In children the lungs are yellowish pink, but the deposition of carbon leads to the surface becoming mottled with patches and fine lines of black in the adult.

Each lung lies free in its own pleural cavity and is only attached by its root to the mediastinum, though in most dissecting room cadavers there are adhesions between the pulmonary and parietal pleura due to pleurisy. When the lungs are fixed *in situ* and their elasticity thereby destroyed, the surfaces bear a number of ridges and grooves corresponding to the irregularities of the surfaces with which they are in contact, and these are retained after the removal of such fixed lungs.

Apex

The apex of the lung extends into the root of the neck 3–5 cm. above the anterior part of the first rib. It lies behind and above the medial third of the clavicle, and is crossed by the subclavian artery and vein which groove it, but are separated from it by the pleura and **suprapleural membrane** [p. 17].

Base

The base of the lung is semilunar in shape and deeply concave to fit the dome of the diaphragm. This concavity is most marked on the right owing to the greater height of the right dome of the diaphragm [Fig. 6]. Because of the concavity of the diaphragmatic surface, it meets the costal surface at the sharp inferior margin [p. 18]. This extends towards the costodiaphragmatic recess of the pleura but does not reach its lower limit, except in forced inspiration. Medially the inferior margin abuts on the pericardium, and is blunt.

Anterior Margin

The anterior margin of the lung is thin and extends into the narrow costomediastinal recess of the pleura. This margin extends antero-inferiorly from the apex to the inferior border of the manubrium sterni, passing

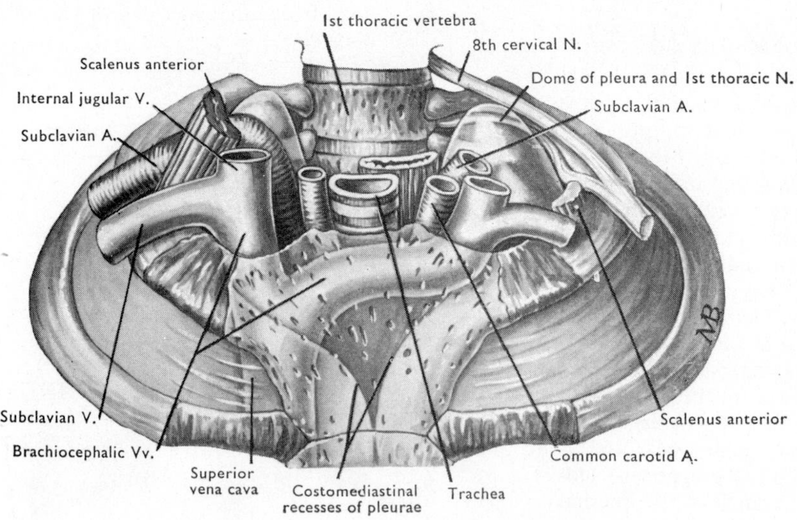

Fig. 31 The superior aperture of the thorax. The anterior margins (costomediastinal recesses) of the pleural sacs and the great veins are shown through the sternum

posterior to the sternoclavicular joint. It then descends vertically to meet the inferior margin opposite the xiphisternal joint. On the left side it is deeply notched by the bulging pericardium posterior to the fifth costal cartilage, and below this extends medially as the **lingula** [FIG. 30]. The **cardiac notch**, so formed, leaves part of the pericardium uncovered by lung.

Posterior Surface

The posterior surface of the lung is thick and rounded and fits into the deep paravertebral gutter. It lies in contact with the costal pleura like the remainder of the costal surface.

Medial Surface

The medial surface lies in contact with the vertebral column (vertebral part) and mediastinum (mediastinal part) and is hollowed out to form the cardiac impression, which is much deeper on the left than on the right lung.

Hilus

The hilus of the lung lies posteriorly in the mediastinal part, near the centre of the medial surface. It is a large depressed area through which structures enter and leave the lung, and it is surrounded by the pleura which is reflected

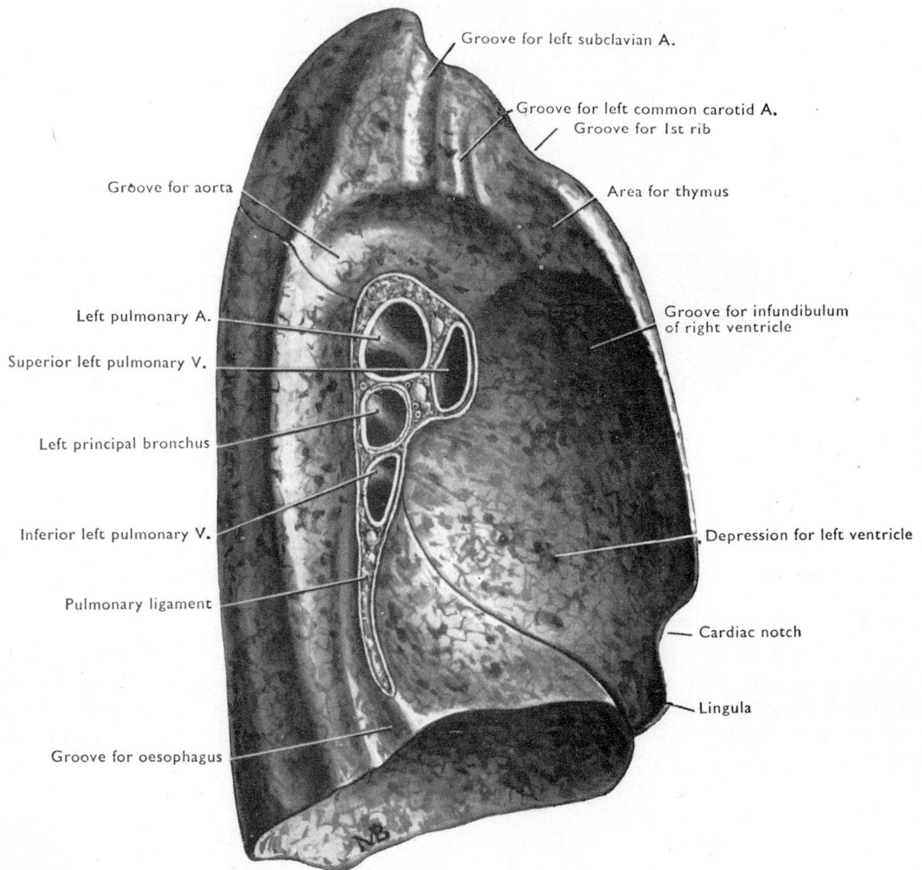

FIG. 32 The medial surface of the left lung hardened *in situ*.

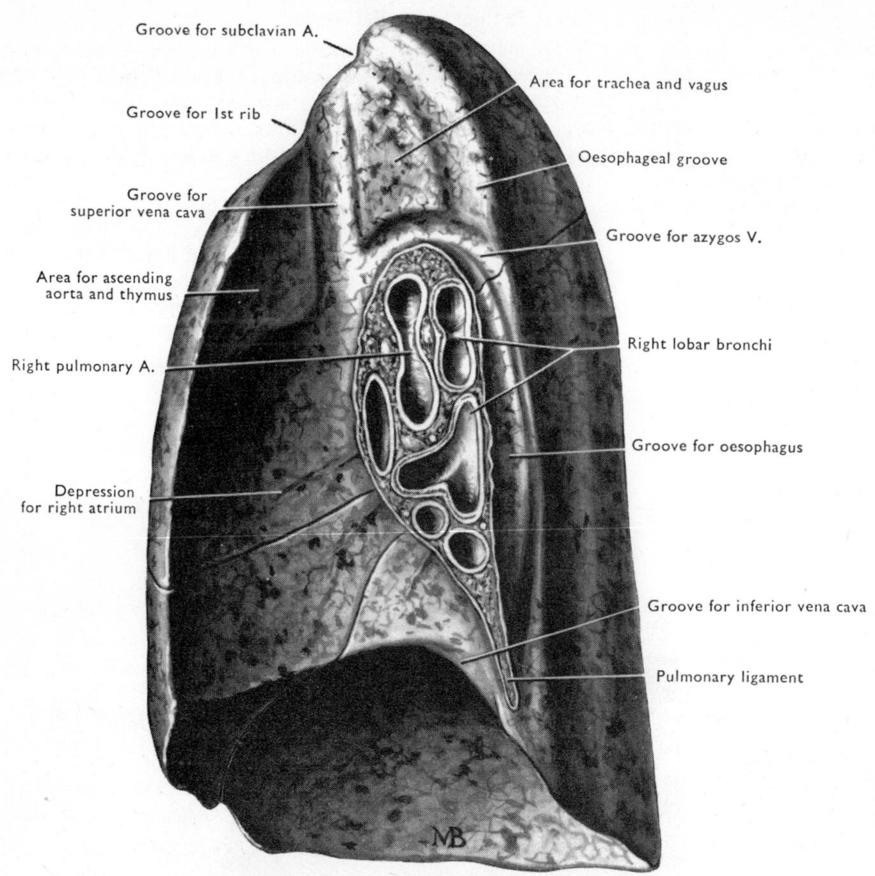

FIG. 33 The medial surface of the right lung hardened *in situ*.

off the lung on to the mediastinum and forms the **pulmonary ligament** inferiorly [FIGS. 32, 33].

Mediastinal Surface of Lung

If the lung is healthy this surface will show markings which are an exact negative of the lateral surface of the mediastinum to which it is applied. With the help of FIGURES 26 and 33, and FIGURES 28 and 32, identify again the structures on the lateral surfaces of the mediastinum and note their relation to the lung by the grooves and depressions which they leave on that structure. Note also that there are certain structures which are too small to leave any impression on the lungs but which are in contact with the mediastinal pleura: (1) the **phrenic nerve** and associated vessels on both sides; (2) the **right vagus** on the trachea, and the **left vagus** crossing the common carotid artery and the aortic arch; (3) the **left superior intercostal vein** crossing the aortic arch; (4) the **thoracic duct** to the left of the oesophagus [FIGS. 49, 59].

ROOTS OF THE LUNGS

All the structures which enter or leave the lung do so through its root, and this is enclosed by a short tubular sheath of pleura which joins the pulmonary and mediastinal parts of the pleura and extends inferiorly from the root as the pulmonary ligament [FIGS. 32, 33].

Each lung root contains: (1) the **principal bronchus** which transmits air to and from the lung; (2) one **pulmonary artery** and superior and inferior **pulmonary veins,** the latter transmit oxygenated blood from the lungs; (3) **lymph vessels** and **nodes** which drain the lung tissue and pulmonary pleura; (4) **bronchial arteries** which carry oxygenated blood to the bronchi and lymph nodes, and which anastomose with the branches of the pulmonary arteries in the lungs; (5) **bronchial veins;** and (6) branches of the vagus and sympathetic trunk which form the **pulmonary plexus** and supply all the structures of the lung. The relative positions of these structures in the lung roots can be seen in FIGURES 32 and 33, and the bronchus can be recognized by the firm, elastic cartilages which lie in its wall and maintain the patency of its lumen despite changes in external pressure. These cartilages are found throughout the bronchial tree, but they never completely encircle the bronchi and so do not prevent the smooth muscle in the walls of these tubes from decreasing their diameter. The single pulmonary artery in the lung root can be differentiated from the two veins both by its position and by the greater thickness of its wall.

LOBES OF THE LUNGS

The **left lung** is divided into two lobes by a deep **oblique fissure** which begins posteriorly opposite the spine of the third thoracic vertebra. It passes antero-inferiorly with a slightly spiral course, to meet the inferior margin close to the sixth costochondral junction. It extends into the lung almost to the hilus, and separates the **inferior** and **superior lobes**. The latter forms the apex and the anterior margin, while the former makes up almost all of the posterior and diaphragmatic surfaces.

The **right lung** is divided by a similar **oblique fissure** which separates the **superior** and **middle lobes** from the **inferior lobe.** A second fissure **(horizontal fissure)** extends from the anterior margin (at the fourth costal cartilage) horizontally backwards to meet the oblique fissure in the mid-axillary line. This fissure separates the wedge-shaped **middle lobe** from the superior lobe.

The pulmonary pleura extends into the fissures of the lungs and allows some degree of movement of the lobes on each other during respiration. The fissures may be obliterated by pleurisy, and infection in the fissures may become localized to form an abscess between the lobes of the lung. Not all the fissures are constantly present, the horizontal fissure being most commonly absent in whole or in part.

The major differences between the two lungs are: (1) the right lung has three lobes; (2) the right lung is shorter than the left, because of the greater height of the right dome of the diaphragm which is elevated by the mass of the liver; (3) the right lung is wider than the left because of the smaller cardiac impression on the right; and (4) the anterior margin of the right lung is vertical, while that of the left is deeply notched by the projecting pericardium; the left superior lobe projecting anteriorly to form the **lingula** below the cardiac notch.

INTRAPULMONARY STRUCTURES

Bronchi

The two principal bronchi, one to each lung, arise from the termination of the trachea and pass inferolaterally to the hilus of the lung. Each pulmonary artery passes transversely into the lung anterior to the corresponding bronchus, while the pulmonary veins descend slightly as they pass from the hilus of the lung to the left atrium. Thus the veins lie in the inferior part of the lung root, while the artery lies in its superior part [FIGS. 32, 33].

Within the lung substance the bronchi divide in a tree-like fashion, and thus each branch supplies a clearly defined sector of the lung. The **principal bronchi** divide into **secondary bronchi** (two on the left and three on the right), and each of these **lobar bronchi** supplies a lobe of the lung. Each lobar bronchus divides into the tertiary branches **(segmental bronchi)**, and these supply sectors of the lungs known as bronchopulmonary segments, each

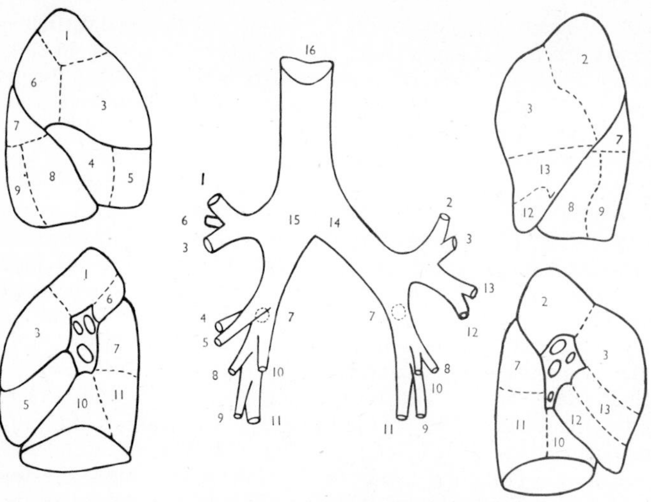

FIG. 34 The bronchi and bronchopulmonary segments. (After Jackson and Huber.) Each segmental bronchus has the same name as the subdivision of the lung supplied by it.

1. Apical.
2. Apicoposterior.
3. Anterior.
4. Lateral.
5. Medial.
6. Posterior.
7. Apical (inferior lobe).
8. Anterior basal.
9. Lateral basal.
10. Medial basal.
11. Posterior basal.
12. Inferior lingular.
13. Superior lingular.
14. Left principal bronchus.
15. Right principal bronchus.
16. Trachea.

of which is a pyramidal subdivision of a lobe having its apex towards the lung root [FIG. 34].

Bronchopulmonary Segments. These are of considerable clinical significance. Thus blockage of a segmental bronchus leads to collapse of the segment supplied by it, and the arrangement of the lung in such segments allows the surgeon to remove diseased parts with minimal disturbance to the surrounding lung tissue.

The general arrangement of the segments can best be understood by reference to FIGURE 34 and by dissecting out the main branches of the bronchi close to the hilus of the lung. The arrangement of the bronchi to the inferior lobe is similar in the two lungs, but the presence of a middle lobe and the earlier division (at the hilus of the lung) of the principal bronchus in the right lung are associated with a different pattern in the superior parts of the two lungs. Thus the **left superior lobar bronchus** is larger than the right and supplies the sector of the left lung corresponding to the superior and middle lobes of the right lung. The upper main branch of the left superior lobar bronchus supplies two segments (**apicoposterior** and **anterior**) which correspond to the three segments of the right superior lobar bronchus (**apical, anterior,** and **posterior**). The lower main branch of the left superior lobar bronchus supplies **superior lingular** and **inferior lingular** segments, and these pass to a sector corresponding to the middle lobe of the right lung, but their arrangement differs from the **lateral** and **medial** segments of the middle lobe bronchus of the right lung.

Blood Vessels

The branches of the **pulmonary artery** distribute venous blood to the lungs, and they follow the bronchi, lying mainly on their posterior surfaces. There is, therefore, a branch of the pulmonary artery to each pulmonary segment. The terminal branches divide into capillaries which form a network in the walls of the alveoli, where gaseous exchange takes place between the blood and the alveolar air.

The **pulmonary veins** drain the oxygenated blood from the lungs to the left atrium of the heart. A main vein emerges from each bronchopulmonary segment, usually on the anterior surface of the corresponding bronchus. There are also veins which run between the segments and on the mediastinal and fissural surfaces of the lungs. The latter may even cross the line of a fissure of the lung when this is incomplete. The artery of the right medial basal segment is frequently a branch of the middle lobe artery, and the corresponding vein usually drains into the vein of the middle lobe.

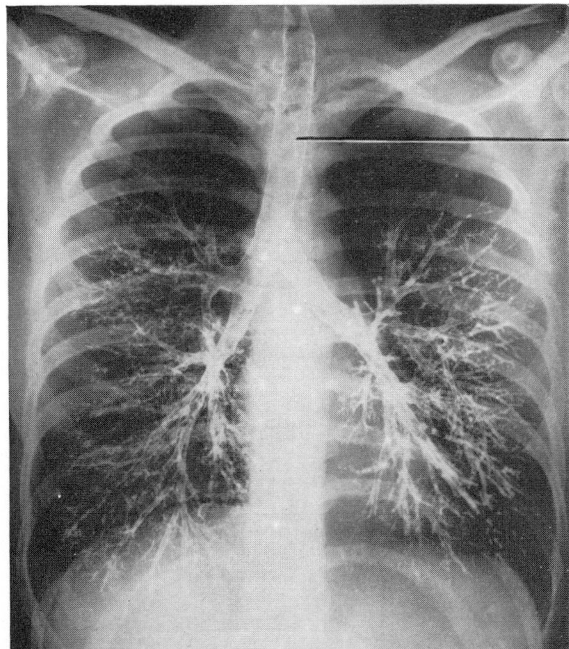

FIG. 35 An anteroposterior radiograph (bronchogram). The trachea and bronchi are outlined by the introduction of X-ray-opaque material. Cf. FIG. 34.

In the left lung repeat the procedure in the same order, and compare the arrangement in the two lungs.

When the posterior surfaces of the bronchi are being cleaned, look for the bronchial arteries. Two are usually present in the left lung and one in the right. Their origins will be seen later. The left bronchial arteries arise from the descending aorta and the right either from the first aortic intercostal artery or the superior left bronchial artery. They are the nutrient vessels of the lung, and some of the blood they transmit is returned through the pulmonary veins, the remainder is returned through the bronchial veins to the azygos and accessory hemiazygos veins on the vertebral bodies.

The **superior** right pulmonary vein drains the superior and middle lobes, and thus corresponds to the superior left pulmonary vein which drains the left superior lobe. Similarly the right and left **inferior** pulmonary veins drain the corresponding inferior lobes.

DISSECTION. When the surface of the lung has been broken at the hilus, it is simple to scrape away the alveolar tissue from the main veins, bronchi, and arteries. In the right lung, begin by cleaning the superior pulmonary vein to demonstrate its tributaries from the superior and middle lobes. Then clean the corresponding bronchi posterior to the veins. Repeat the procedure with the inferior pulmonary vein and corresponding bronchi, noting the small, grey or black pulmonary lymph nodes which lie in the angles formed by the bifurcations of the bronchi.

When the bronchi have been cleaned, follow the branches of the right pulmonary artery. Note that they correspond to the branches of the bronchi and lie mainly on their posterior surfaces.

Lymph Vessels and Nodes of Lung

The lymph vessels of the lung cannot be demonstrated in dissecting room specimens, but the nodes are very obvious because of their black colour and the dense connective tissue which binds them to the structures in the lung. A **superficial plexus** of lymph vessels lies deep to the pulmonary pleura, and drains to the bronchopulmonary lymph nodes in the hilus of the lung by passing over the surfaces of the lung. This plexus communicates with the deep lymph vessels which begin on the terminal air ducts and pass with the bronchi and blood vessels. They drain through **pulmonary nodes** situated in the bifurcations of the bronchi, to the **bronchopulmonary nodes** in the angles between the stem and first branches of the principal bronchus. Thence the lymph passes to the nodes on the principal bronchi, in the angle between the two bronchi (**inferior tracheobronchial nodes**), and to those between each bronchus and the lateral aspect of the trachea (**superior tracheobronchial nodes**). From the tracheobronchial nodes the lymph either drains through the **right bronchomediastinal trunk** to the right

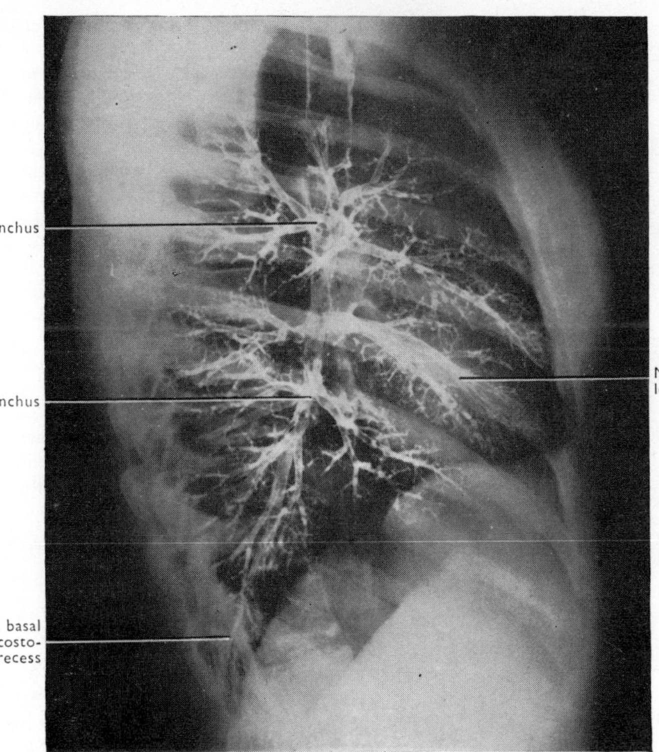

FIG. 36 A lateral radiograph to show the right bronchial tree by the introduction of X-ray-opaque material.

brachiocephalic vein, or through the thoracic duct or **left bronchomediastinal trunk** on the left side. Some of the lymph on both sides may pass to the lower deep cervical nodes, and the tracheobronchial nodes communicate with the other mediastinal nodes.

Enlargement of the bronchopulmonary nodes may be visible in radiographs as an increase in the density of the shadow caused by the lung root; a simple enlargement is smooth and lobular.

DISSECTION. Find the left vagus on the aortic arch. Follow its recurrent laryngeal branch inferior to the arch and the ligamentum arteriosum, a short fibrous cord which extends from the root of the left pulmonary artery to the aortic arch immediately anterior to the recurrent laryngeal nerve. Identify again the cardiac nerves on the aortic arch. Trace them into the concavity of the arch where they join a plexus of nerve fibres and ganglion cells, the superficial cardiac plexus. Identify this and note branches radiating from it to the heart and great vessels.

Superficial Cardiac Plexus

This is the anterior extremity of a complicated plexus of nerve fibres and cells which extends from the bifurcation of the trachea to the concavity of the arch of the aorta. It sends branches to the heart and lungs. The superficial part receives the superior cervical cardiac branch of the left sympathetic trunk and the inferior cervical cardiac branch of the left vagus. The remaining cardiac branches of these two structures on both sides pass to the deep part of this system, and their oblique, descending course is the result of the caudal displacement of the heart and lungs during development. From the superficial part, branches pass to the heart on the pulmonary trunk, and to the left pulmonary plexus.

ANTERIOR MEDIASTINUM

[FIG. 37]

This is a narrow cleft posterior to the body of the sternum. It contains the remains of the thymus, which extends inferiorly from the anterior part of the superior mediastinum to the level of the third or fourth costal cartilage. Together with some loose, fatty tissue the thymus separates the great vessels and the superior part of the pericardium from the pleura and sternum [FIGS. 39, 49, 59].

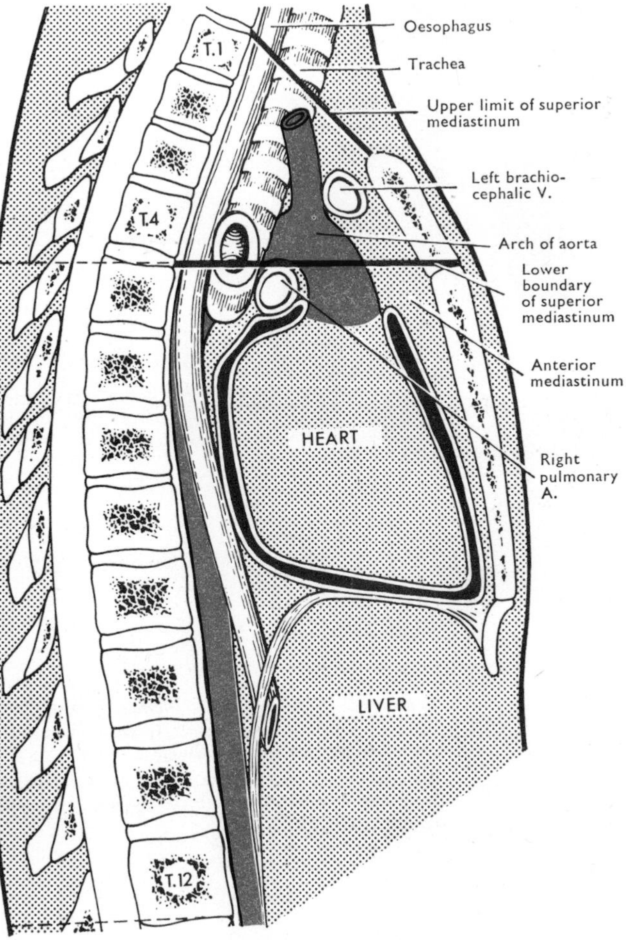

FIG. 37 A diagram of a median section through the thorax to show the general distribution of the structures in the mediastinum. The heart in the pericardium forms the middle mediastinum, while the anterior and posterior mediastina lie between it and the sternum and vertebral column respectively. Note that the posterior mediastinum also extends inferiorly between the diaphragm and the vertebral column.

Thymus

In the child this is a bilobed mass of lymphoid tissue. It develops as a bilateral structure from the third pharyngeal pouches of the embryo in common with the **inferior parathyroid glands,** and subsequently descends with the pericardium from the neck into the thorax. Thus it may retain a fibrous connexion with one or both of the inferior parathyroid glands in the neck. In the foetus and new-born [FIG. 38] the thymus is nearly as large as the heart, and continues to grow until puberty, but involutes thereafter. In the adult it is usually reduced to two strips which consist of lymphoid and fibrous tissue infiltrated with fat, but the extent and rate of its involution are very variable.

The functions of the thymus are not entirely clear, but it is known to produce large numbers of lymphocytes as a result of the very rapid division of its constituent cells in the young animal. If the thymus is removed from mice at birth, they usually die after a few weeks with a profound reduction in the number of circulating lymphocytes,

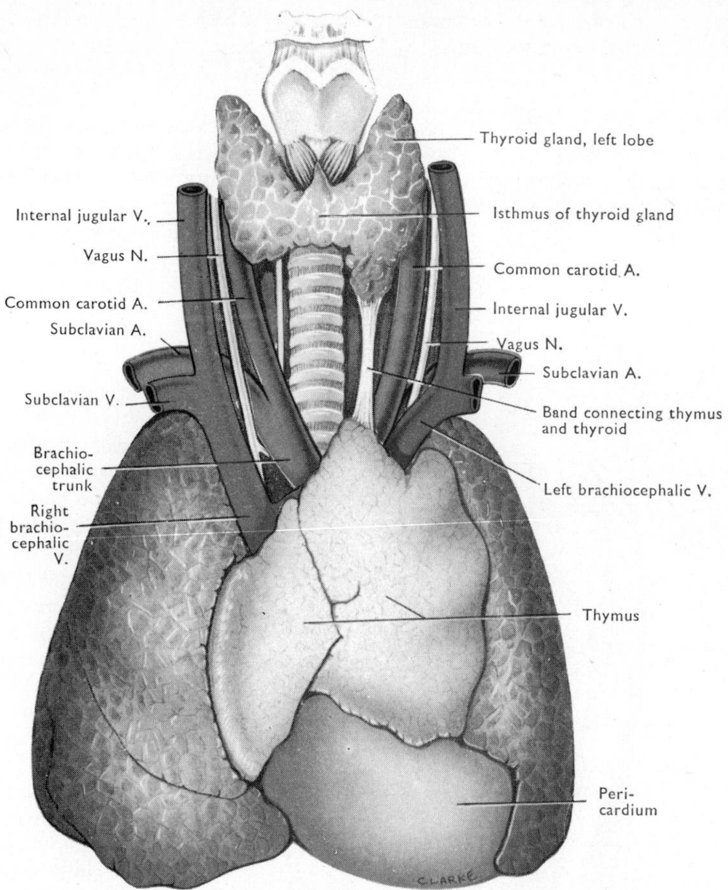

FIG. 38 The thyroid gland and thymus in a full-term foetus.

and a failure of the other lymphoid tissues to develop. This may be due partly to the failure of thymus lymphocytes to populate the other lymphoid tissues, but more especially is the result of the absence of a hormone produced by the thymus. This hormone stimulates the formation of lymphocytes in the other lymphoid tissues, and thus makes available the cells which can produce antibodies to foreign proteins and other antigens, a feature which is not present before birth.

DISSECTION. Clean the thymus as far as possible, and separate it from the pericardium, turning it superiorly. Note any blood vessels passing to the thymus. The veins run superiorly on its deep surface and enter the left brachiocephalic vein posterior to the manubrium of the sternum, while the arteries come from the internal thoracic vessels and occasionally from the arch of the aorta.

MIDDLE MEDIASTINUM

Pericardium

The pericardium is a serous bag, akin to the pleura, and the heart appears to be invaginated into it from above and behind. It consists of three layers: (1) an outer fibrous layer which is

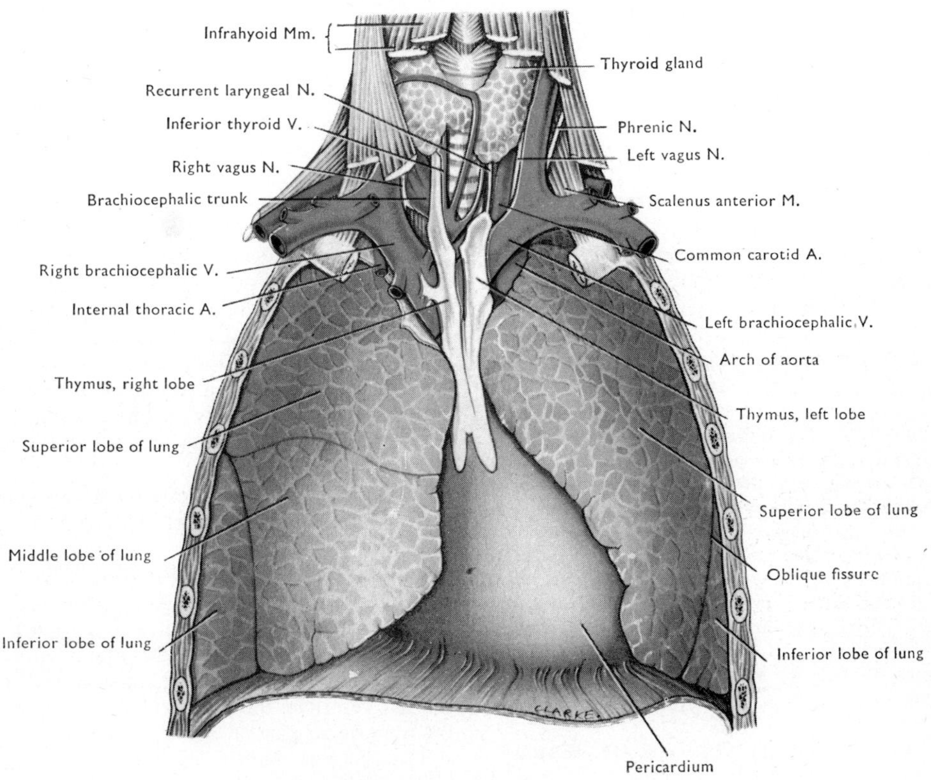

FIG. 39 The thyroid gland and thymus in the adult.

lined by (2) the parietal layer of serous pericardium, while the enclosed heart is covered by (3) the visceral layer of serous pericardium. The apposed surfaces of **serous pericardium** are smooth, having a mesothelial lining, and are separated by a thin film of moisture which allows them to slide freely on each other, thus facilitating the movements of the heart within the pericardium. The two layers of serous pericardium are continuous with each other around the great vessels entering and leaving the heart, and at the same sites the fibrous pericardium fuses with the connective tissue surrounding the vessels.

Fibrous Pericardium. This is a conical fibrous sac which is pierced at its **apex** by the aorta, pulmonary trunk, and superior vena cava. Its **base** rests on the diaphragm (which separates it from the liver and fundus of the stomach) and is fused with its central tendon, but is separated from it laterally by a little areolar tissue. On the right side the central tendon of the diaphragm and base of the pericardium are pierced by, and fused with, the **inferior vena cava**.

The pericardium lies posterior to the body of the sternum and the cartilages of the second to sixth ribs. It is separated from these by the lungs and pleurae, except: (1) in the median plane, where two condensations of fibrous tissue connect it to the superior and inferior parts of the body of the sternum (**sternopericardial ligaments**); and (2) where the left pleura deviates to the left, the pericardium is directly in contact with the sternum and transversus thoracis muscle. To the left of this, the pericardium is covered by the anterior extremity of the pleural sac into which the cardiac notch of the left lung extends only on deep inspiration.

The lateral surfaces and the lateral parts of the posterior surface of the pericardium are in contact with the corresponding mediastinal pleura, and the pulmonary veins pierce the pericardium on the line of meeting of these two surfaces. The median part of the posterior surface is in contact with the oesophagus and descending aorta, both of which separate it from the vertebral column.

DISSECTION. Make a vertical cut through each side of the pericardium immediately anterior to the line of the phrenic nerve. Join the lower ends of these two incisions by a transverse incision through the pericardium approximately 1 cm. above the diaphragm. Turn the flap of pericardium upwards, and examine the pericardial cavity. Determine the superior attachment of the flap to the superior vena cava, aorta, and pulmonary trunk, and divide it close to this attachment, leaving a narrow strip of pericardium attached to the vessels so that its position can be identified later [Fig. 40].

STERNOCOSTAL SURFACE OF HEART [FIG. 40]

The greater part of this surface is formed by the **right ventricle** and the **right atrium.** Because of the rotation of the heart [p. 22] the left ventricle and left atrium lie more posteriorly, but form a small strip of the sternocostal surface on the left, including the apex of the heart. The right and left atria, though separated internally by a septum, have muscular walls which are directly continuous, and together they form a U-shaped structure which lies postero-inferior to the ascending aorta and the pulmonary trunk. The **auricles** of the atria, form the ends of the U, and partially overlap the anterior surfaces of these vessels, appearing on the sternocostal surface. The right atrium extends further anteriorly than the left and also forms part of the sternocostal surface.

The **atria** lie posterosuperior to the ventricles and are separated from them by the deep **coronary sulcus,** part of which passes obliquely across the sternocostal surface from the root of the ascending aorta to the junction of the **right margin** of the heart (formed by the right atrium) with the diaphragmatic surface. Inferior to the sulcus is the **ventricular part** of the sternocostal surface. This ends below and to the left in the **apex of the heart,** and is divided by the **anterior interventricular groove** into a right two-thirds formed by the right ventricle, and a left third formed by the left ventricle. The groove is marked by a line of fat which contains the anterior interventricular branch of the left coronary artery and the great cardiac vein, and it marks the line along which the **interventricular septum** meets the sternocostal surface.

Superiorly and to the left the sternocostal surface of the **right ventricle** narrows to become continuous with the pulmonary trunk through its upper, funnel-shaped **infundibulum.**

The **left border** of the sternocostal surface is more convex than the right and is almost entirely formed by the thick, bulging wall of the left ventricle, the left auricle appearing in the uppermost part.

The **inferior border** of the sternocostal surface is sharp, and is wedged between the dipahragm and the anterior wall of the thorax. It is formed almost entirely by the right ventricle.

Transverse Sinus of Pericardium. This aperture connects the two sides of the pericardial cavity posterior to the ascending aorta and pulmonary trunk and anterosuperior to the atria. It can be demonstrated by placing a finger anterior to the lowest part of the superior vena cava and pushing it to the left, posterior to the ascending aorta. The finger appears on the left between the pulmonary trunk and the left auricle. With the finger in the sinus, pass a flexible probe through the right pulmonary artery till it appears through the cut end of the left pulmonary artery. The probe lies posterosuperior to the finger in the transverse sinus, while the atria lie postero-inferior [FIG. 43].

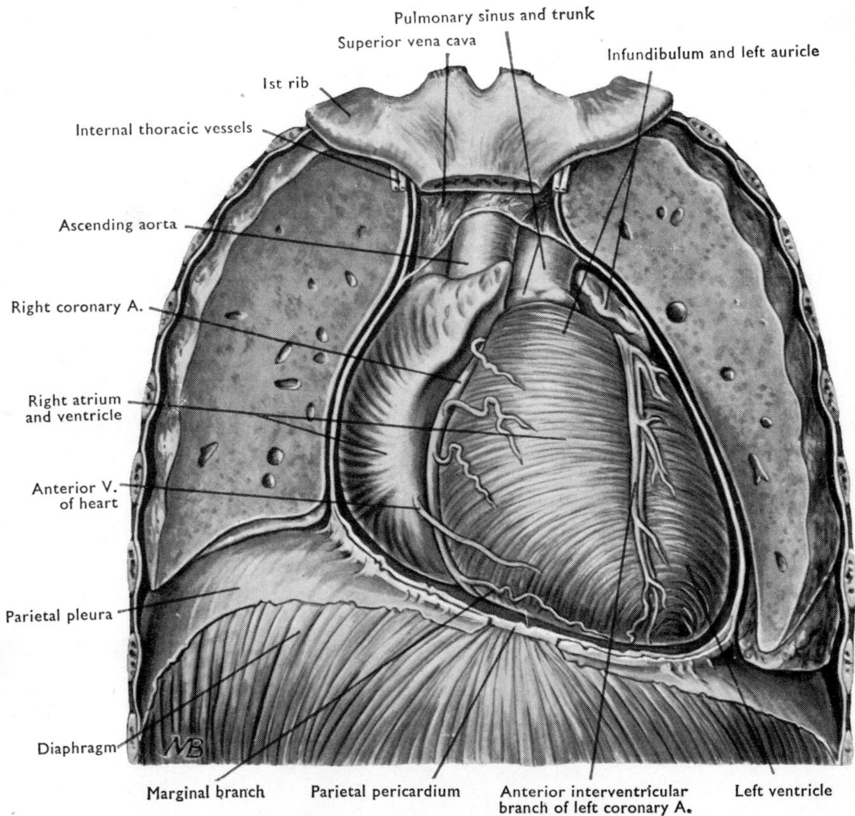

FIG. 40 The sternocostal surface of the heart *in situ.* The front of the pericardium has been removed together with the anterior parts of both lungs.

The transverse sinus thus lies between the arterial and venous ends of the heart. It is the remnant of an aperture in the dorsal mesocardium (a fold of pericardium which connects the originally straight heart tube to the dorsal wall of the pericardial cavity). The aperture is caught between the arterial and venous ends of the heart when they are approximated as the heart folds on its middle (ventricular) section [FIGS. 22–25]. The transverse sinus thus separates a sleeve of pericardium surrounding the great arteries from a similar sleeve enclosing the entering veins.

Oblique Sinus of Pericardium. Pass the fingers of one hand between the diaphragmatic pericardium and the heart, and note that there is no attachment of the heart to the diaphragm except at the extreme right where the inferior vena cava pierces the diaphragm and immediately enters the right atrium. The apex of the heart lies free in the pericardial cavity. Lift the heart forwards and pass the fingers superiorly behind the heart to the left of the inferior vena cava; they now lie in a blind pouch of the pericardial cavity (oblique sinus of the pericardium) posterior to the left atrium. The lateral walls of this pouch are formed by the reflexion of the parietal pericardium on to the posterior wall of the left atrium [FIG. 51] over the veins entering the heart. These veins consist of two pulmonary veins on each side with the two venae cavae superior and inferior to the right pulmonary veins.

With two fingers in the oblique sinus, pass a seeker through each of the right and left pulmonary veins in turn, and note that as it passes into the left atrium the seeker can be felt immediately lateral to the oblique sinus. Press the fingers superiorly into the blind extremity of the oblique sinus, and note that a finger in the transverse sinus is separated from the tips of the fingers in the oblique sinus by a small quantity of tissue; this is the superior margin of the left atrium [FIG. 43] immediately inferior to the pulmonary arteries.

Serous Pericardium

The serous pericardium is the thin, elastic layer of tissue which covers the heart (visceral layer or epicardium) and lines the fibrous, parietal pericardium. The apposed surfaces

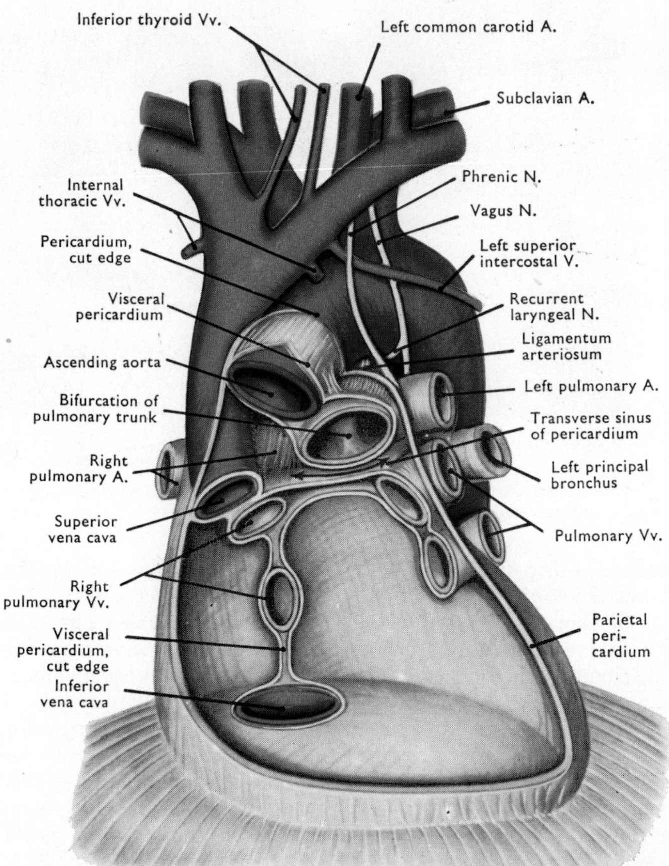

FIG. 41 The pericardium and great vessels after removal of the heart. The arrow lies in the transverse sinus of the pericardium, and the posterior wall of the oblique sinus lies between the right and left pulmonary veins.

of these two parts are covered by a slippery layer of simple squamous epithelium.

The arrangement of the serous pericardium, which has been inspected above, can best be understood if it is appreciated that the heart is enclosed in a sleeve of visceral pericardium [FIG. 25]. One end of the sleeve surrounds the aorta and pulmonary trunk, while the other end surrounds the entering veins. The transverse sinus separates the ends of the sleeve where they become continuous with the parietal pericardium. The venous end of the sleeve is complicated by being partially separated into right and left halves by the intrusion of the oblique sinus of the pericardium into it from below. The only part of the surface of the heart which is not covered with serous pericardium is the superior margin of the left atrium which lies between the oblique and transverse sinuses in the part of the venous sleeve which joins the right and left walls of the oblique sinus and closes that sinus superiorly [FIG. 43].

DISSECTION. Strip the visceral pericardium from the sternocostal surface of the heart, and scrape away the fat from the ventricular surface. This will expose the anterior interventricular branch of the left coronary artery lying with the great cardiac vein in the anterior interventricular groove. Note the branches that the artery gives to both ventricles and to the interventricular septum on which it lies, and trace it inferiorly till it curves on to the diaphragmatic surface of the heart close to the apex. Follow the artery and vein superiorly till they disappear inferior to the left auricle [Fig. 40].

Remove the fat from the coronary sulcus, and take care not to destroy a number of small veins (anterior cardiac veins) which pass across the sulcus from the right ventricle to enter the right atrium directly. In the depths of the sulcus, identify the right coronary artery and follow it superiorly to its origin from a swelling (right aortic sinus) at the root of the ascending aorta deep to the right auricle. Trace the artery inferiorly to the point at which it turns on to the posterior surface of the heart. Note the branches to the right ventricle and atrium and especially one which arises close to the origin of the artery and passes over the left surface of the auricle towards the superior vena cava; this supplies part of the atrium and the sinu-atrial node.

Clean the myocardium and note the general direction of its fibres.

Remove any remaining fragments of intercostal muscles from the downturned flap of anterior thoracic wall, and replacing it in position, note the relation of the various parts of the sternocostal surface of the heart to the sternum and costal cartilages.

SURFACE ANATOMY OF HEART [FIG. 42]

The **superior border** of the heart, formed by the upper margins of the atria, is mainly hidden by the aorta and the pulmonary trunk. It extends from the lower border of the left second costal cartilage (approximately 1·5 cm. from the margin of the sternum) to the upper border of the third right costal cartilage close to the margin of the sternum. A line joining these two points also marks out the position of the pulmonary arteries which lie along the superior margin of the heart.

The **right border** of the heart, formed by the right atrium, extends from the right end of the superior border to a point on the right sixth costal cartilage 1–2 cm. from the margin of the sternum. This border is slightly convex to the right.

The **inferior border** of the heart, formed mainly by the right ventricle, extends from the inferior extremity of the right border to a point (**apex of the heart**) in the fifth left intercostal space immediately medial to a vertical line dropped through the mid-point of the clavicle (mid-clavicular line). Normally this border is slightly concave inferiorly, but in any condition leading to hypertrophy of the right ventricle (*e.g.*, increased pulmonary arterial pressure) it becomes convex and gives the heart a globular shape.

The **left border** is marked by a line, convex to the left, joining the left ends of the superior and inferior borders. It is formed mainly by the left ventricle, the left auricle forming a small part of this border superiorly.

The **coronary sulcus** lies on a line joining the sternal ends of the third left and sixth right costal cartilages.

The great **orifices** of the heart and the **valves** which guard them will be seen when the heart opposite the fourth intercostal space.

The positions given above are only approximate because the heart is a mobile organ and its shape and position are subject to considerable variation in relation to changes in intrathoracic pressure and the height of the diaphragm during respiration. Thus if a deep breath is taken and expiration is attempted against a closed mouth and nose, the high intrathoracic pressure reduces the amount of venous blood returning to the heart which consequently narrows, while the low position of the diaphragm also tends to elongate the heart. The converse effect can be produced by attempting to inspire against a closed nose and mouth after full expiration [Figs. 6, 7].

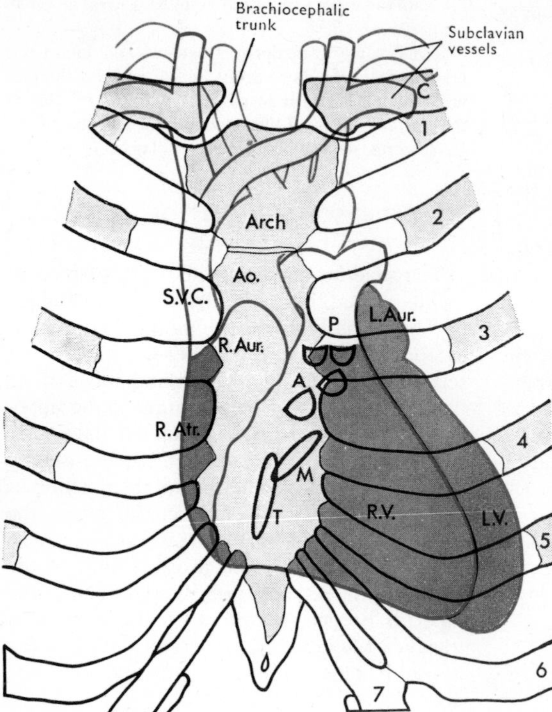

Fig. 42 The relation of the heart and great vessels to the anterior wall of the thorax.

1-7. Ribs and costal cartilages.
A. Aortic valve.
Ao. Ascending aorta.
C. Clavicle.
L.Aur. Left auricle.
L.V. Left ventricle.
M. Left atrioventricular (mitral) orifice.
P. Valve of pulmonary trunk.
R.Atr. Right atrium.
R.Aur. Right auricle.
R.V. Right ventricle.
S.V.C. Superior vena cava.
T. Right atrioventricular (tricuspid) orifice.

is opened, but they lie on a line parallel and slightly inferior to the coronary sulcus. Thus the **pulmonary orifice** lies opposite the sternal end of the left third costal cartilage. The **aortic orifice** lies posterior to the left margin of the sternum opposite the third intercostal space. The **left atrioventricular** (mitral) **orifice** lies posterior to the left half of the sternum opposite the fourth costal cartilage, while the **right atrioventricular** (tricuspid) **orifice** lies posterior to the middle of the sternum

Diaphragmatic Surface of Heart

This slightly concave surface is formed entirely by the ventricles, and the line of separation of these is marked by the **posterior interventricular groove** which may only be visible as a line of fat. It contains the posterior interventricular branch of the right coronary artery and the middle cardiac vein, and demonstrates that the **left ventricle** forms the left two-thirds of this surface [Fig. 65].

Base of Heart

This is the posterior or vertebral surface of the heart which is formed entirely by the atria, principally the left atrium. The base is separated from the diaphragmatic surface by the posterior part of the **coronary sulcus,** and this contains parts of the right and left coronary arteries and a large vein, the **coronary sinus,** which enters the right atrium to the left of the inferior vena cava [Figs. 43, 51].

Coronary Arteries [Figs. 40, 44, 55, 65]

Only parts of these arteries can be seen at the present stage of the dissection. The coronary arteries are the nutrient arteries of

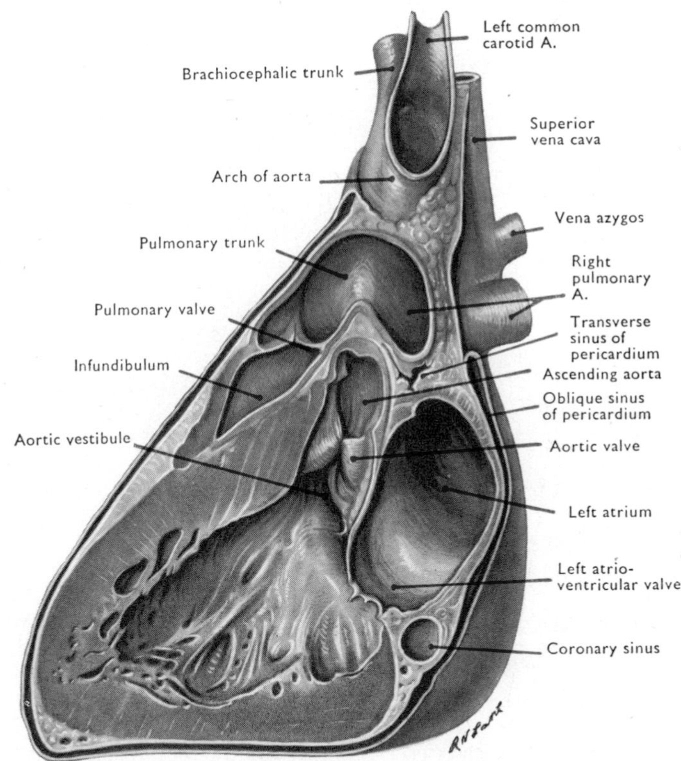

FIG. 43 A sagittal section through the heart and pericardium.

the heart, and are greatly enlarged vasa vasorum. They arise from two of the three dilatations (sinuses) at the root of the aorta, the right coronary artery from the right sinus, and the left from the left sinus.

The **right coronary artery** passes forwards between the superior part of the infundibulum and the auricle of the right atrium, and turns inferiorly in the coronary sulcus to the inferior part of the right margin of the heart. Here it gives off the **marginal branch** [FIG. 40] then turns to the left in the posterior part of the coronary sulcus, giving off its largest branch (**posterior interventricular**) along the posterior interventricular groove towards the apex, and terminates to the left of this by giving branches to the left atrium and ventricle [FIGS. 55, 65]. It supplies the roots of the aorta and pulmonary trunk, a large part of the right ventricle, all of the right atrium, and parts of the posterior and inferior surfaces of the left atrium and ventricle respectively. The posterior interventricular branch also supplies small branches to the inferior part of the interventricular septum. These vessels anastomose with the corresponding branches of the anterior interventricular branch of the left coronary artery in the septum.

The **left coronary artery** runs to the left around the posterior surface of the pulmonary trunk, inferior to the left auricle. It then divides into a large anterior interventricular branch and a circumflex branch. The **anterior interventricular branch** [FIG. 40] runs towards the apex in the anterior interventricular groove, and supplies both ventricles and the antero-

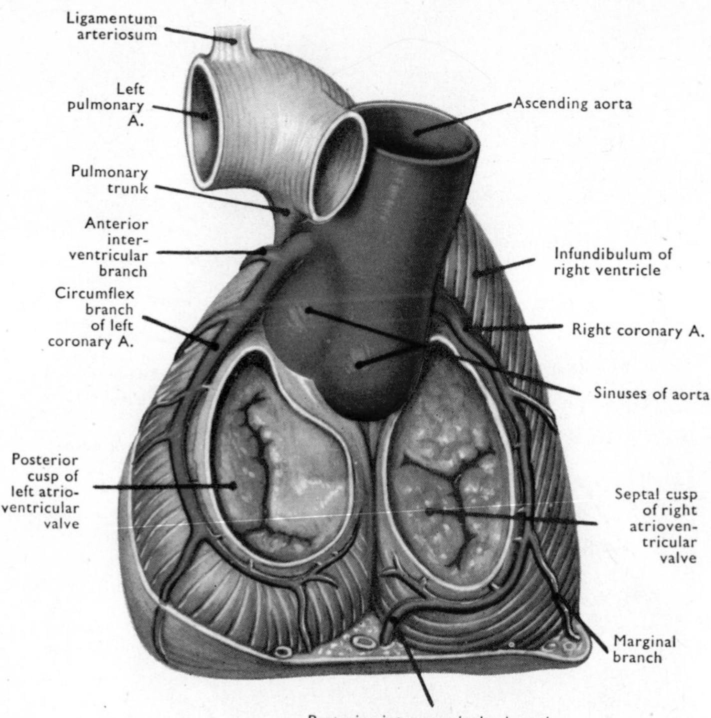

FIG. 44 The base of the ventricular part of the heart after removal of the atria. The right coronary artery usually extends further to the left than in this specimen; cf. FIG. 55. The sternocostal surface is to the right.

superior part of the interventricular septum. The **circumflex branch** curves postero-inferiorly to the right in the coronary sulcus, and terminates to the left of the posterior interventricular groove by giving branches to the left ventricle and atrium [FIG. 65].

The coronary arteries are the only arterial supply to the heart, and though they anastomose to a slight extent, particularly in the interventricular septum, this is inadequate to compensate for the blockage of any but the smallest branches, particularly when the arteries are already diseased. Such blockage, due to clotting of the blood within the arteries (coronary thrombosis), therefore usually leads to death of the affected muscle fibres and their replacement with fibrous tissue if the individual survives.

Veins of Heart

The major parts of the venous drainage are dealt with later, but it is possible to follow the **great cardiac vein** with the anterior interventricular artery to the left extremity of the coronary sulcus, and to see the **anterior cardiac veins** draining directly from the anterior surface of the right ventricle into the right atrium across the coronary sulcus [FIGS. 40, 45]. The **small cardiac vein** may also be seen running with the marginal artery along the inferior margin of the heart to enter the posterior part of the coronary sulcus with the right coronary artery.

The **middle cardiac vein** may also be seen running with the posterior interventricular artery. This vein drains into the coronary sinus (q.v.) together with all the other cardiac

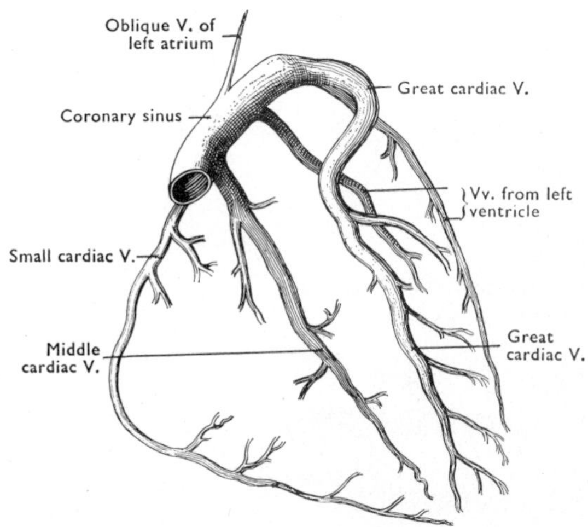

FIG. 45 A diagram of the tributaries of the coronary sinus.

veins with the exception of the anterior cardiac veins and certain small venous channels which lie in the walls of the heart and open directly into its chambers, the **venae cordis minimae.**

Nerves of Heart

The nerves come from the cardiac plexuses situated on the bifurcation of the trachea. The nerve fibres are of two kinds: (1) **sympathetic fibres** which arise in the ganglion cells of the cervical and upper thoracic ganglia of the sympathetic trunk; (2) **parasympathetic fibres** which arise in the ganglion cells of the cardiac plexuses and in scattered ganglia along the blood vessels of the heart. Some of the sympathetic supply the coronary arteries, and tend to produce vasodilatation, but both groups innervate the heart. On stimulation the sympathetic increase the heart rate, while the parasympathetic slow it. The nerve fibres tend to run with the coronary vessels thus forming the right and left **coronary plexuses,** but they also run independently, and many accompany the conducting tissue of the heart (q.v.).

CHAMBERS OF HEART

The chambers of the heart and the valves which separate them are best displayed with the heart *in situ.* This is achieved by making a series of coronal sections through the heart approximately parallel to the sternocostal surface [FIGS. 46, 56, 62]. As these slices are made, the sternum and costal cartilages should be folded back into position from time to time so that the relation of the parts of the heart to the anterior thoracic wall may be confirmed. Also the slices may be replaced so that the relative positions of the parts of the heart can be determined.

DISSECTION. The first coronal slice lies immediately anterior to the ascending aorta. Lay a knife transversely across the anterior surface of the ascending aorta in a coronal plane with the edge pointing inferiorly, and cut in this direction towards the anterior part of the diaphragmatic surface of the heart. The knife should cut obliquely into the anterior surface of the pulmonary trunk, and pass inferiorly into the right atrium a short distance anterior to the entry of the superior vena cava, posterior to the right auricle. Continue the cut through the right surface of the right atrium to meet the diaphragm where the right coronary artery turns into the posterior part of the coronary sulcus. Carry the incision through the left surface of the heart to the apex in the same plane, passing immediately anterior to the left auricle. When these cuts have been made, lift the sternocostal surface of the heart anteriorly, and divide the interventricular septum down to the anterior part of the diaphragmatic surface in the same plane. Join the right and left cuts through the anterior part of the diaphragmatic surface, immediately posterior and parallel to the marginal artery. Remove the anterior surface of the heart. Clean any blood clot from the chambers of the heart, taking care not to damage either the cusps of the right atrioventricular valve or of the pulmonary valve at the root of the pulmonary trunk. The right atrium, atrioventricular orifice and valve (tricuspid), the right ventricle, infundibulum, pulmonary valve and trunk are now exposed and should be studied on both surfaces of the cut.

Right Atrium [FIGS. 46, 47]

The right atrium consists of two parts: (1) a smooth-walled posterior part which receives the great veins (superior and inferior venae cavae and the coronary sinus) and represents

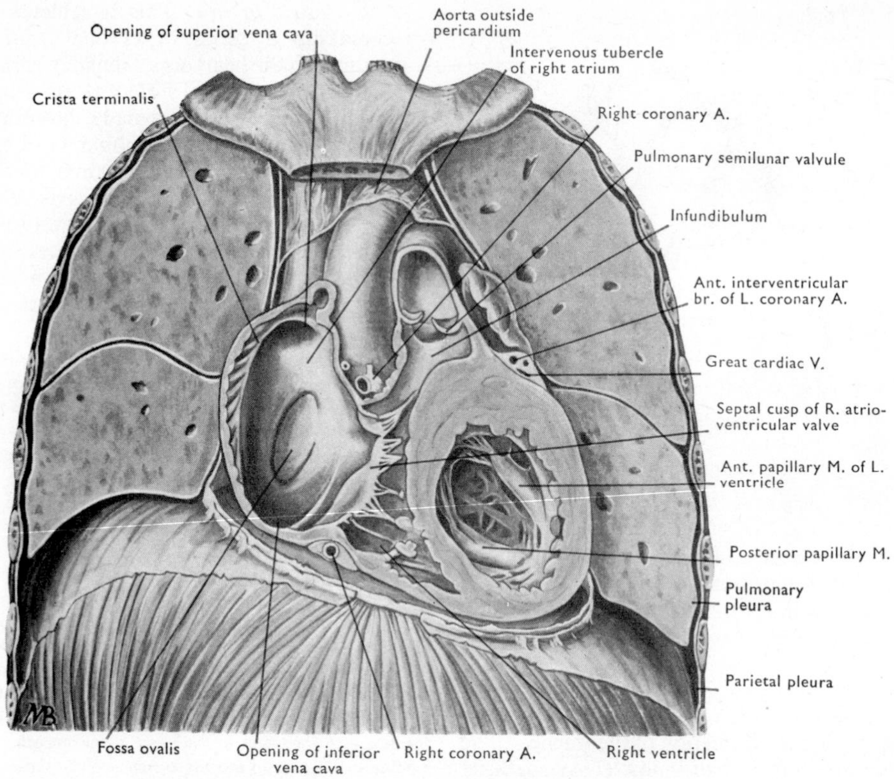

FIG. 46 The heart *in situ.* A drawing of the parts of the heart exposed by the first coronal section. See dissection instructions, and FIG. 40.

the confluence of the veins, or sinus venosus, of the embryo; (2) an anterior part which is ridged with more or less parallel muscle bundles (**musculi pectinati**) which extend into the auricle. The two parts are separated on the right by an internal vertical ridge (**crista terminalis**) and a corresponding external groove (**sulcus terminalis**). The crista terminalis begins superiorly, anterior to the opening of the superior vena cava, and extends to a point, anterior to the opening of the inferior vena cava. Here it becomes continuous with a sharp ridge (**valve of the inferior vena cava**) which sweeps superiorly on the posteromedial wall of the atrium in line with the left wall of the inferior vena cava. This ridge fades out on the posteromedial wall of the atrium, but appears to be continuous with the superior curved margin (**limbus fossae ovalis**) of an oval fossa (**fossa ovalis**) which lies on this wall of the right atrium approximately midway between the openings of the venae cavae. The crista terminalis and the valve of the inferior vena cava represent the remains of the right of two venous valves which guard the opening of the sinus venosus into the right atrium in the embryo, before the sinus is absorbed into the wall of the atrium. The posteromedial wall of the right atrium is the **interatrial septum** [FIG. 62], and the fossa ovalis is the remnant of the **foramen ovale** of the foetus through which the inferior vena caval blood passed to the left atrium, carrying the oxygenated placental blood to that chamber. The floor of the fossa is formed by the thin flap (**septum primum** of the interatrial septum) of the valvular foramen ovale. The limbus is the free margin of the rigid **septum secundum** which, assisted by the valve of the inferior vena cava, directs the inferior caval blood into the left atrium when the pressure in that atrium is low due to the small volume of blood passing through the lungs and entering the left atrium through the pulmonary veins. This difference in pressure in the two atria in intra-uterine life allows the flow of inferior caval blood to force the septum primum to the left away from the septum secundum, and thus keep the foramen ovale open. When the pressures in the two atria are equalized by the establishment of a full pulmonary circulation after birth, the septum primum is applied to the left side of the septum secundum and subsequently fuses with it, obliterating the foramen ovale. Thus any persistent part of the foramen is found between the floor and limbus of the fossa ovalis, **under** cover of the latter.

Note that the openings of the superior and inferior venae cavae are not in the same straight line, but are slightly angled to each other. Thus the flow of inferior caval blood is directed towards the fossa ovalis, while the superior caval stream passes towards the right atrioventricular orifice, anterior to the inferior caval flow. The angulation between the two streams is marked by the **intervenous tubercle** [FIGS. 46, 48], a slight angulation of the wall of the atrium superior to the fossa ovalis. This arrangement produces an effective separation of the two streams during intra-uterine life.

Superior Vena Cava

This vein is formed by the union of the right and left brachiocephalic veins behind the sternal end of the first right costal cartilage, and it

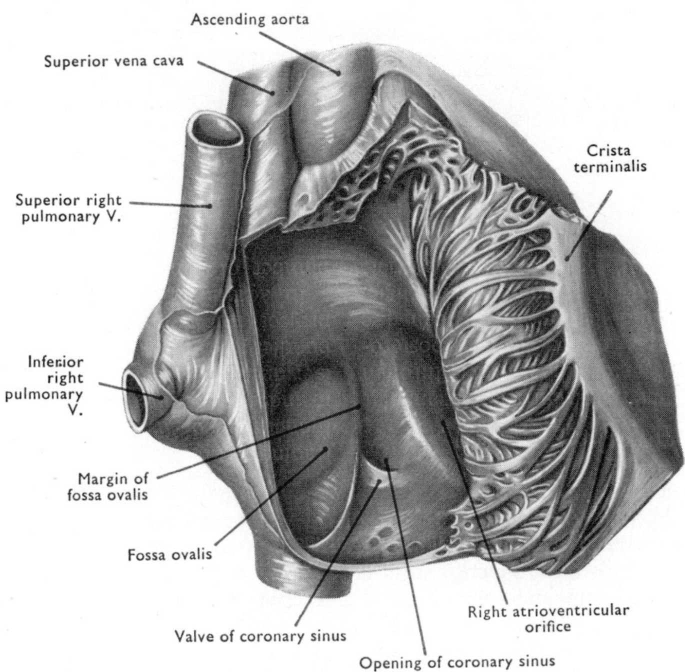

FIG. 47 The interior of the right atrium exposed by turning its right and anterior walls to the left.

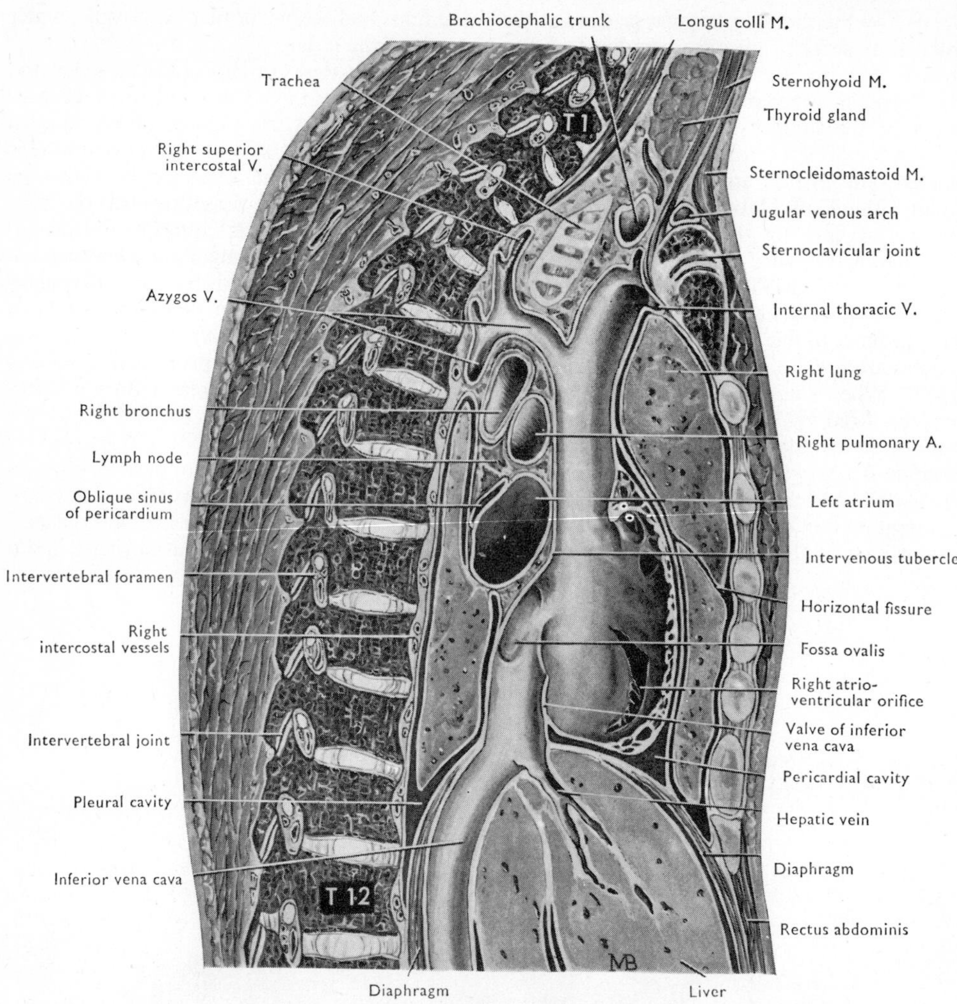

FIG. 48 A sagittal section through the thorax and upper abdomen along the line of the superior and inferior venae cavae. The remainder of this section is shown in FIG. 116.

ends by entering the superior part of the right atrium at the level of the third right costal cartilage close to the sternum. The **azygos vein** [FIG. 26] arches over the superior surface of the right lung root and enters the posterior surface of the superior vena cava at its mid-point, just before it enters the fibrous pericardium. Thus the superior vena cava drains all the blood from the head and neck, upper limbs, and the walls of the thorax and upper part of the abdomen.

The superior vena cava lies on the right of the superior mediastinum, anterolateral to the trachea and posterolateral to the ascending aorta in the middle mediastinum. The phrenic nerve intervenes between it and the right pleura which partially surrounds the right surface of the superior vena cava.

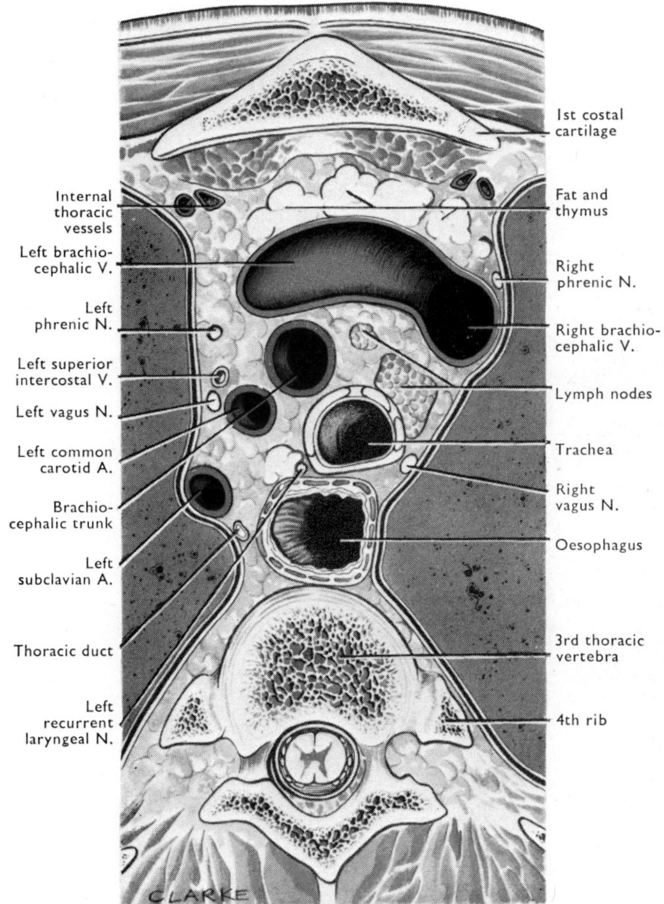

FIG. 49 A horizontal section through the thorax at the level of the third thoracic vertebra.

The inferior half of the vein lies in the pericardium beside the ascending aorta and partially overlapped by the right auricle. It is immediately anterior to the superior half of the right lung root, but is separated from the phrenic nerve and pleura by the pericardium. The close association of the vein with the lung root and its contained pulmonary veins [FIG. 50] makes it possible for an abnormal pulmonary vein to drain directly into the superior vena cava from the right lung.

Inferior Vena Cava [FIGS. 48, 71]

The intrathoracic part of this vein is very short (<2 cm.). It pierces the **central tendon of the diaphragm** approximately at the level of the eighth thoracic vertebra, and enters the postero-inferior part of the right atrium at the level of the sixth chondrosternal joint, immediately after piercing the pericardium. The right pleura and lung are wrapped round its right surface, on which lies the phrenic nerve, and they extend posterior to it, partially separating it from the vena azygos and the greater splanchnic nerve.

Coronary Sinus [FIGS. 45, 47, 51, 65]

This vein enters the right atrium immediately posterior to the right atrio-ventricular orifice, and its blood is directed towards that orifice by the **valve** of the coronary sinus which lies immediately to the right of the opening of the sinus. The superior extremity of the valve of the inferior vena cava is to the right of the valve of the coronary sinus and separates it from the fossa ovalis.

The **anterior cardiac veins** pierce the anterior wall of the right atrium. **Venae cordis minimae** enter the atrium through small, irregularly scattered openings which are difficult to identify.

The right atrioventricular orifice lies in the antero-inferior part of the right atrium, and opens into the postero-inferior part of the right ventricle. The orifice is guarded by the three cusps of the right atrioventricular (tricuspid) valve [FIG. 55].

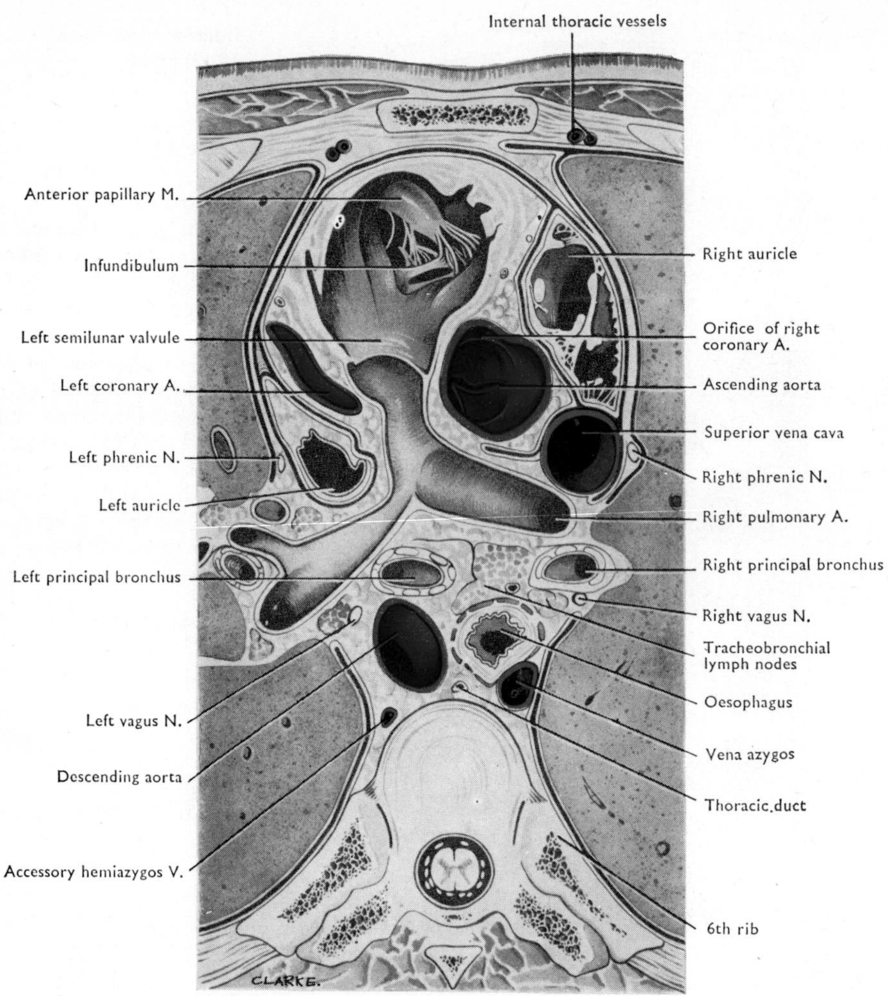

FIG. 50 A horizontal section through the thorax at the level of the intervertebral disc between the fifth and sixth thoracic vertebrae.

Right Ventricle [FIGS. 46, 53, 57, 67]

The cavity of the right ventricle is triangular in outline. Blood enters the ventricle through the **atrioventricular orifice** at the postero-inferior angle, and leaves it through the **pulmonary orifice** at the posterosuperior angle. The smooth-walled part of the ventricle leading to the posterosuperior angle is the funnel-shaped **infundibulum,** while the remainder of the internal surface of the ventricle is ridged by a number of irregular muscle bundles and ridges (**trabeculae carneae**) which project from its walls.

In addition to the trabeculae carneae, a number of conical muscle masses **(papillary**

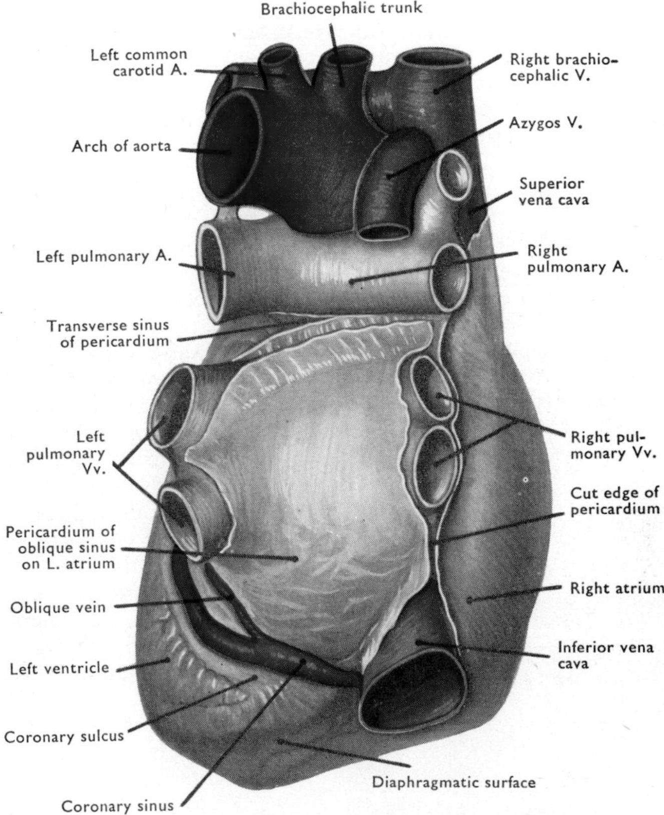

FIG. 51 The posterior surface of the heart and great vessels.

muscles) project from the walls of the ventricle. These are surmounted by tendinous strands (**chordae tendineae**) which pass to the margins and ventricular surfaces of the cusps of the right atrioventricular valve; the chordae tendineae of one papillary muscle pass to the adjacent parts of two cusps. Thus when the papillary muscles contract, together with the rest of the ventricular muscle, they tend to draw the cusps together and prevent them being forced back into the atrium as the intraventricular pressure rises. This prevents the valve turning outside in, and increases the efficiency of the ventricular contraction by preventing much of the contractility being used up in ballooning the cusps into the atrium.

Papillary Muscles. In the right ventricle there are usually three: (1) attached to the inferior wall, a large **posterior papillary muscle** which sends chordae tendineae to the **posterior** and **septal cusps** of the valve; (2) attached to the anterior wall, a larger **anterior papillary muscle** distributed to the anterior and posterior cusps; (3) attached to the septum, a number of small **septal papillary muscles** distributed to the anterior and septal cusps. Occasionally the anterior and posterior muscles are divided into a number of smaller projections.

Septomarginal Trabecula [FIGS. 53, 67]. One

of the trabeculae carneae crosses the cavity of the ventricle from the septum to the anterior papillary muscle. This septomarginal trabecula probably plays no part in preventing distension of the ventricle, but it carries the right crus of the **atrioventricular bundle** (conducting tissue of the heart, q.v.) and this ensures early contraction of the papillary muscle so that the chordae tendineae are already taut by the time the ventricular contraction as a whole is starting.

In transverse section the right ventricle is crescentic in shape because the thick muscle of the interventricular septum bulges to the right. The difference in thickness of the muscle of the two ventricles is directly related to the work done by each; the right ventricle only having to overcome the relatively slight resistance of the lungs (pulmonary systolic arterial pressure is 25–35 mm. Hg), while the left has to maintain a much higher arterial pressure (120 mm. Hg systolic) to achieve the systemic circulation. Thus in any condition which increases the pulmonary arterial resistance there is a compensatory hypertrophy of the right ventricular wall.

Right Atrioventricular Orifice [Figs. 46, 57]. This is approximately 2·5 cm. in diameter, and is surrounded by a fibrous ring which gives attachment to the cusps of the right atrioventricular valve. This ring is part of the **fibrous skeleton** of the heart which surrounds both atrioventricular orifices and also the pulmonary and aortic orifices. It gives attachment to the cusps of all the valves and effectively interrupts the conduction of impulses from the atrial to the ventricular muscle except through the atrioventricular bundle which perforates the fibrous tissue at the postero-inferior part of the interventricular septum. This feature permits the delay which exists between the onset of the atrial and the ventricular contracti onso The cut edge of the fibrous ring cand n seenethbe surface of the heart section [Fig. 54].

Right Atrioventricular (Tricuspid) Valve. The three **cusps** of this valve are named from their position: **anterior,** which separates the atrioventricular foramen from the infundibulum; **septal,** which is applied to the interventricular septum; **posterior,** which lies on the inferior wall of the right ventricle. The posterior and anterior cusps are more nearly horizontal than the vertical position which their names suggest. The margin and ventricular surface of each cusp has the attachment of the chordae tendineae, while the atrial surface. over which the blood flows, is smooth.

Pulmonary Orifice. This orifice lies superiorly at the apex of the infundibulum. It is surrounded by a thin

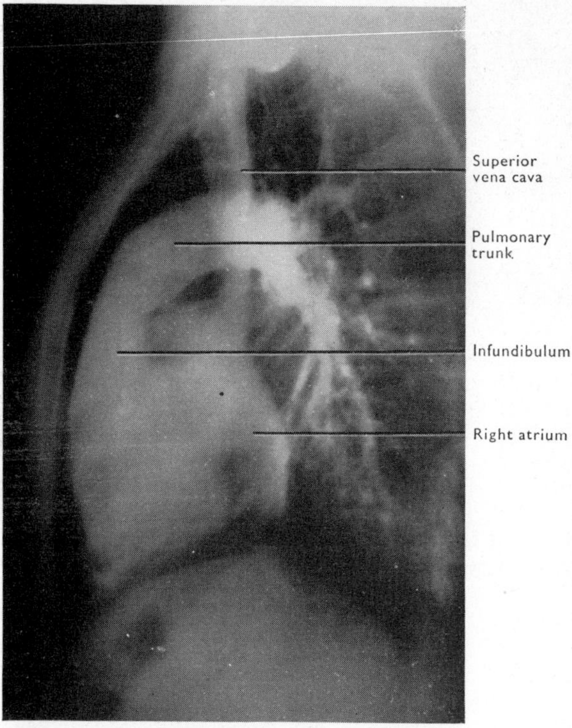

Fig. 52 A lateral radiograph of the thorax taken during the passage of contrast material through the heart. In this phase the superior vena cava, right heart, and the pulmonary trunk and arteries are filled.

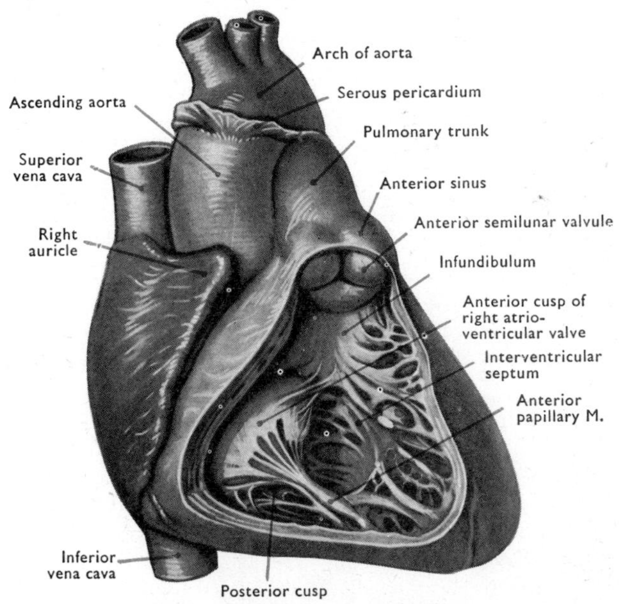

FIG. 53 The interior of the right ventricle exposed from in front.

fibrous ring which gives attachment to the valvules of the pulmonary valve internally and to the ventricular muscle antero-inferiorly, and is continuous with the wall of the pulmonary trunk posterosuperiorly.

Valve of Pulmonary Trunk. This consists of three **semilunar valvules** [FIG. 55] each of which is deeply concave on its arterial surface, and consists of a thin layer of fibrous tissue covered on each surface with a layer of endothelium. The fibrous tissue is thickened along the free and fixed margins of each valvule, especially at the centre of the free margin where it forms a small rounded peak, the **nodule** of the semilunar valvule. The thin, crescentic edges on each side of the nodule are the **lunules** of the valvule. The semilunar valvules are forced apart by the ejection of blood from the contracting ventricle. As this ceases, the elastic recoil of the pulmonary trunk and arteries forces the blood back towards the ventricle, ballooning out each valvule so that the free margins are forced together to form a Y-shaped arrangement of ridges radiating to the wall of the trunk from the nodules pressed together at the centre. The valvules are named **anterior, right** and **left** [FIG. 46]. Opposite each valvule the wall of the pulmonary trunk is slightly dilated [FIG. 53] to form a **sinus** of the pulmonary trunk.

Pulmonary Trunk [FIGS. 40, 43, 46, 60]

This great artery begins at the superior extremity of the infundibulum, anterior and to the left of the ascending aorta, and separated from the sternal end of the third left costal cartilage by the pericardium, pleura and lung. It is approximately 5 cm. long and half as wide, and winds round the left side of the ascending aorta to end in the concavity of the aortic arch by dividing into **right and left pulmonary arteries** behind the sternal end of the second left costal cartilage. In its upper part it is separated from the superior margin of the left atrium by the transverse sinus of the pericardium, and it is enclosed, with the ascending aorta, in a sheath of serous pericardium. The right and left coronary arteries are in contact with it at its origin [FIG. 55].

DISSECTION. To make the second slice through the heart [Fig. 56], begin superiorly by cutting half through the aorta at the junction of its ascending part with the arch, and also through the anterior half of the superior vena cava. Turn the edge of the knife inferiorly, and cut longitudinally through the middle of both vessels parallel to the first slice. Carry this cut inferiorly through the right atrium, left auricle, and left ventricle as far as a horizontal line passing through the membranous atrioventricular septum. This can be identified as a small depression on the left wall of the right atrium approximately 1·5 cm. anterior to the opening of the coronary sinus. From the horizontal line passing through the lower part of the membranous septum, continue the cut downwards and forwards to meet the first cut at the inferior surface of the heart.

This slice removes the anterior walls of the ascending

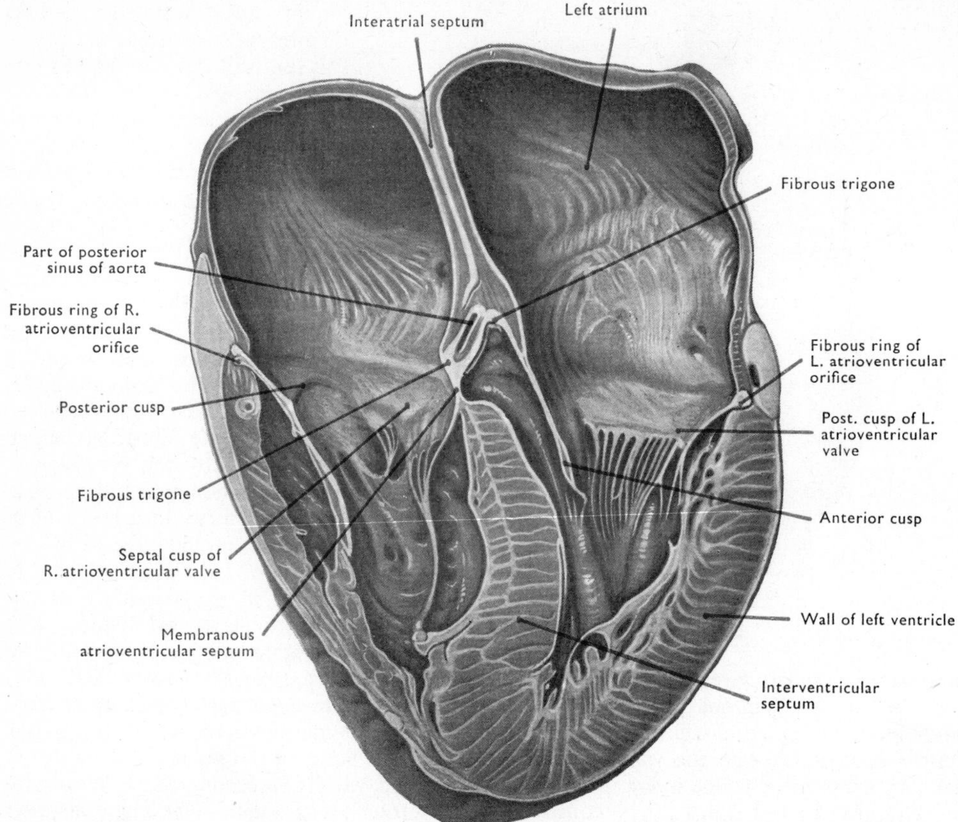

FIG. 54 A section through the heart to show the interventricular and interatrial septa and the fibrous rings that surround the orifices.

aorta, superior vena cava, and left ventricle, the lower part of the pulmonary trunk and the infundibulum, the left auricle and part of the wall of the right atrium. It leaves sufficient of the right ventricle and atrioventricular valve for orientation purposes, and demonstrates the positions of all the valves of the heart when taken in conjunction with the previous slice. The anterior interventricular branch of the left coronary artery is divided at its origin, but the stem of the left coronary artery and the beginning of its circumflex branch can be exposed by removing the loose fatty tissue between the root of the ascending aorta and the base of the left auricle.

Remove any blood clot from the left ventricle, but be careful not to damage the papillary muscles and chordae tendineae in the ventricle. This exposes the ventricular end of the left atrioventricular channel and the smooth-walled aortic vestibule passing superiorly and to the right from the ventricle to the aortic valve. Note that the membranous atrioventricular septum forms part of the right wall of the aortic vestibule, the posterior wall of which is the anterior surface of the anterior cusp of the left atrioventricular (mitral) valve.

Remove blood clot from the aorta and superior vena cava to expose the origin of the left coronary artery and the opening of the azygos vein.

Left Ventricle [FIGS. 54, 56, 57]

The cavity of the left ventricle is longer than that of the right. It is circular in transverse section, and its walls are very much thicker

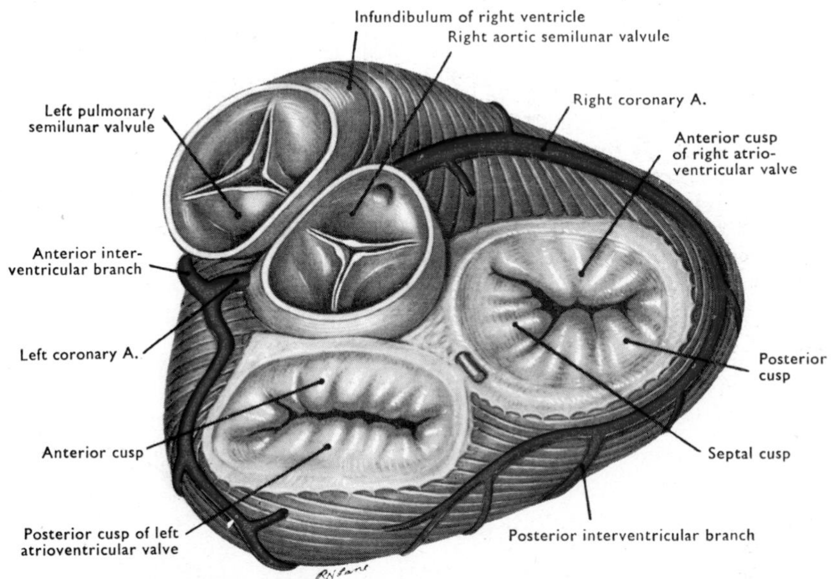

FIG. 55 The base of the ventricular part of the heart with the atria and great vessels removed. The atrioventricular bundle is shown piercing the right fibrous trigone.

than those of the right ventricle. The internal surfaces of the walls are covered with a dense mesh of trabeculae carneae, which are finer and more numerous than those in the right ventricle. They are particularly marked at the apex, but the surfaces of the septum and the upper part of the anterior wall are comparatively smooth.

Papillary Muscles. There are two large papillary muscles, **anterior** and **posterior** [FIG. 46]. The former is attached to the anterior part of the left wall, while the latter arises from the inferior wall more posteriorly. The chordae tendineae from each papillary muscle pass to both cusps of the left atrioventricular (mitral) valve.

Aortic Vestibule. The smooth walls of this part of the ventricle are partly fibrous, except anteriorly and to the left where the ventricular muscle reaches up to the aortic valve.

Aortic Orifice. This orifice lies in the right posterosuperior part of the ventricle, and, like the pulmonary orifice, is surrounded by a fibrous ring to which the valvules of the aortic valve are attached. Pass a finger between the cusps of the mitral valve, and note that the anterior cusp is all that separates the posterior part of the aortic orifice from the left atrioventricular orifice. Thus the anterior cusp of the mitral valve separates the stream of blood entering the ventricle from the outflowing stream to the aorta, and is smooth on both surfaces.

Aortic Valve. The structure of this valve is in all respects similar to the pulmonary valve, except that the valvules are thicker and differently placed, and the aortic sinuses are larger. The valvules are named posterior, right and left [FIG. 55].

Interventricular Septum. The greater part of this septum is thick and muscular, but its posterosuperior part is thin and membranous [FIGS. 54, 56] where it is connected with the fibrous rings which surround the atrioventricular and arterial orifices.

The interventricular septum is placed

obliquely, with its anterior border to the left and its inferior border to the right. The right surface faces forwards and to the right and bulges into the right ventricle [FIG. 46]. The muscular part extends from the inferior border of the heart immediately to the right of the apex to join the membranous part immediately inferior to the attachment of the septal cusp of the tricuspid valve.

The **membranous part** of the interventricular septum attaches the muscular interventricular septum [FIG. 56] to the right wall of the aortic orifice and to the muscular wall of the right atrium applied to the aorta. Anteriorly the membranous part ends at a point inferior to the right valvule of the aortic valve, and posteriorly at the anterior surface of the anterior cusp of the mitral valve. The membranous part forms the right wall of the aortic vestibule, and the septal cusp of the tricuspid valve is attached anteroposteriorly along the right surface close to the inferior margin. Thus the upper part forms a membranous atrioventricular septum, while the inferior part (below the attachment of the septal cusp of the tricuspid valve) is the membranous interventricular septum. The membranous part of the septum is developed from the same tissue that forms the valves of the heart, and since it develops separately from the muscular part of the septum, it may be deficient and leave an interventricular or

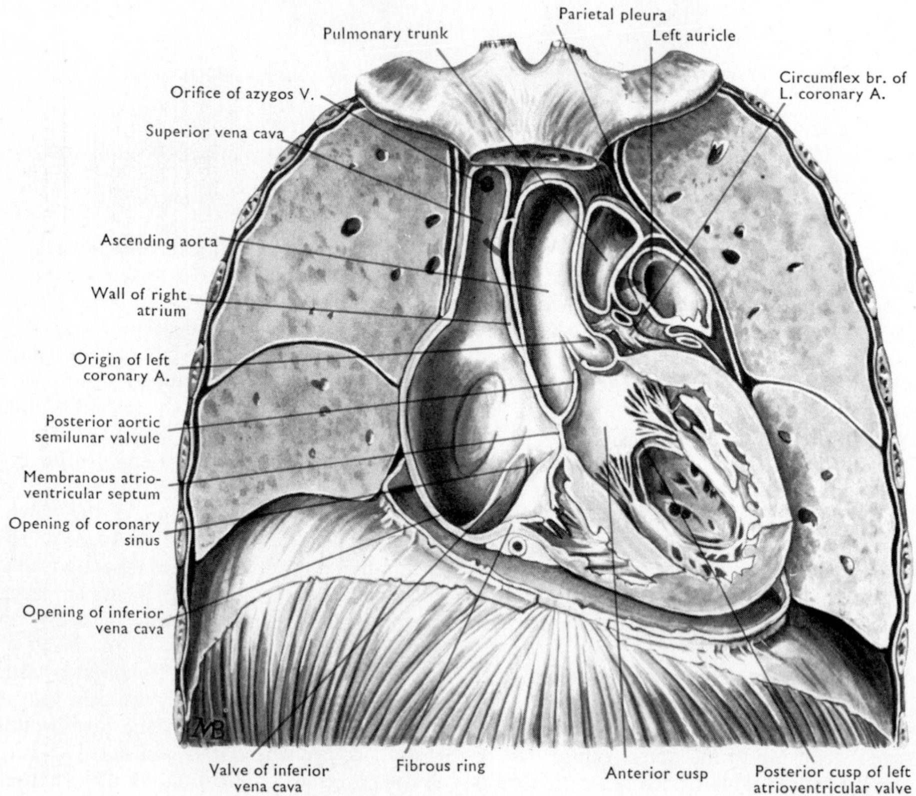

FIG. 56 The heart *in situ*. A drawing of the parts of the heart exposed by the second coronal section. See dissection instructions and FIG. 46. The arrow lies in the transverse sinus of the pericardium.

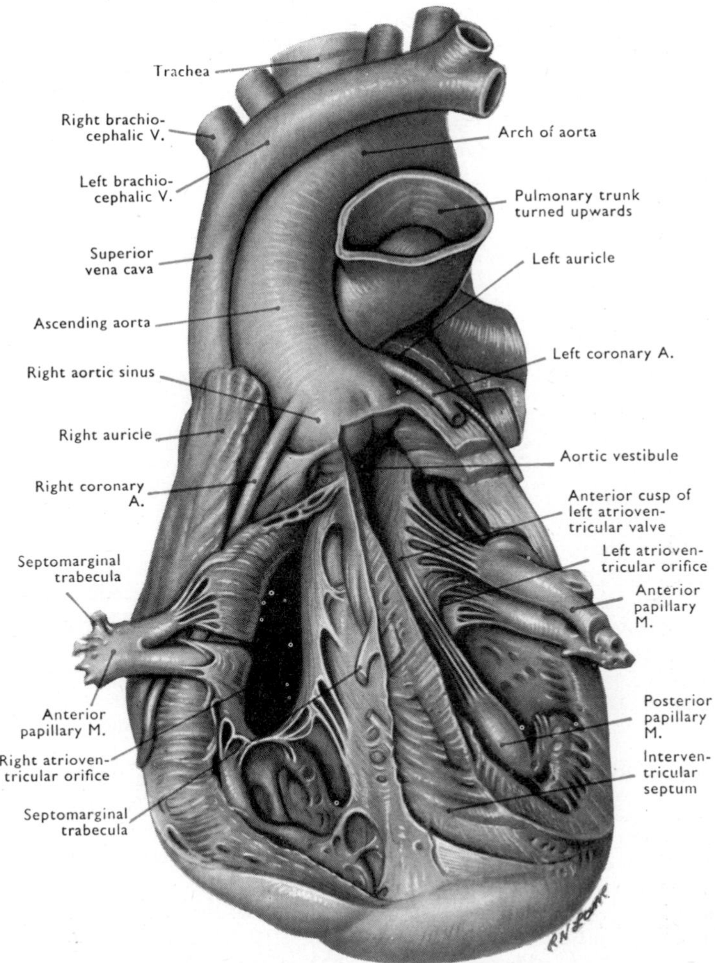

FIG. 57 A dissection of the ventricles of the heart. The root of the aorta has been exposed by separating the pulmonary trunk from the right ventricle and turning the trunk upwards.

atrioventricular foramen. The presence of such an interventricular foramen, if large, inevitably means that the pressures in both ventricles are the same and there is consequently a hypertrophy of the right ventricular wall.

THE AORTA

The aorta arises from the aortic orifice of the left ventricle behind the third left intercostal space at the margin of the sternum, and it ends on the anterior surface of the fourth lumbar vertebra by dividing into the right and left common iliac arteries.

ASCENDING AORTA
[FIGS. 42, 46, 56, 60, 63]

This is the first part of the aorta. It runs upwards, with a slight inclination forwards and to the right, to join the arch of the aorta behind the right half of the sternal angle. It is enclosed in a sheath of serous pericardium with the pulmonary trunk, and has four dilatations of its wall: (1) the three **aortic sinuses** at its root; (2) a slight swelling of the right border of the ascending aorta, the **bulb of the aorta.** This is the part of the wall which receives the full thrust of the blood discharged from the left ventricle, and is a common site for the formation of an aortic aneurysm.

The ascending aorta begins between the left atrium and the infundibulum with the right atrium on its right side. It ascends anterior to the right pulmonary artery and right bronchus, with the superior vena cava to the right and the pulmonary trunk inclining posteriorly on its left surface. It is separated from the sternum by pericardium, pleural sac, lung, and remains of the thymus. The vasa vasorum of the ascending aorta arise principally from the left coronary artery, a branch of which ascends on its left side sending circumferential branches around the aorta at regular intervals. A branch from the right coronary artery may also be present.

THE SUPERIOR MEDIASTINUM

DISSECTION. If the upper limbs have been dissected and the clavicles divided, proceed to divide the first ribs immediately anterior to the subclavian veins and turn the manubrium of the sternum superiorly to uncover the superior mediastinum. If the upper limbs have not been dissected, make two drill holes through the middle one third of each clavicle approximately 1–2 cm. apart. Cut the clavicles between these holes with a fine saw, divide the first ribs with bone forceps as above, and turn the manubrium sterni upwards, together with the medial thirds of the clavicles and the first costal cartilages. After the dissection of the superior mediastinum, the cut ends of the clavicles may be drawn together by a wire passed through the drill holes.

Clean the superior part of the superior vena cava and the brachiocephalic veins forming it. Identify the inferior thyroid, internal thoracic, and left superior intercostal veins, and follow them into the brachiocephalic veins [Fig. 41]. Displace the brachiocephalic veins and clean the parts of the aortic arch not already seen from the left side, together with the branches arising from its convex surface. Identify again the nerves on the left surface of the arch of the aorta [p. 63] and follow them superiorly between the left common carotid and subclavian arteries.

Follow the left vagus to the concavity of the aortic arch and note again the recurrent laryngeal branch hooking round the arch. Clean the superior part of the pulmonary trunk and its branches as far as possible. Note the fibrous strand (ligamentum arteriosum) which joins the superior surface of the root of the left pulmonary artery to the concavity of the aortic arch, and confirm that the left recurrent laryngeal nerve hooks round its posterior surface.

Brachiocephalic Veins

Each of these veins begins posterior to the medial end of the corresponding clavicle by the union of the internal jugular and subclavian veins, and they end by uniting to form the superior vena cava posterior to the lower border of the first right costal cartilage [Figs. 31, 42, 49].

The **right brachiocephalic vein** has a short, vertical course immediately lateral to the brachiocephalic trunk, with the **phrenic nerve** posterolateral to it. The left brachiocephalic vein passes obliquely downwards and to the right, posterior to the upper part of the manubrium sterni, and crosses the left common carotid artery and the brachiocephalic trunk at their origin [Figs. 4, 37, 41, 49, 58].

Tributaries. In addition to the inferior thyroid and internal thoracic veins, each brachiocephalic vein receives the vertebral and highest intercostal veins. The **right** vein also drains the lymph trunks from the right side of the head and neck, upper limb, and part of the thorax, and these may combine in different ways before entering the vein. The **left** brachiocephalic vein also receives the thoracic duct, the left bronchomediastinal lymph trunk, the left superior intercostal vein, and some mediastinal veins.

ARCH OF AORTA

[Figs. 28, 41, 42, 59]

The arch begins posterior to the right half of the sternal angle. It passes posteriorly with a slight inclination and convexity to the left, while arching superiorly into the inferior part

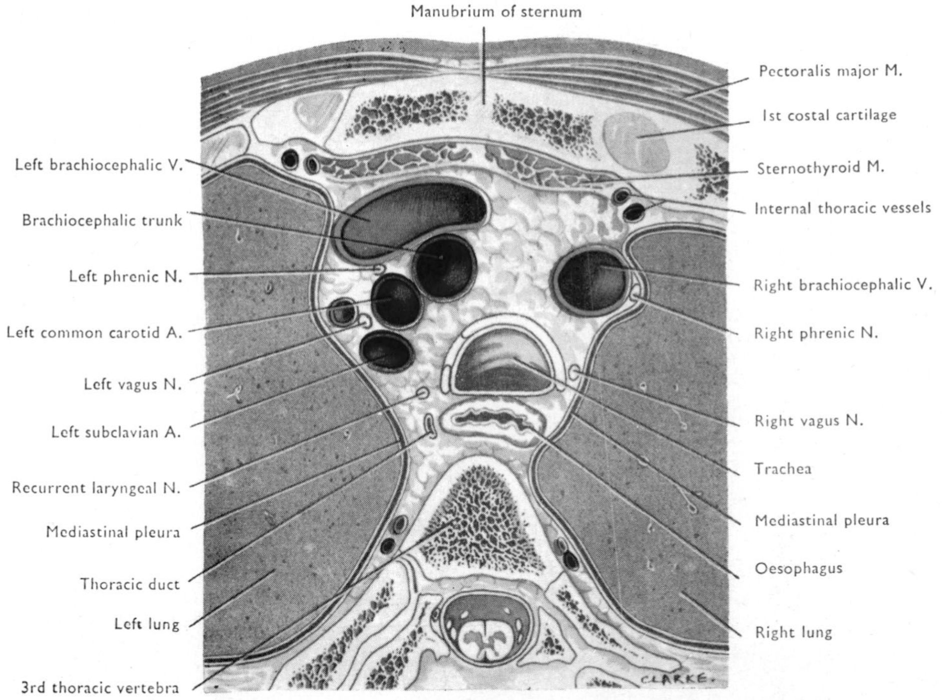

FIG. 58 A horizontal section through the thorax at the level of the third thoracic vertebra.

of the superior mediastinum. The convexity to the left is caused by it arching from the front of the trachea over the left side of that structure and of the oesophagus to join the descending aorta on the left of the disc between the fourth and fifth thoracic vertebrae in the same horizontal plane as its origin. The superficial surface of the arch is in contact anteriorly with the remains of the thymus, and is crossed by the left brachiocephalic vein near the roots of its branches. Further posteriorly the phrenic nerve, the cervical cardiac branches of the left vagus (inferior) and sympathetic (superior), the vagus itself, and the left superior intercostal vein cross its left surface.

The inferior or concave surface of the arch curves over the structures passing to the root of the left lung. It is in contact with the bifurcation of the pulmonary trunk and the left pulmonary artery, and also with the left bronchus [FIG. 69]. In addition, the ligamentum arteriosum passes from the root of the left pulmonary artery to the arch, and the left recurrent laryngeal nerve passes posterior to the ligament to reach the groove between the trachea and oesophagus medial to the arch. The superficial cardiac plexus [p. 38] lies inferior to the arch on the ligamentum arteriosum.

Branches of Arch

Brachiocephalic Trunk. This artery, the largest of the three branches, begins behind the centre of the manubrium sterni [FIG. 42], anterior to the trachea and posterior to the left brachiocephalic vein. It passes superolaterally to reach the right side of the trachea and end posterior to the upper margin of the right sternoclavicular joint by dividing into the right common carotid and right subclavian

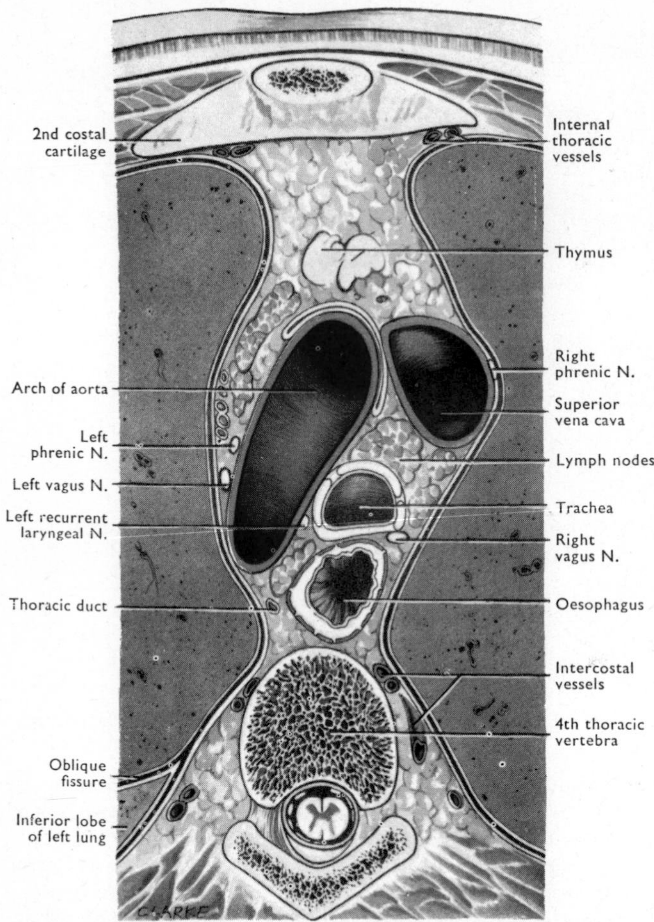

FIG. 59 A horizontal section through the thorax at the level of the fourth thoracic vertebra.

to the left sternoclavicular joint, on the left side of the trachea.

Left Subclavian Artery. It arises from the posterior part of the aortic arch, and is, therefore, both further to the left and more posterior than the other branches. Thus it grooves the medial side of the left lung and lies lateral to the trachea. It ascends vertically, and therefore runs obliquely across the left side of the trachea, recurrent laryngeal nerve, oesophagus, and thoracic duct, all of which curve anteriorly with the vertebral column. It enters the neck some distance posterior to the sternoclavicular joint, and arching laterally, grooves the anterior surface of the cervical pleura and the apex of the lung [FIGS. 28, 32].

Pulmonary Arteries

These arteries will be exposed more clearly in the next dissection, but their position should be confirmed now.

The **right pulmonary artery** [FIGS. 41, 51, 62] begins in the concavity of the arch

arteries, anterior to the dome of the pleura. It may give rise to the small **thyroidea ima artery,** which ascends on the front of the trachea to the isthmus of the thyroid gland.

Left Common Carotid Artery. This artery arises from the convexity of the arch immediately to the left of the brachiocephalic trunk, and follows almost the same course as that trunk but on the left side. It ascends anterior to the left subclavian artery [FIGS. 28, 58] close to the left pleura with the left vagus and phrenic nerves, and enters the neck posterior

of the aorta anterior to the left bronchus. It passes to the right and slightly downwards, anterior to the oesophagus and right principal bronchus, and posterior to the ascending aorta and superior vena cava. Close to the lung root it gives off the branch which accompanies the right superior lobar bronchus.

The **left pulmonary artery** lies inferior to the posterior part of the aortic arch [FIG. 62], and passes posteriorly and to the left across the left bronchus and the descending thoracic aorta to the lung root.

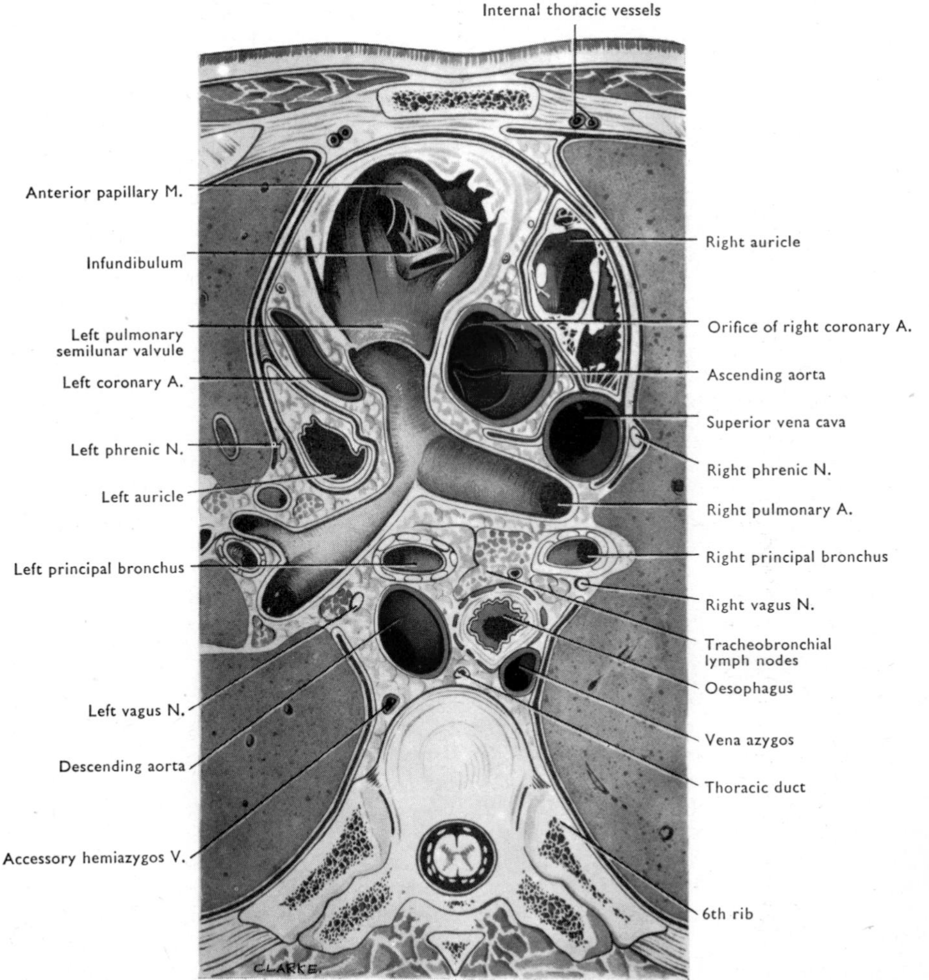

FIG. 60 A horizontal section through the thorax at the level of the intervertebral disc between the fifth and sixth thoracic vertebrae.

Ligamentum Arteriosum. This is a short fibrous band that connects the superior surface of the root of the left pulmonary artery with the inferior surface of the arch of the aorta, distal to the origin of the left subclavian artery. The **left recurrent laryngeal nerve** passes posterior to the ligament, and the **superficial cardiac plexus** lies on it. The ligament has no significance in the adult, but it is the remnant of a wide channel (the **ductus arteriosus**, FIG. 61) which is of profound importance during foetal life. There are serious consequences if it fails to close in the early postnatal phase.

During intra-uterine life, the lungs have no function since oxygenation of the foetal blood occurs in the placenta, the oxygenated blood being returned to the foetal heart through the

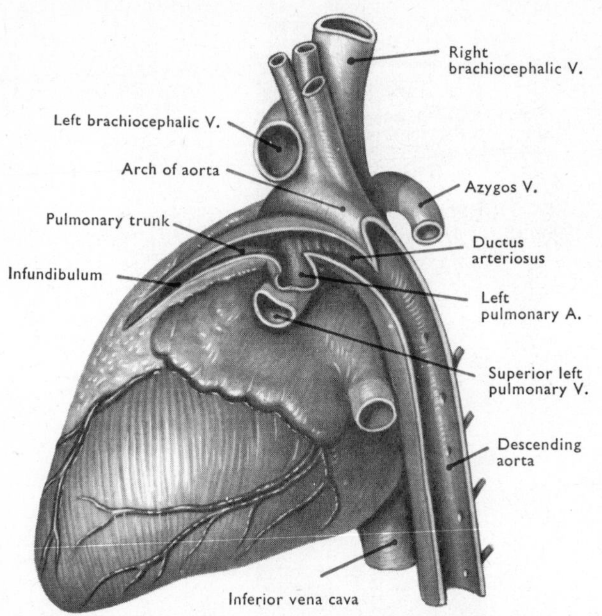

FIG. 61 A dissection of the heart and great vessels of a foetus. Note the direct connexion of the pulmonary trunk with the aorta through the ductus arteriosus, a shunt which allows the blood in the pulmonary trunk to by-pass the lungs in the foetus.

umbilical vein and the inferior vena cava. This blood, mixed with the venous blood from the lower limbs and abdomen in the inferior vena cava, passes directly through the **foramen ovale** [p. 50] in the interatrial septum into the left atrium. Thence it is passed to the left ventricle and pumped principally to the head and neck and upper limbs through the aorta and the branches of its arch, a smaller quantity passing into the descending aorta.

The venous blood drained from the head and neck, upper limbs, and the walls of the thorax passes into the right atrium via the superior vena cava, and is directed by that vessel through the right atrioventricular orifice into the right ventricle. Thence it is pumped into the pulmonary trunk, but only a tiny fraction passes through the pulmonary arteries to the lungs, the majority is carried through the **ductus arteriosus** into the posterior part of the arch of the aorta. Here it enters the descending aorta, and mixing with part of the blood from the left ventricle, is distributed to the rest of the body and to the placenta.

The fact that the blood in the pulmonary trunk enters the aorta rather than passing into the lungs, indicates that the pressure is higher in the pulmonary trunk than in the descending aorta, and that the peripheral resistance in the unexpanded lungs is greater than that in the aortic territory. This also means that the pressure in the right ventricle of the foetus is not significantly different from that in the left, a feature which accounts for the fact that there is not the same difference in thickness of the muscular walls of the two ventricles as there is in the adult.

The small amount of blood passing through the lungs of the foetus accounts for the low pressure in the left atrium which facilitates the passage of the inferior vena caval blood through the foramen ovale into the left atrium.

At birth the lungs expand with the first breaths, the peripheral resistance of the pulmonary circulation drops suddenly, and blood from the pulmonary trunk flows freely through the lungs to the left atrium. This raises the pressure in the left atrium to that in the right, and thus prevents the flow of blood from the right atrium to the left and closes the valvular **foramen ovale,** the walls of which subsequently fuse. The sudden drop in pulmonary arterial pressure leads to a flow of blood from the aorta to the pulmonary artery along the ductus arteriosus, but this is arrested by the contraction of the muscular wall of the ductus arteriosus which is usually complete within the first week after birth. Thus the pulmonary and systemic circulations are separated, and this becomes permanent with the obliteration of the lumen of the ductus arteriosus and its replacement with fibrous tissue to form the **ligamentum arteriosum.** This is not usually complete until the end of the first year of life.

If the ductus arteriosus fails to close, the pressure in the pulmonary circulation remains as high as that in the systemic circulation. Thus the reduction in thickness of the right ventricular wall which normally occurs in early postnatal life does not take place, the heart becomes globular in shape, and the persistent pulmonary hypertension has serious effects on the functions of the heart and lungs.

DISSECTION. Turn the ventricular part of the heart anteriorly to expose the diaphragmatic surface. As far as possible clean the vessels on this surface. In particular identify and clean the posterior interventricular artery and the middle cardiac vein running with it. Follow the former posteriorly and to the right and attempt to demonstrate its continuity with the right coronary artery, the cut end of which lies in the coronary sulcus.

The third slice [Fig. 62] through the heart is made parallel to the first. It demonstrates the left atrium, the left atrioventricular orifice, the posterior cusp of the mitral valve, the interatrial septum, and the pulmonary arteries. Begin at the apex of the heart approximately 1·5 cm. posterior to the previous section, and carry the knife posterosuperiorly through the left ventricular wall parallel to and between the cusps of the mitral valve, splitting the papillary muscles longitudinally and passing through the left atrioventricular orifice. Continue the incision through the left side of the heart, cutting through the base of the left auricle and between the left and anterior walls of the left atrium. Carry the incision through the bifurcation of the pulmonary trunk, and then anteriorly through the arch of the aorta anterior to the ligamentum arteriosum and the left common carotid artery. On the right side the incision should pass immediately anterior to the openings of the coronary sinus and inferior vena cava and through the middle of

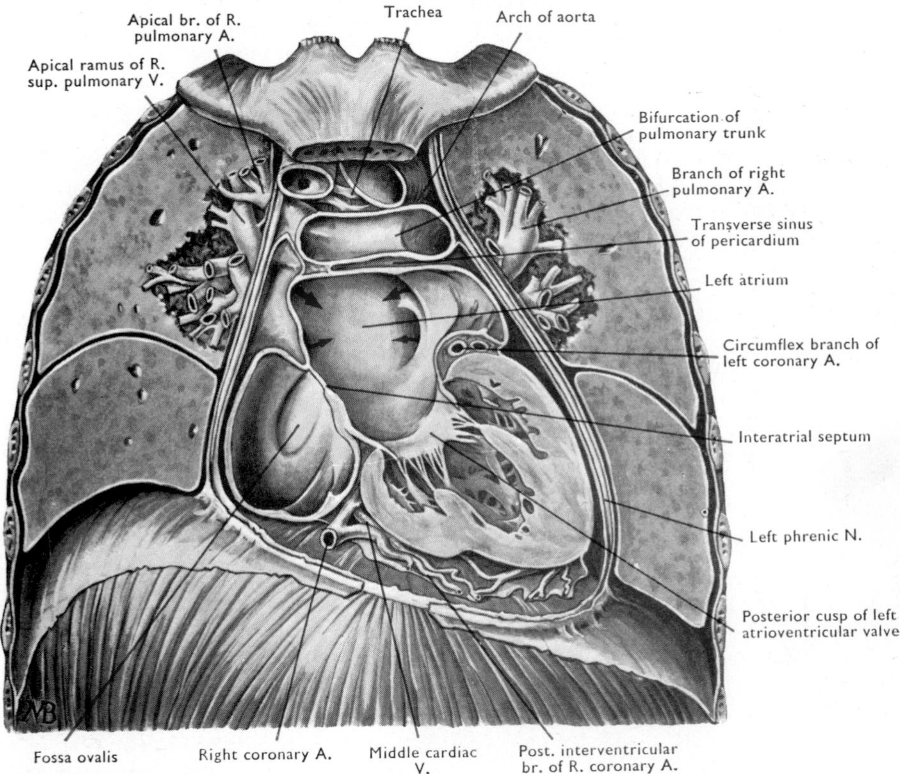

FIG. 62 The heart *in situ*. A drawing of the parts of the heart exposed by the third coronal section. See dissection instructions and FIG. 56. The arrows emerge from the pulmonary veins, and the branches of the right coronary artery have been removed from the last slice and left on the diaphragm.

the fossa ovalis. It should then pass upwards, immediately posterior to the superior vena cava, to the level of entry of the azygos vein into the superior vena cava. Then cut forwards through the superior vena cava and remove the slice.

Clean any blood clot from the left atrium and pulmonary veins, and also from the pulmonary arteries and the arch of the aorta. Identify and clean the cut ends of the right coronary artery, of the circumflex branch of the left coronary artery, and of the veins which accompany them in the right and left extremities of the coronary sulcus. Confirm the arrangement of the pulmonary veins [Figs. 32, 33 and p. 44].

Left Atrium [FIGS. 43, 62, 63]

The left atrium lies posteriorly and forms virtually the entire base of the heart, though its long, narrow auricle projects forwards and partly overlaps the beginning of the pulmonary trunk. On each side, two pulmonary veins, superior and inferior, enter the upper half of the left atrium close to the lateral margins of the posterior surface, the superior veins slightly anterior to the inferior veins.

The sternocostal surface of the left atrium is covered by the ascending aorta and the pulmonary trunk, and the pulmonary arteries course along its superior margin, while the coronary sinus runs transversely along its inferior margin [FIGS. 51, 65] in the coronary sulcus.

Interior of Left Atrium [FIGS. 43, 64]. This is almost entirely smooth, musculi pectinati being confined to the auricle. There is, however, a prominent muscular ridge which projects into the atrium anterior to the left pulmonary veins, so that the openings of these veins are scarcely visible from in front [FIG. 62].

The interatrial septum is clearly visible [FIG. 62]. Note that it slopes posteriorly and to the right so that a considerable part of the left atrium lies posterior to the right atrium, and that only the postero-inferior part of the right atrium, immediately superior to the entry of the inferior vena cava, forms part of the posterior surface (base) of the heart.

Orifices of Left Atrium. The orifices of the pulmonary veins have been seen already. Neither they nor the openings of the venae çordis minimae are guarded by valves.

The **left atrioventricular orifice** lies at the antero-inferior part of the left atrium. It is the orifice through which the oxygenated pulmonary venous blood is discharged into the left ventricle. It is smaller (2 cm.) than the right atrioventricular orifice and usually only admits the tips of two fingers.

The **left atrioventricular** (mitral) **valve** has two obliquely set cusps. The larger anterior cusp lies anterior and to the right of the posterior cusp. The cusps

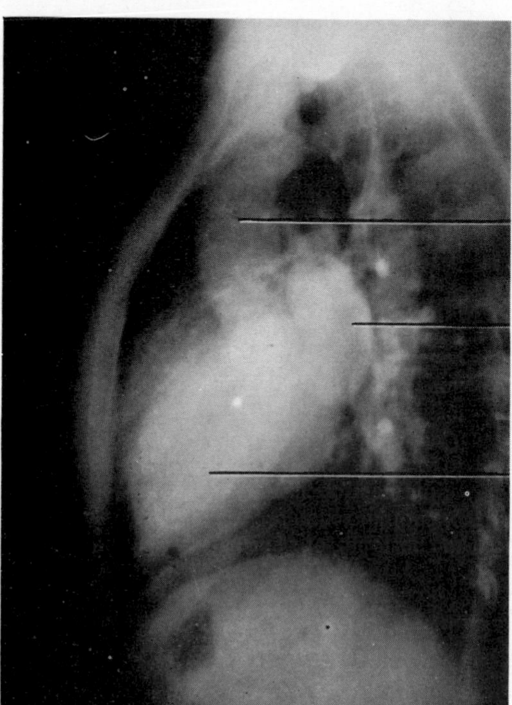

FIG. 63 A lateral radiograph of the thorax taken during the passage of contrast material through the heart. In this phase the left heart and part of the aorta are filled.

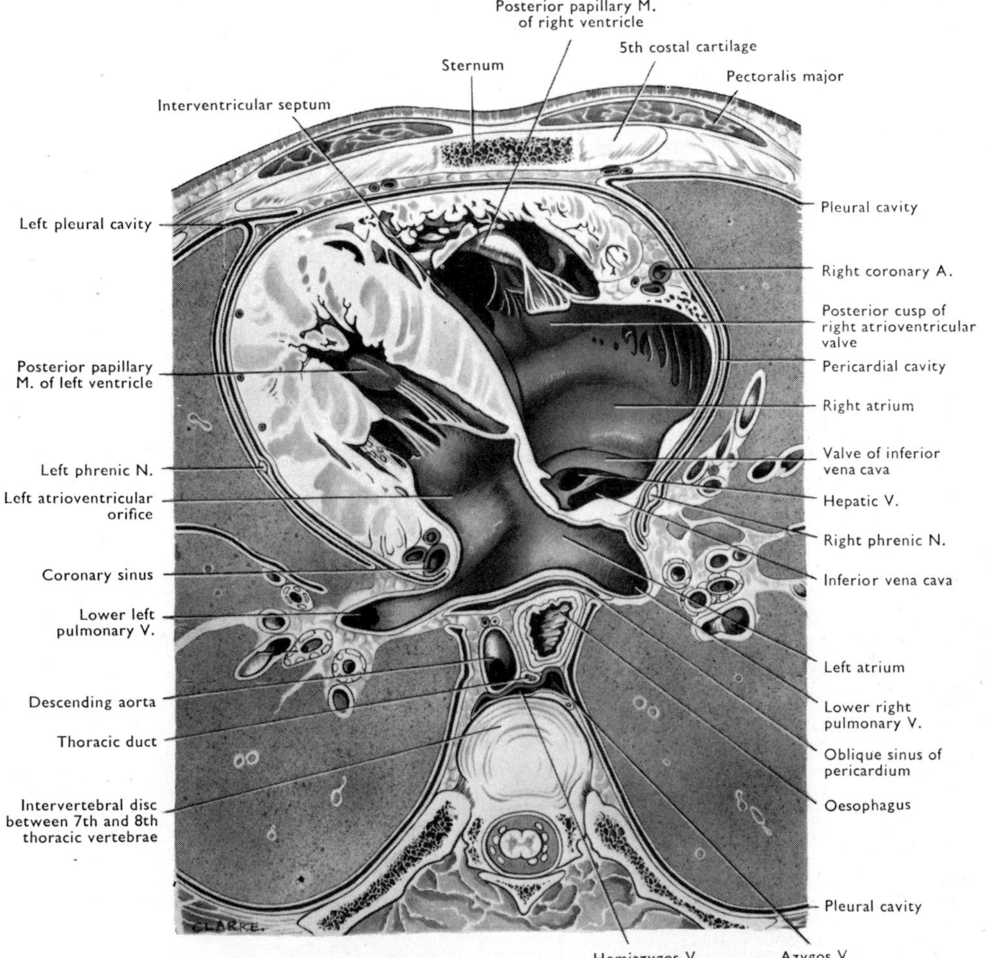

FIG. 64 A horizontal section through the thorax at the level of the intervertebral disc between the seventh and eighth thoracic vertebrae.

of the valve are attached to that part of the fibrous skeleton of the heart which surrounds the left atrioventricular orifice [FIG. 54], and their apices project into the ventricle. The margins and ventricular surfaces of the cusps receive the **chordae tendineae** of the **papillary muscles,** those from the anterior muscle passing to the anterior or left halves of the two cusps, while those from the posterior muscle pass to the posterior or right halves. The attachment of chordae tendineae to the ventricular surface of the **anterior cusp** is much less extensive than to the ventricular surface of the posterior cusp. That surface of the anterior cusp forms the posterior wall of the **aortic vestibule** and has blood flowing over it during ventricular systole; its posterior surface has blood flowing over it during atrial systole.

DISSECTION. Divide the pulmonary veins and the inferior vena cava within the pericardial cavity. Lift up the ventricular part of the heart and identify and divide the layers of pericardium which are reflected over and between these veins [Fig. 41] and which form the walls of the oblique sinus of the pericardium. This frees the remainder of the heart from the pericardium and allows an examination of the oblique sinus and of the posterior surface of the heart.

Identify the coronary sulcus on the posterior surface of the heart. Remove the visceral pericardium which covers this sulcus, and clean the coronary sinus lying in it together with the terminal branches of the coronary arteries. Note that the right coronary artery supplies a considerable part of the diaphragmatic surface of the left ventricle and that the branches of the two coronary arteries do not anastomose in the coronary sulcus. Identify and follow the oblique vein of the left atrium [Fig. 65] towards the anterior surface of the inferior left pulmonary vein.

Coronary Sinus [Figs. 51, 65]

This large sinus drains all the venous blood from the heart, except that which enters the cavities directly through the anterior cardiac veins and the venae cordis minimae. The coronary sinus runs from left to right in the posterior part of the coronary sulcus, and opens into the right atrium immediately to the left of the orifice of the inferior vena cava. The coronary sinus receives the **great cardiac vein** [Fig. 45] at its left extremity, and the small and middle cardiac veins at its right extremity immediately before it enters the right atrium. The **middle cardiac vein** runs with the posterior interventricular branch of the right coronary artery, while the **small cardiac vein** runs to the left in the posterior part of the coronary sulcus with the right coronary artery.

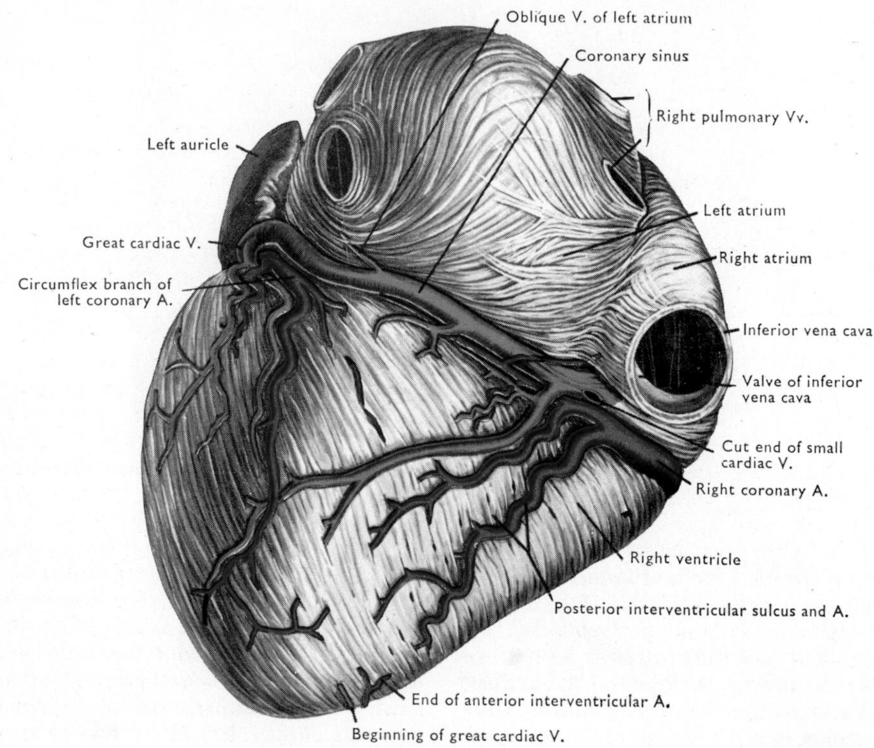

Fig. 65 A dissection of the diaphragmatic surface of the heart.

The **oblique vein of the left atrium** is the remnant of the left common cardinal vein of the embryo, and thus corresponds to the part of the superior vena cava (inferior to the entry of the azygos vein) formed from the right common cardinal vein. Thus if a left superior vena cava persists in its entirety, its inferior part replaces the oblique vein and enters the coronary sinus. Both the oblique vein and the coronary sinus are partly covered by cardiac muscle on their posterior aspects.

STRUCTURE OF WALLS OF HEART

The walls of the heart consist of a layer of cardiac muscle covered externally with serous pericardium (**epicardium**), and lined internally with endocardium. Both these layers are composed of connective tissue covered with endothelium which produces a surface relatively free from friction. The **endocardium** plays a major role in the formation of the flaps of the valves, and is continuous with a similar lining in the arteries and veins.

Myocardium

The cardiac muscle is a striated type of muscle composed of a large number of short muscle cells joined end to end at intercalated discs. Some of the cells branch so that this muscle forms a mesh through which electrical impulses can spread freely from cell to cell and thus over the entire myocardium, except where the muscular continuity is broken by the presence of the fibrous skeleton which separates the atria and ventricles.

It is difficult to dissect the muscle fibres in a heart which has been sliced, but the direction of the fibres can be determined by stripping off the muscle layer by layer.

Atrial Muscle. (1) The most **superficial fibres** run transversely round both atria. They are best marked close to the coronary sulcus. (2) A **deeper layer** of fibres which passes anteroposteriorly across each atrium from the fibrous atrioventricular ring. These tend to become continuous with the transverse fibres at the coronary sulcus, and with the third group round the entry of the veins. (3) **Anular fibres** which loop round the orifices of the veins and become continuous with groups (1) and (2) [FIG. 65].

Ventricular Muscle. (1) **Superficial fibres** which sweep spirally (clockwise as seen from the apex) around the surfaces of both ventricles from the fibrous atrioventricular rings towards the apex of the opposite ventricle. At the apex of each ventricle they form a whorl, and sinking deeply, end in the **papillary muscles** of the ventricle opposite to the atrioventricular ring from which they arise. (2) A **deeper,** horizontal layer of muscle. These fibre bundles form S-shaped loops which begin and end in association with the papillary muscles of the two ventricles. One loop of the S passes at least partly round each ventricle, and the intermediate limb lies in the interventricular septum. Only some of these S-shaped bundles have loops of equal length, the length of one loop tending to be inversely proportional to the other.

Conducting System of Heart [FIGS. 66, 67]

This system consists of specialized muscle fibres. These are responsible: (1) for initiating the normal heart beat (**sinu-atrial node**); (2) for transmitting the stimulating impulse from the atria to the ventricles through the fibrous skeleton of the heart with a delay which is sufficient to allow the atrial contraction to be complete before the ventricles begin to contract (**atrioventricular node** and **trunk of atrioventricular bundle**); and (3) for conducting the stimulating impulse through the ventricular muscle so that it contracts appropriately (**trunk** and **crura** of the atrioventricular bundle).

Microscopically the nodes are composed of interlacing muscle cells which are considerably thinner and less heavily striated than ordinary cardiac muscle fibres. They are separated by a considerable amount of fibro-elastic tissue, and have a number of sympathetic and parasympathetic nerve cells and nerve fibres associated with them.

Sinu-atrial Node. This is a small collection of the specialized muscle tissue, which lies in the wall of the right atrium at the superior end of the **crista terminalis** on the right of the opening of the superior vena cava [FIG. 66].

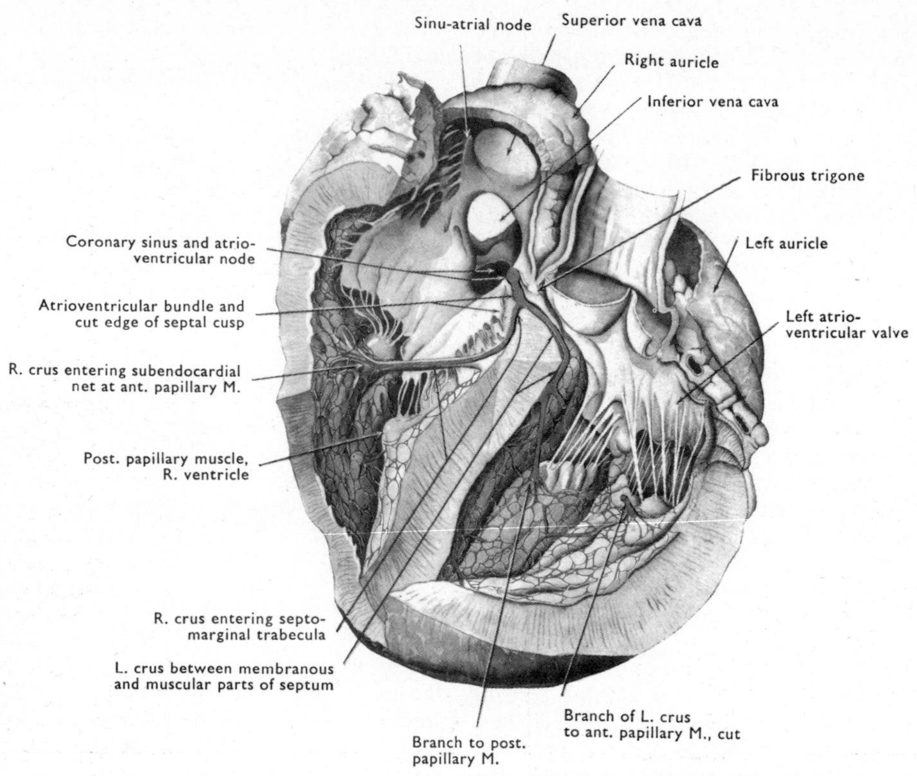

FIG. 66 The conducting system of the sheep's heart as seen in an injected specimen.

It appears to initiate the impulse which causes atrial contraction and spreads through the atrial net of muscle without any special conducting tissue. Although the node initiates contraction of the atria in the absence of nerves, the rate of firing can be altered by nervous stimulation, being accelerated by sympathetic stimulation and slowed or even stopped by vagal stimulation through the **cardiac plexuses.** It should be appreciated also that cardiac muscle has the inherent capacity for rhythmic contraction and that the rate is normally dictated by the sinu-atrial node. Destruction of that node leads to a slower rate of heart beat, which may often be initiated by the atrioventricular node.

Atrioventricular Node. This is composed of the same kind of tissue as the sinu-atrial node. It lies in the antero-inferior part of the interatrial septum, immediately above the opening of the coronary sinus. It receives impulses from the atrial muscle with which it is directly continuous and transmits them through the **atrioventricular bundle** and its branches (crura), and this part of the system conducts at a much slower rate (0·2 m./sec.) than the atrial muscle (1 m./sec.).

Atrioventricular Bundle. The **trunk**, composed of thin, pale muscle fibres, passes antero-inferiorly from the atrioventricular node to pierce the **fibrous atrioventricular ring** (right fibrous trigone, FIGURE 55) and reach the posterior part of the membranous interventricular septum. Here it runs along the edge of the muscular interventricular septum, immediately inferior to the line of attachment of the

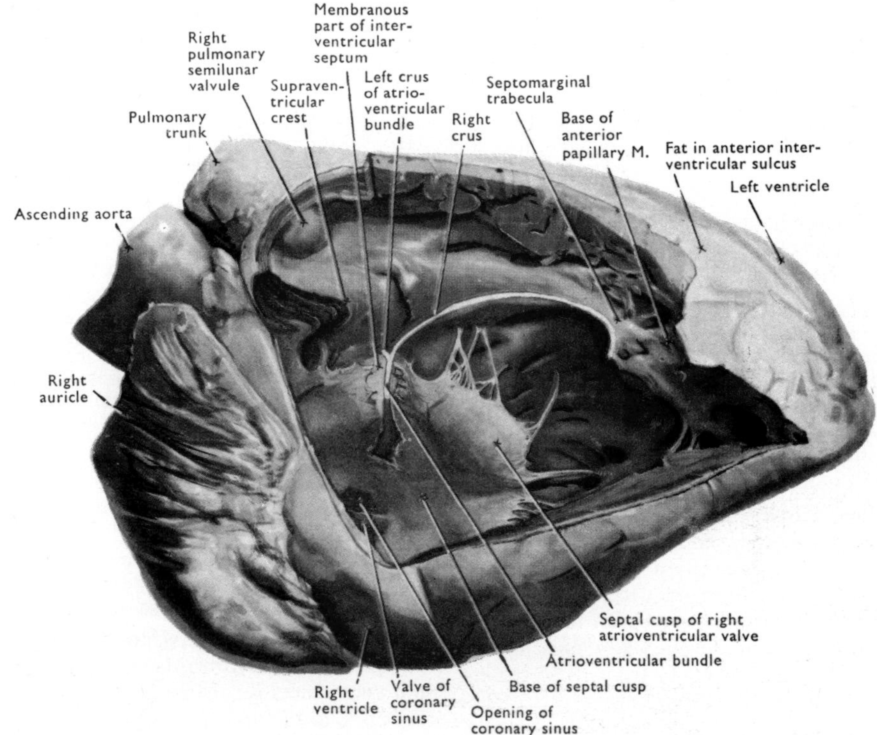

FIG. 67 A dissection of the right ventricle to show the course and division of the trunk of the atrio-ventricular bundle and the course of its right crus.

septal cusp of the tricuspid valve, and divides into right and left crura which descend, one on each side of the interventricular septum [FIG. 66] beneath the endocardium. The **right crus** passes towards the septal end of the **septo-marginal trabecula,** and giving branches to the septum and posterior papillary muscle, enters the trabecula and runs in it to the anterior papillary muscle. It supplies this muscle and spreads out on the wall of the right ventricle.

The **left crus** pierces the interventricular septum between its membranous and muscular parts, and descends to the posterior papillary muscle, giving some fine strands across the cavity of the ventricle to the anterior papillary muscle. Branches of this crus also spread out to form a subendocardial net.

The trunk and its crura are difficult to see in the human heart for the muscle fibres it contains are not sufficiently different from the other muscle fibres, but they are readily visible in the foetus and young child and in the sheep and calf. In the latter the fibres of the sub-endocardial net are very large and pale (**Purkinje fibres**) and contain much glycogen. The entire extent of the trunk, its crura, and the subendocardial net are ensheathed in connective tissue, and this sheath may be injected to demonstrate the course of these bundles.

DISSECTION. Detach the septal cusp of the tricuspid valve and expose the membranous atrioventricular septum. Clean away the endocardium on the postero-inferior edge of the muscular interventricular septum and attempt to identify the trunk of the atrio-ventricular bundle, which passes anterosuperiorly on it and divides into its two crura. Attempt to follow the

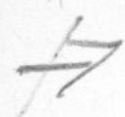

crura to the septomarginal trabecula and the posterior papillary muscle respectively. As the parts of this system can rarely be seen in a satisfactory manner in the dissecting room hearts, it is desirable to obtain a sheep's heart in which it is relatively simple to display the trunk and crura of the bundle.

Action of Heart

It should now be possible to understand the sequence of events which comprise the cardiac cycle. The **sinu-atrial node** initiates the stimulating impulse which spreads rapidly over the atrial muscle and causes it to contract, the anular fibres around the veins partially constrict these orifices and inhibit the reflux of blood into the veins. The impulse reaches the **atrioventricular node,** and is transmitted (with delay) principally to the papillary muscles, but also throughout the ventricles. Thus the **papillary muscles** are the first to contract and tighten the chordae tendineae so that the atrioventricular valves are in a condition to withstand the pressure developed by ventricular contraction. Also, since most of the ventricular muscles reach the papillary muscles, the impulse spreads outwards from these regions to the rest of the ventricular muscle. The spread of the impulse through the ventricular muscle is very rapid, and the contraction of the ventricular muscle, which follows it, begins at almost the same time throughout the different parts of the ventricle, but the septum and apex contract fractionally earlier than the base of the ventricles, and this tends to give a directional thrust of the contained blood towards the great arteries.

DISSECTION. Remove the pulmonary arteries by dividing the ligamentum arteriosum and separating them from the pleura. This exposes the tracheal bifurcation and the main bronchi. Before cleaning these structures, follow the left recurrent laryngeal nerve to the medial aspect of the arch of the aorta, and note the branches which it gives to the deep cardiac plexus on the anterior aspect of the tracheal bifurcation. As the recurrent laryngeal nerve turns superiorly it runs close to, or even in the same sheath as, the superior cervical cardiac branch of the left vagus and the middle and inferior cervical cardiac branches of the left sympathetic trunk, all of which descend medial to the aortic arch into the deep cardiac plexus. Note the branches which leave the deep cardiac plexus along the bronchi and towards the heart. Clean the bronchi and the inferior part of the trachea.

THORACIC PART OF TRACHEA

The trachea is a wide tube (10–12 cm. long) which is kept patent by a series of U-shaped bars of cartilage embedded transversely in its fibro-elastic wall. The posterior surface is flat [Fig. 59] where it is applied to the oesophagus and the ends of the cartilage bars are united by plain muscle and elastic fibrous tissue. The thoracic part lies in the median plane of the superior mediastinum, and is 5–6 cm. long. It divides at the level of the sternal angle, opposite the interval between the third and fourth thoracic spines. This position is not fixed, but descends, even to the level of the sixth thoracic vertebra, by stretching of the elastic trachea on inspiration.

The thoracic part of the trachea is nearly surrounded by blood vessels. Inferiorly the **arch of the aorta** crosses the anterior and left surfaces of the trachea [Fig. 59], while the **azygos vein** arches forwards on its right surface, both structures separating it from the pleura. Superior to the arch of the aorta, the anterior surface of the trachea is separated from the left brachiocephalic vein by the diverging **brachiocephalic trunk** and the **left common carotid artery** [Fig. 58], the latter passing with the left subclavian artery and the phrenic and vagus nerves along the left surface of the trachea. In the angle between the brachiocephalic trunk and the left common carotid artery, the inferior thyroid veins and the thyroidea ima artery lie on the anterior surface of the trachea. The right surface of the trachea, superior to the azygos vein, is separated from the pleura only by the vagus nerve [Fig. 27], while the posterior surface lies on the oesophagus and the left recurrent laryngeal nerve, the latter sending branches to both.

Bronchi

Each principal bronchus passes inferolaterally into the hilus of the corresponding lung in line with the inferior lobar bronchus.

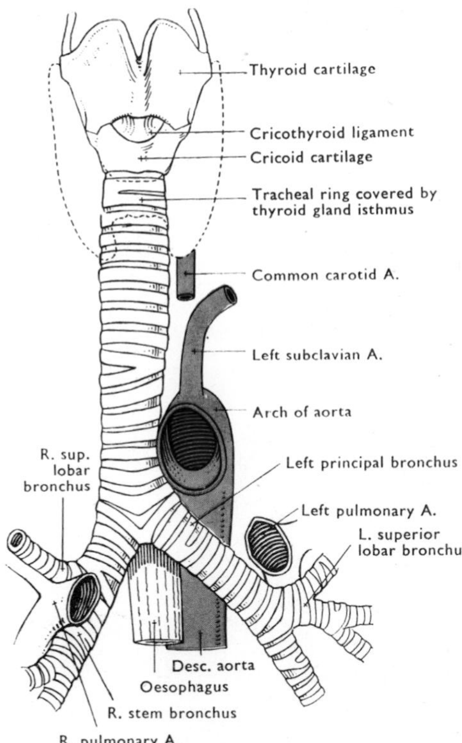

FIG. 68 The larynx, trachea, and bronchi. The thyroid gland is shown by a broken line.

The extrapulmonary parts of the principal bronchi are kept open by U-shaped cartilaginous bars similar to those in the trachea, and are therefore flattened posteriorly. The intrapulmonary parts of the bronchial tree are supported by irregularly placed cartilages and tend to be cylindrical in shape.

Right Principal Bronchus. This bronchus is approximately 2·5 cm. long. It is wider and more vertical than the left, and hence foreign bodies drawn into the trachea tend to enter it and lodge in one or other of its branches, usually in the right inferior lobar bronchus. When this happens, the air distal to the block is rapidly absorbed, and thus the lung tissue in the territory of the occluded bronchus collapses and becomes solid.

This bronchus passes posterior to the ascending aorta, superior vena cava, and the right pulmonary artery. It is formed anterior to the oesophagus and has the azygos vein on its posterior and superior surfaces. The first branch, **right superior lobar bronchus,** arises immediately medial to the hilus of the lung where the pulmonary artery passes anterior to the bronchus.

Left Principal Bronchus. This bronchus is more horizontal than the right. It is nearly 5 cm. long, both because of the greater distance from the tracheal bifurcation to the hilus of the left lung and because the first branch, **left superior lobar bronchus**, arises within the lung substance [FIG. 35].

The left pulmonary artery separates this bronchus from the left atrium anteriorly, and the upper left pulmonary vein is anterior at the hilus [FIG. 69]. The arch of the aorta is superior, and the oesophagus and descending aorta posterior to it.

Both bronchi have the corresponding bronchial vessels and pulmonary plexus on their posterior surfaces.

Deep Cardiac Plexus

This plexus lies on the lowest part of the trachea, posterior to the arch of the aorta. It consists of interlacing nerve fibres from the parasympathetic (vagus) and sympathetic systems, together with a few groups of ganglion cells most of which belong to the parasympathetic system.

Nerve fibres reach it: (1) through all the cervical cardiac branches of the sympathetic trunks (except the left superior) and cardiac branches of the second, third, and fourth thoracic ganglia of both sympathetic trunks, and (2) through the cervical cardiac branches of both vagi (except the inferior left), the thoracic cardiac branch of the right vagus, and the cardiac branches of both recurrent laryngeal nerves.

The deep cardiac plexus is continuous with the superficial cardiac plexus on the ligamentum arteriosum [p. 63], and together they send **efferent fibres:** (1) to the atria directly, and to the rest of the heart through the **coronary plexuses,** and (2) to the lungs over

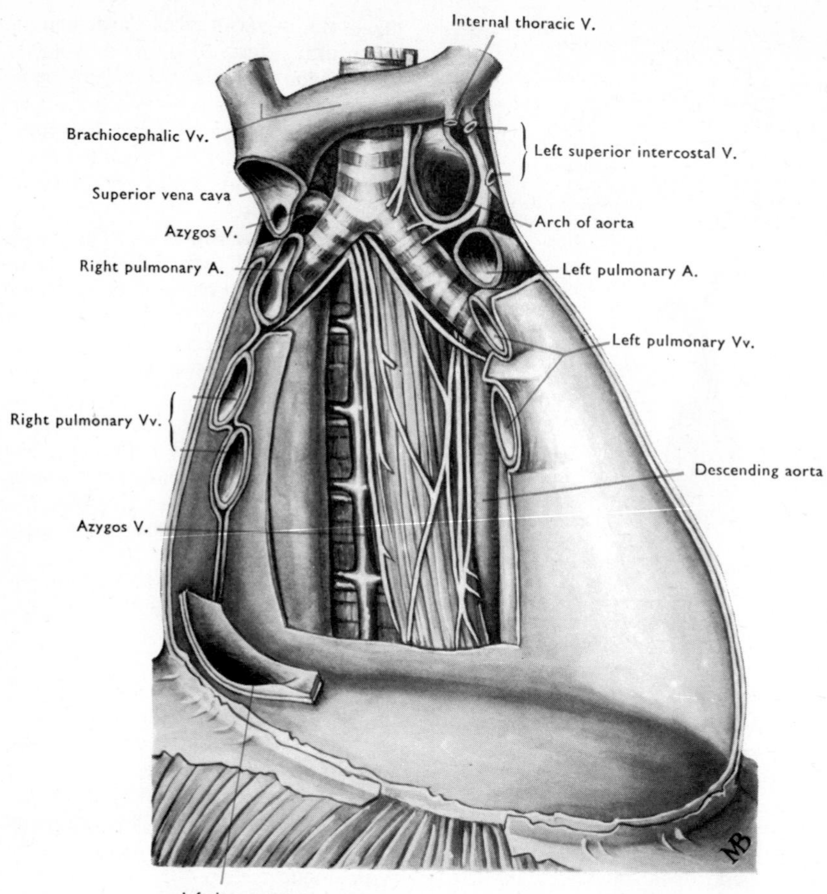

FIG. 69 A dissection of the upper part of the posterior mediastinum after removal of the heart and posterior wall of the pericardium. See also FIG. 70.

the anterior surfaces of the lung roots (**anterior part of pulmonary plexus**).

The cardiac plexuses are of considerable importance in the control of the heart and respiration, and they transmit sensory as well as efferent fibres [p. 38]. The **sensory fibres** transmit impulses from pressure receptors in the aortic arch, superior vena cava and elsewhere, and also impulses from the heart which are responsible for producing the pain of ischaemic disease of the heart. The former pass with the vagus, while the latter enter the spinal medulla through the upper thoracic ganglia of the sympathetic trunk.

DISSECTION. Remove the posterior surface of the parietal pericardium between the right and left pulmonary veins. This uncovers the anterior surface of the oesophagus in the posterior mediastinum. Immediately to the right of the oesophagus and posterior to the beginning of the right bronchus, find the right vagus leaving the pulmonary plexus as one or more nerve trunks [Fig. 70]. At the same position on the left margin of the oesophagus, find the corresponding parts of the left vagus nerve. Follow both vagi on to the

oesophagus and note how their branches unite to form the oesophageal plexus. Clean both the plexus and the oesophagus.

To the right of the oesophagus clean the azygos vein and its tributaries, and deep to the right half of the oesophagus find and clean the thoracic duct. On the left of the oesophagus clean the anterior surface of the descending aorta. As far as possible follow these structures inferiorly through the posterior mediastinum. If necessary, turn the trachea upwards to expose the oesophagus in the superior mediastinum.

THORACIC PARTS OF VAGUS NERVES

Right Vagus

It runs postero-inferiorly on the right surface of the trachea, at first medial to the pleura and then to the arch of the azygos vein. Posterior to the right bronchus, it divides into a number of branches, **posterior part of the pulmonary plexus,** which pass towards the lung and also join the right and left pulmonary

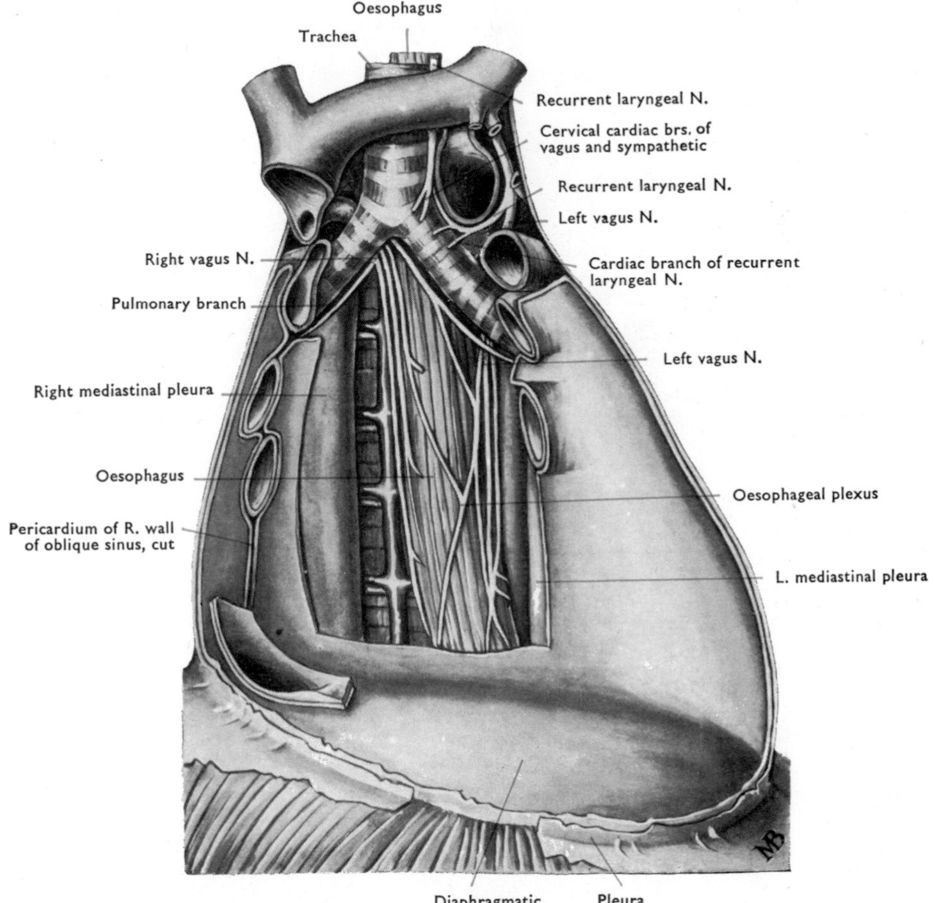

FIG. 70 A dissection of the upper part of the posterior mediastinum after removal of the heart and posterior wall of the pericardium. See also FIG. 69.

plexuses anterior [Fig. 70] and posterior to the oesophagus.

Branches. (1) A **cardiac branch** arises on the right of the trachea and descends over it to the deep cardiac plexus. (2) Branches to the bronchi and lung through the **pulmonary plexus.** (3) Branches to the oesophagus and pericardium through the **oesophageal plexus.**

Left Vagus

This nerve descends to the left side of the arch of the aorta between the left common carotid and subclavian arteries. At the inferior border of the arch it curves medially,

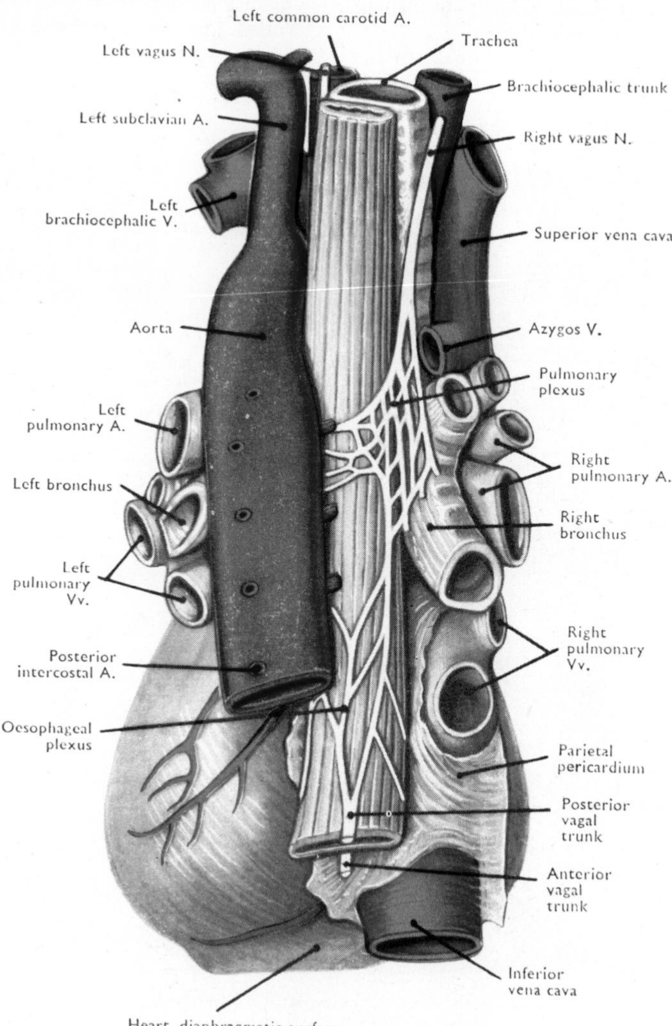

Fig. 71 The posterior aspect of the heart and of the structures in the superior mediastinum and the upper part of the posterior mediastinum.

gives off the left recurrent laryngeal nerve [FIG. 70] and breaks up into branches (**left pulmonary plexus**) posterior to the left bronchus. At the lower border of the root of the left lung it emerges as one or more branches which pass on to the oesophagus to form part of the **oesophageal plexus.**

The **left recurrent laryngeal nerve** curves medially round the inferior border of the aortic arch, posterior to the ligamentum arteriosum, and ascends through the superior mediastinum in the groove between the left sides of the trachea and the oesophagus, to both of which it gives branches. Inferomedial to the arch of the aorta it gives branches to the deep cardiac plexus.

Pulmonary Plexus

The major, **posterior part** of this plexus lies behind each lung root. The nerve fibres reach it from branches of both vagus nerves and from the second, third, and fourth thoracic ganglia of the sympathetic trunk. The smaller, **anterior part** is formed by nerve fibres from the cardiac plexus together with branches of the corresponding vagus which arise above the lung root. Both parts of the plexus supply the structures in the lung root, the lung (including the smooth muscle of the bronchi) and the visceral pleura.

Oesophageal Plexus [FIG. 70]

This plexus surrounds the oesophagus, and consists of fibres of both vagi which mingle in it, together with sympathetic fibres that join it from the **greater splanchnic nerve.** This plexus supplies fibres to the oesophagus, the

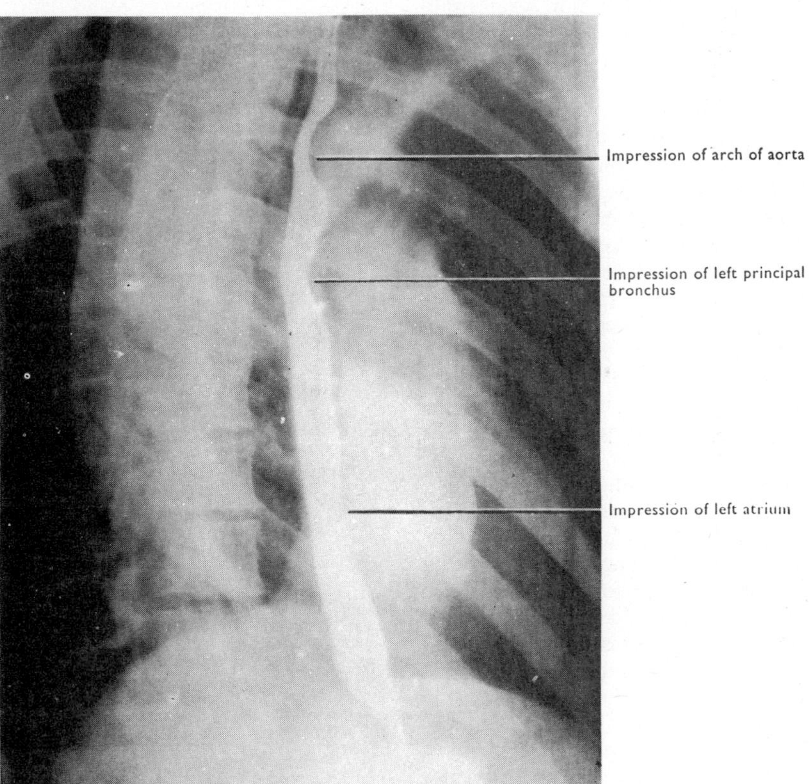

FIG. 72 A right oblique radiograph of the thorax with the oesophagus filled with barium.

pericardium, and the parietal pleura, and its component bundles unite to form the anterior and posterior **vagal trunks** on the inferior part of the oesophagus. These trunks pass through the oesophageal opening in the diaphragm and become the anterior and posterior **gastric nerves.** Each of these trunks and nerves contains fibres from both vagi and from the sympathetic.

OESOPHAGUS

[FIGS. 26, 28, 49, 59, 60, 64, 70, 73]

The oesophagus extends from the pharynx in the neck through the superior and posterior mediastina to pierce the diaphragm at the level of the tenth thoracic vertebral body (or ninth thoracic spine) 2–3 cm. to the left of the median plane. It enters the thorax between the trachea and the vertebral column, slightly to the left of the median plane. As it leaves the superior mediastinum it lies posterior to the left principal bronchus and left pulmonary artery. Inferior to this it is immediately posterior first to the pericardium, which separates it from the left atrium, and then to the posterior part of the diaphragm. At the seventh thoracic vertebral body it inclines still further to the left. Here it is separated from the vertebral column by the descending thoracic aorta which passes to the median plane before entering the abdomen at the level of the twelfth thoracic vertebra, posterior to the diaphragm.

The structures which are posterior to the oesophagus are those lying directly on the vertebral column, *i.e.*, the longus colli, the azygos vein, the thoracic duct (q.v.), the upper six or seven right posterior intercostal arteries, and the descending thoracic aorta.

The *right side* of the oesophagus is close to the right pleura, except where the arch of the vena azygos intervenes, and where the inferior part of the oesophagus deviates to the left and indents the left pleura and lung [FIG. 32].

The *left side* of the oesophagus is close to the left pleura above the arch of the aorta, but the thoracic duct and the upper part of the left subclavian artery intervene. The arch and descending parts of the aorta lie on the left of the oesophagus to the level of the seventh thoracic vertebra.

The left recurrent laryngeal nerve is anterior to the oesophagus in the superior mediastinum, while the oesophageal plexus surrounds it in the posterior mediastinum.

The oesophagus is compressed: (1) by the arch of the aorta; (2) where it passes posterior to the **left principal bronchus;** and (3) where it

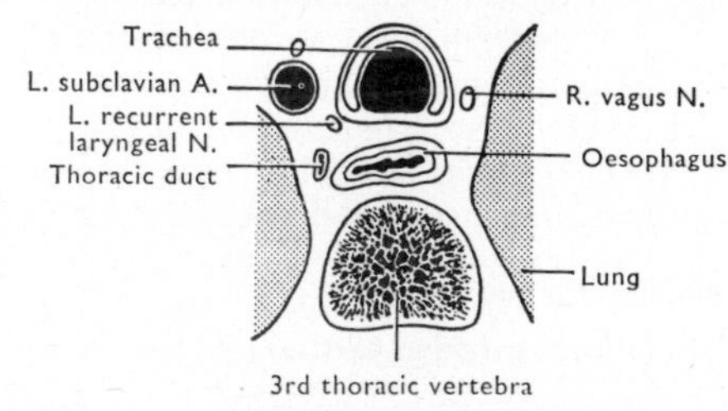

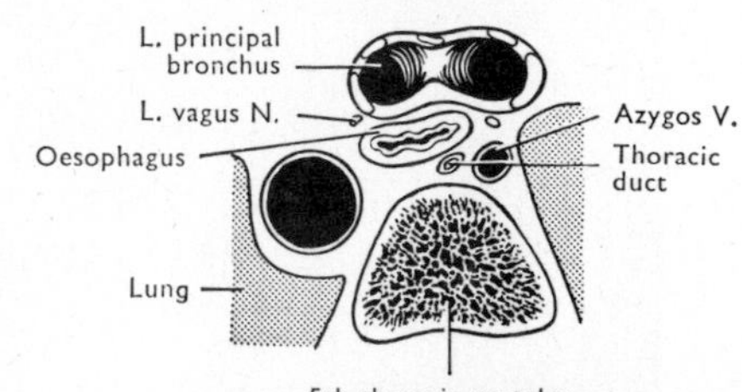

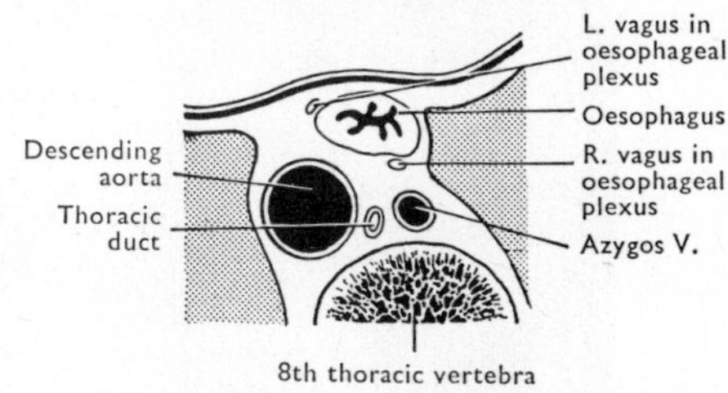

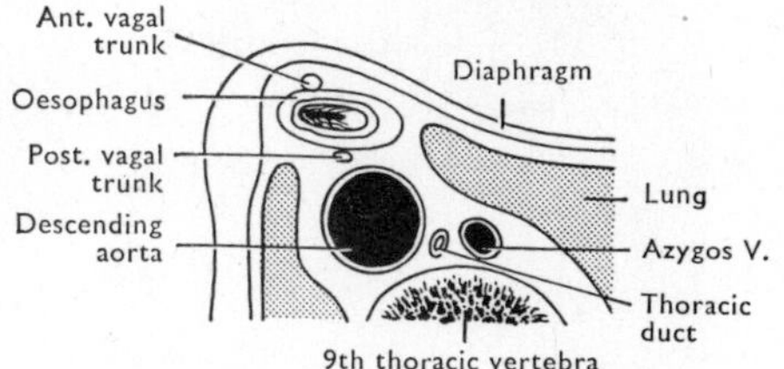

FIG. 73 Outline drawings of four sections through the oesophagus at different thoracic levels.

perforates the diaphragm. These sites may be shown as narrowings of the lumen in oblique radiographs following a barium swallow [FIG. 72]. If the left atrium is dilated it indents the shadow of the oesophagus in such radiographs.

Structure. The lining of the oesophagus is the mucous type of **stratified squamous epithelium.** It lies on a thick layer of areolar tissue in which are longitudinal bundles of muscularis mucosae, and it is thrown into folds by contraction of the outer muscular layers. The **muscle** layers (outer longitudinal and inner circular) are mainly longitudinal in the superior part where they are composed entirely of **striated muscle fibres,** but contain progressively more circular fibres in the middle third, where striated and smooth muscle fibres are mixed, and in the lower third the fibres are exclusively of **smooth muscle** and predominantly circular in direction. There is no special development of circular muscle fibres to form a sphincter in the wall of the oesophagus either at the diaphragmatic aperture or at the entry into the stomach. The presence of striated muscle in the superior part ensures the rapid transport of the bolus through that part which is applied to the trachea.

The mucous membrane contains very few glands, though a few deep mucous glands lie in the submucosa close to the diaphragm, and there may be islands of gastric type mucous membrane in the inferior part of the oesophagus.

The oesophagus is surrounded by loose areolar tissue which allows it to expand freely during the swallowing of a bolus.

DESCENDING AORTA
[FIGS. 28, 50, 64, 71, 73]

This continuation of the arch of the aorta begins on the left side of the fourth thoracic intervertebral disc. It descends through the posterior mediastinum between the left pleura, and the thoracic duct and azygos vein on the right. At first posterior to the left lung root and then to the posterior surface of the pericardium, it deviates anteriorly and to the right behind the oesophagus, and continues on the anterior surface of the vertebral column, behind the inferior part of the diaphragm. It enters the abdomen posterior to the dorsal edge of the diaphragm at the level of the twelfth thoracic vertebra. It lies on the vertebral column, the hemiazygos veins, and its own intercostal and subcostal branches.

Branches. From the anterior surface: (1) two **left bronchial arteries,** from the superior of which the right bronchial artery may arise [p. 84]; (2) several **oesophageal branches** direct to the oesophagus; and (3) a number of small branches which supply the fat and lymph nodes of the mediastinum, the pericardium, and inferiorly the diaphragm. Nine pairs of **posterior intercostal** (q.v.) and one pair of **subcostal arteries** arise from the posterior surface.

THORACIC DUCT
[FIGS. 60, 73, 75]

This small, vein-like structure conveys most of the lymph of the body to the blood stream. This includes the lymph from the intestines (chyle) which contains a considerable amount of fat in the form of fine droplets, and this gives it a milky appearance after a meal.

DISSECTION. Clean the upper part of the thoracic duct to its termination.

The thoracic duct arises from the **cisterna chyli,** an elongated lymphatic sac which lies on the first and second lumbar vertebrae between the aorta and the right crus of the diaphragm. There may be a similar sac which lies posterior to the aorta. This carries lymph from the left side to join the thoracic duct where it leaves the cisterna chyli to pass into the thorax applied to the right surface of the aorta. It ascends through the posterior mediastinum between the descending aorta and the azygos vein, at first posterior to the diaphragm and then behind the oesophagus. At the fifth thoracic vertebra it crosses obliquely to the left side of the oesophagus and ascends on this to the root of the neck in contact with the arch of the aorta and the left pleura. In the root of the neck it arches laterally and then downwards

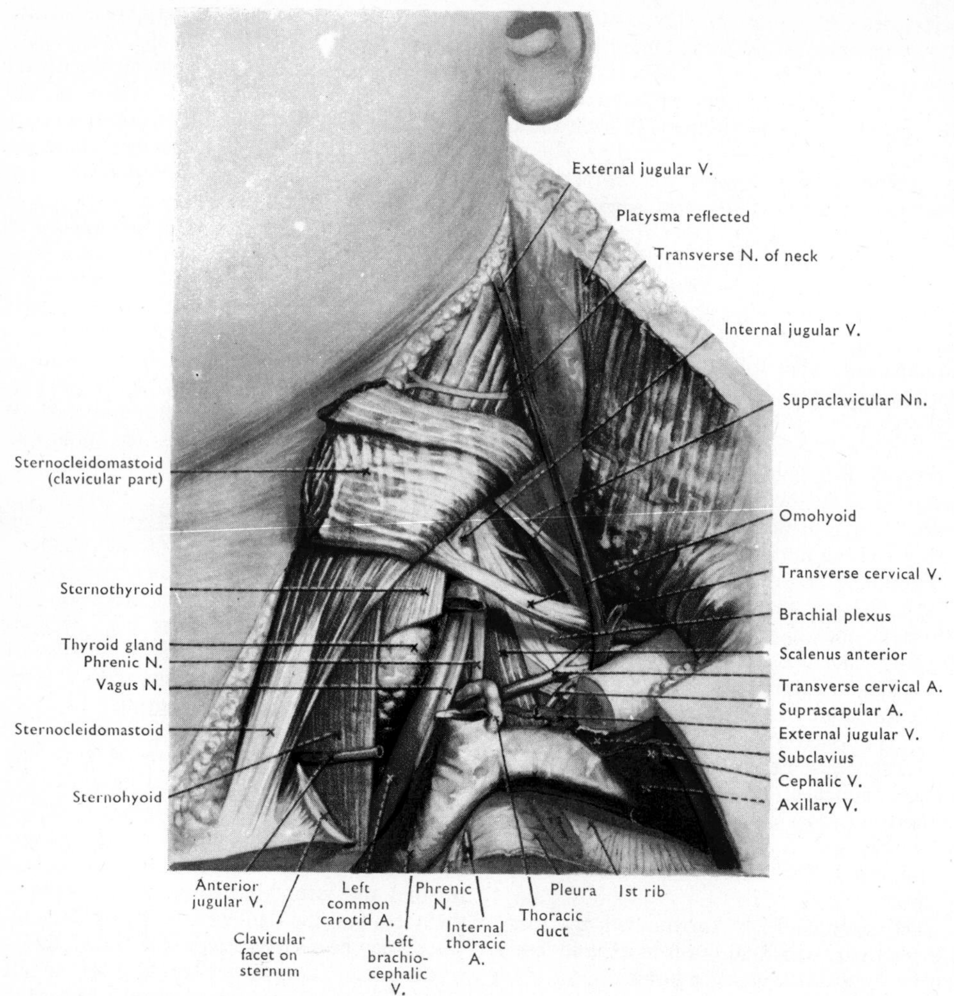

FIG. 74 A dissection of the root of the neck to show the termination of the thoracic duct. Cf. FIG. 16.

(between the carotid sheath anteriorly and the vertebral vessels and subclavian artery posteriorly) to enter the angle of junction of the internal jugular and subclavian veins [FIG. 74].

The thoracic duct is frequently double through part of its course. It contains many valves, the last of which lies a short distance from its termination.

Tributaries. The cisterna chyli receives the right and left lumbar lymph trunks which drain lymph from the lower limbs, the lower part of the anterior abdominal wall, the pelvis, and posterior abdominal wall, including the gonads, kidneys, and suprarenal glands. It also receives the intestinal lymph trunks, and hence the lymph from the abdominal contents, except the superior part of the liver which drains through the diaphragm to **mediastinal** or **parasternal nodes**. The thoracic duct also receives all the lymph vessels which run with

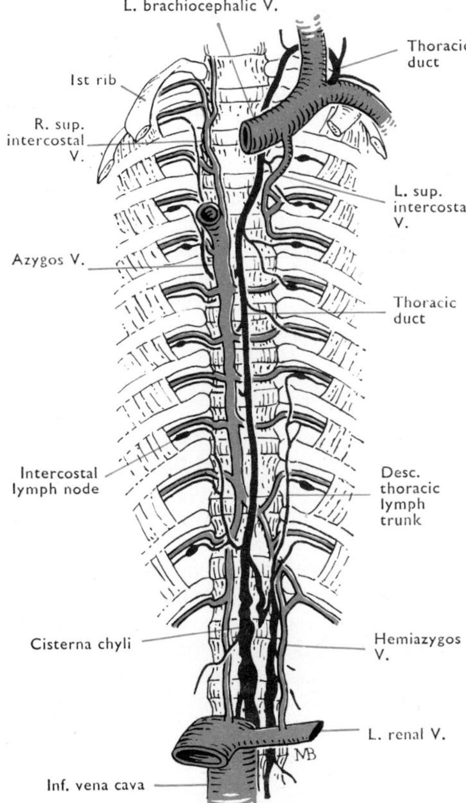

FIG. 75 The thoracic duct and posterior intercostal veins. In this case no accessory hemiazygos vein is present and the number of venous communications across the midline is greater than usual.

the posterior intercostal vessels [FIG. 75] and frequently the left **jugular** and **subclavian trunks** close to its termination. Thus it drains the posterior thoracic wall and parietal pleura, and the lymph from the left side of the head and neck and the left upper limb. It rarely receives the left bronchomediastinal lymph trunk, but when it does it also drains the left lung, left side of the heart, and a large part of the mediastinum, though normally it merely drains the oesophagus and the posterior parts of the pericardium and diaphragm. The **bronchomediastinal trunk** usually enters the left brachiocephalic vein independently, as may the left jugular and subclavian trunks.

Right Lymphatic Duct

This vessel is occasionally formed by the union of the right jugular, right subclavian, and right bronchomediastinal trunks, but it is more usual for the jugular and subclavian trunks to unite and enter the right veins at the same position as the thoracic duct on the left.

The **right bronchomediastinal trunk** corresponds to the left vessel, but also drains the upper part of the right lobe of the liver. It usually enters the right brachiocephalic vein, but even if it unites with the jugular and subclavian trunks of the right side, the vessel so formed has a much smaller field of drainage than the thoracic duct.

Lymph Nodes of Thorax

1. The **parasternal nodes** lie with the internal thoracic vessels. They drain the upper part of the anterior abdominal wall, the adjacent part of the anterior thoracic wall, including the medial part of the mammary gland, and the anterior part of the diaphragm. This corresponds to the distribution of the internal thoracic artery.
2. **Intercostal lymph nodes** lie in the posterior parts of the intercostal spaces and drain to the thoracic duct [FIG. 75].
3. **Phrenic nodes.** These lie near the attachment of the phrenic nerve to the diaphragm and of the diaphragm to the anterior thoracic wall.
4. The **posterior mediastinal lymph nodes** lie along the descending aorta and drain the posterior mediastinum (including the diaphragm, pericardium, and oesophagus) to the thoracic duct.
5. The **tracheobronchial nodes** lie on the thoracic trachea and the principal bronchi. They drain these structures and receive lymph from the lungs.
6. **Bronchopulmonary lymph nodes** lie in the hilus of the lung and in the bifurcations of the bronchi. They drain the lung tissue and the visceral pleura.
7. The **anterior mediastinal lymph nodes** lie

beside the left brachiocephalic vein, and they drain the heart, pericardium, and thymus.

The **bronchomediastinal lymph trunk** is formed, on each side, by the junction of efferent lymph vessels from the parasternal, tracheobronchial, and anterior mediastinal nodes.

Lymph from the lungs carries phagocytes which have ingested carbon particles deposited on the walls of the alveoli from the inspired air. Many of these remain in the lung giving it its mottled appearance, the rest reach the lymph nodes which become laden with carbon particles.

DISSECTION. Complete the cleaning of the posterior intercostal vessels and the intercostal nerves. Follow the left posterior intercostal veins to the hemi-azygos and accessory hemiazygos veins. Clean these veins and note their communications with the azygos vein.

Posterior Intercostal Arteries

One posterior intercostal artery passes to each intercostal space. The first two spaces are supplied by the **highest intercostal artery** which arises from the costocervical trunk at the neck of the first rib. It descends lateral to the sympathetic trunk, anterior to the necks of the first and second ribs, and the eighth cervical and first thoracic ventral rami passing to the brachial plexus [FIG. 15].

The remaining posterior intercostal arteries arise from the posterior surface of the descending thoracic aorta (the right vessels being longer than the left because of the asymmetrical position of the aorta) and the superior four ascend obliquely to their intercostal spaces. The first right aortic intercostal usually supplies the **right bronchial artery.** The aortic intercostal arteries lie on the periosteum of the vertebral bodies and are posterior to all the other structures (*e.g.*, azygos vein, thoracic duct, sympathetic trunk). As each enters the intercostal space it passes superior to the intercostal nerve, gives off its dorsal branch, and runs between the nerve and the vein to enter the costal groove near the angle of the rib [FIG. 9].

The **dorsal branch** passes posteriorly (medial to the superior costotransverse ligament) with the dorsal ramus of the spinal nerve. Each dorsal branch sends a spinal branch through the corresponding intervertebral foramen to supply the contents of the vertebral canal.

The **subcostal arteries** are the last pair of branches of the descending thoracic aorta. They accompany the twelfth thoracic ventral rami (**subcostal nerves**) along the inferior borders of the twelfth ribs, and enter the abdomen by passing posterior to the origin of the diaphragm from the lateral arcuate ligament (q.v.)

Intercostal Nerves

These are the ventral rami of the upper eleven thoracic nerves, and they pass laterally between the internal intercostal membrane and the pleura to disappear between the intercostal muscles [p. 10] as the most inferior element of the intercostal neurovascular bundle.

The greater part of the ventral ramus of the **first thoracic nerve** passes superolaterally in front of the neck of the first rib to join the brachial plexus. The **intercostal branch** is small and passes obliquely across the inferior surface of the first rib to enter the first space close to the costal cartilage. *It has no cutaneous branches.*

The ventral ramus of the **second thoracic nerve** usually sends a branch to join the brachial plexus. This is commonly small, but may be large, in which case the large lateral cutaneous branch of the second intercostal nerve (**intercostobrachial**) is small or absent.

The **subcostal nerve** passes with the subcostal artery into the abdominal wall. Its lateral cutaneous branch passes inferiorly over the iliac crest to supply skin in the gluteal region.

Posterior Intercostal Veins

The **highest** crosses the neck of the first rib to join the corresponding brachiocephalic vein. The **second** and **third** unite to form the right and left **superior intercostal veins.** The right descends to enter the azygos vein, while the left crosses the arch of the aorta to the left brachiocephalic vein, but may enter the accessory hemiazygos vein.

The remaining veins enter the **azygos vein** on the right, while the arrangement on the left is variable and depends on the number of veins crossing the midline to join the azygos vein. Usually the fourth to eighth left posterior intercostal veins enter the **accessory hemiazygos vein,** which descends with the aorta to the eighth thoracic vertebra and crosses the midline to join the azygos vein. It may be replaced by a number of separate veins crossing the vertebral column individually [FIG. 75].

The **hemiazygos vein** arises in the abdomen from the posterior surface of the left renal vein. It enters the thorax through the left crus of the diaphragm, receives the subcostal and remaining posterior intercostal veins, and crosses the vertebral column, posterior to the aorta and thoracic duct, to join the azygos vein.

THE JOINTS OF THE THORAX

DISSECTION. In the portion of the sternum with the costal cartilages and parts of the ribs attached, identify the sternal, sternocostal, interchondral, and costochondral joints. Clean the ligaments on the surfaces of these, and then remove a thin slice from the anterior surface of each to expose the interior.

Sternal Joints

The **manubriosternal joint** lies at the sternal angle. It is a secondary cartilaginous joint at which the cartilage covered ends of the manubrium and body of the sternum are united by a **fibrous disc** in which there may be a cavity. It is strengthened by thickened, longitudinal periosteal fibres in front and behind, and the importance of this joint in respiration is indicated by the failure of the manubrium and body of the sternum to unite except occasionally in old age. This contrasts with the earlier (childhood to 21 years) fusion of the four pieces of the body of the sternum which, prior to this, are united to each other and to the xiphoid process (xiphisternal joint) by hyaline cartilage, the latter joint being ossified in middle life.

Sternocostal Joints

Seven pairs of costal cartilages articulate with the margins of the sternum. The first **costal cartilages** are directly united to the manubrium, and the only movement between the first ribs and the manubrium is due to the flexibility of the costal cartilages. This cartilage begins to calcify and ossify at the end of growth, with consequent loss of mobility, thus indicating that the manubrium and first ribs must move virtually as one piece on their costovertebral joints.

The **second** to **seventh** sternocostal joints are synovial in type and each has a fibrous capsule which is strengthened anteriorly and posteriorly by a **radiate sternocostal ligament,** the fibres of which diverge from the costal cartilage to the part of the sternum with which each costal cartilage articulates. The second sternocostal joint is double owing to the presence of an **intra-articular sternocostal ligament** which is attached to the fibrous disc of the manubriosternal joint. Some of the other joints also may be double, and the seventh costal cartilage may have no synovial joint with the sternum.

Interchondral Joints

These are small synovial joints between the adjacent margins of the costal cartilages of the sixth to ninth ribs, while that of the tenth is a fibrous joint. They give some rigidity to the costal margin while allowing sliding movements between the costal cartilages.

Costochondral Joints

At these joints each cartilage fits into a pit on the end of the bony rib and is fused with it.

DISSECTION. Clean the ligaments that attach the heads of the ribs to the vertebral bodies and intervertebral

discs, and the ligaments that join the ribs to the transverse processes [Fig. 77]. Remove the anterior parts of the capsules of the joints of the heads of the ribs, and identify the intra-articular ligament if present. Then remove the ribs entirely by cutting the various ligaments, and compare the articulations of the heads and tubercles at the various levels.

COSTOVERTEBRAL JOINTS [FIGS. 77, 78]

Most of these joints are complex and consist of two separate articulations: (1) the **head** of the rib with the adjacent parts of its own vertebral body, the vertebra above, and the intervertebral disc between, and (2) the articular part of the **tubercle** of the rib with the transverse process of its own vertebra. The presence of these two separate articulations forces the rib to move round an axis which passes through both of them, and thus they act as a hinge, the axis of which passes inferolaterally and can only be changed if the tubercle is able to slide supero-inferiorly on the transverse process. The articular facets on the transverse processes of the upper thoracic vertebrae are shallow, spherical sockets which face anteriorly and do not allow such sliding movement, while those on the lower vertebrae are flatter, tend to face more superiorly, and permit this movement to a slight degree.

The exceptions to this general arrangement are: (1) the heads of the *first* and *last three ribs* articulate only with their own vertebral bodies, and (2) the *last two ribs* do not articulate with the transverse process, and therefore have a much freer range of movement.

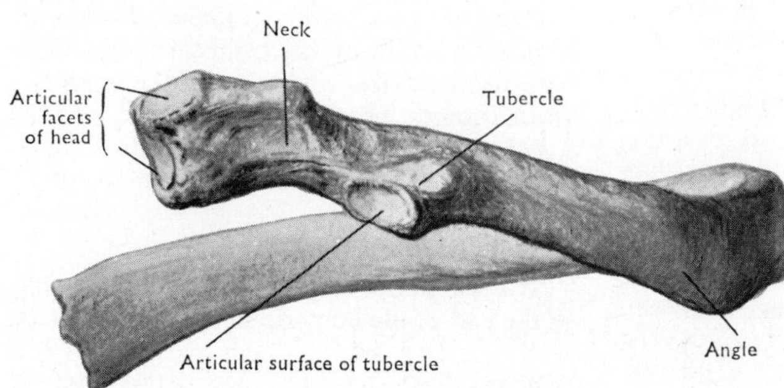

FIG. 76 The fifth right rib seen from behind.

The **heads** of the ribs which articulate with two vertebrae do so by two bevelled facets each of which forms a separate synovial joint with the lateral surface of a vertebral body [FIG. 84]. These two joints are separated by the **intra-articular ligament** which is attached to the intervertebral disc; a feature which is not present in the single joints of the ribs which articulate with one vertebra only. The joints are surrounded by an **articular capsule** and are strengthened anteriorly by the **radiate ligament** of the head. The upper and lower bands of this ligament pass to the two vertebral bodies, the intermediate band to the intervertebral disc.

The **costotransverse joint** is surrounded by an articular capsule which is strengthened laterally by the **lateral costotransverse ligament.** This joins the non-articular part of the tubercle to the tip of the transverse process. In addition the joint is stabilized by: (1) the **costotransverse ligament** from the back of the neck of the rib to the anterior surface of the transverse process, and (2) the **superior costotransverse ligament** which joins the crest of the neck of the rib to the transverse process above. The anterior fibres of the latter run superolaterally and the posterior fibres run superomedially. The aperture between this ligament and the vertebral column transmits the dorsal ramus of the spinal nerve and the dorsal branch of the intercostal artery.

Movements of Ribs [FIGS. 5, 78]

These have been described already [p. 6] but the salient points are: (1) The two **first ribs,** together with the manubrium sterni, move as one piece on the first thoracic vertebra, their joints with which lie in the same transverse plane and form a complex, single hinge. Because the first ribs pass obliquely downwards and forwards, raising the manubrium increases the anteroposterior diameter of the superior aperture, and the pure vertical

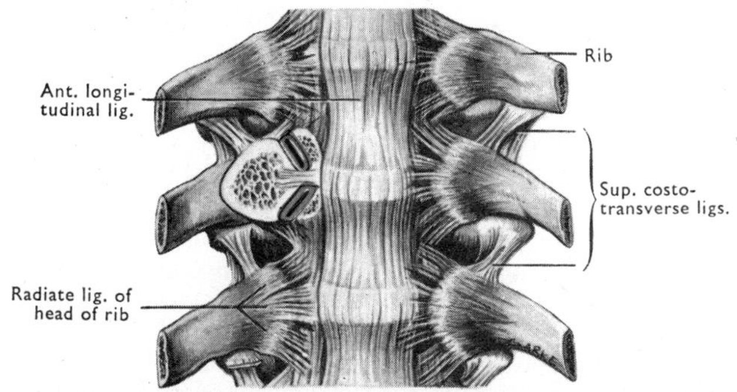

FIG. 77 The anterior longitudinal ligament and costovertebral joints from in front. One joint has been opened by an oblique slice through the head of the rib.

movement produces no lateral pressure on the structures passing over the first rib into the upper limb. (2) The **true ribs,** when raised, not only increase the anteroposterior diameter of the thorax and carry the body of the sternum anteriorly with them in the same manner as the movement of the first ribs, but since they also move outwards on their obliquely placed posterior hinge, they increase the transverse diameter; a feature which is allowed for in the true ribs by the angulation of the flexible costal cartilages. (3) In the **false ribs,** the tubercles slide posteriorly on the flat articular surfaces, thus tending to swing the anterior ends of the ribs outwards. This movement is additional to the simple elevation of the ribs, and it adds to the increased transverse diameter of the thorax and resists the tendency of the diaphragm to draw the costal margin inwards.

JOINTS AND LIGAMENTS OF VERTEBRAL COLUMN

If the head and neck has been or is being dissected, it is possible to see all the features of the vertebral ligaments after the dissectors of the head and neck have removed the spinal medulla (Vol. 3, pp. 30–38, 139). If the head and neck has still to be dissected, the display of the structures should be delayed until this is done, since a clear picture can be obtained from the following description and illustrations, provided the appropriate macerated vertebrae are studied at the same time.

Intervertebral Discs

The vertebral bodies are united by intervertebral discs which consist of many concentric layers of strong collagenous fibrous tissue (**anulus fibrosus**) that run between the cartilage layers which cover the superior and inferior surfaces of the bodies. The alternate layers of collagen run at an angle to each other, and together they surround an internal mass of gelatinous material (the **nucleus pulposus**). This is held under pressure by the anulus and lies slightly nearer the posterior than the anterior surface of the disc [FIG. 80]. The discs allow a certain amount of movement around the nucleus

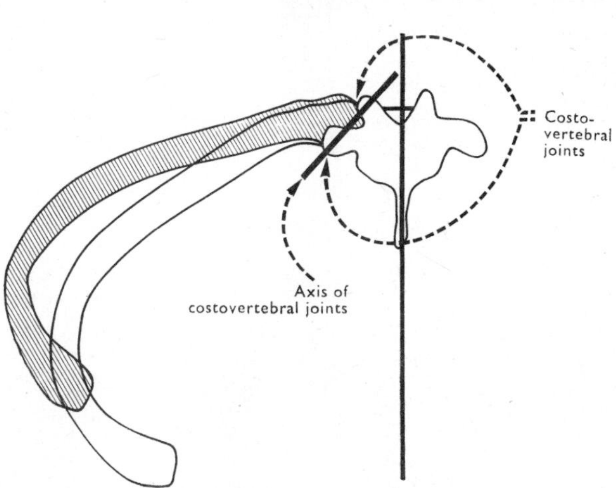

FIG. 78 An upper thoracic vertebra and rib viewed from behind. The shaded outline of the rib represents its position in inspiration, while the clear outline shows the position in expiration, movement taking place around the axis of the two costovertebral joints. Note that the axis of the two joints ensures that the transverse diameter of the thorax is increased on inspiration.

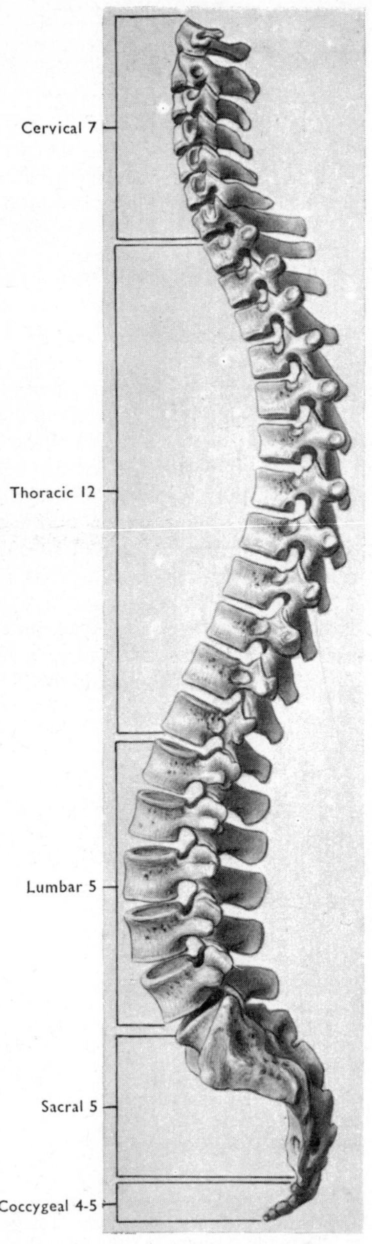

FIG. 79 The left surface of the vertebral column.

pulposus in any direction, but the direction which is possible in any region is determined by the nature of the articular facets on the vertebral arches, while the amount of movement is controlled by the thickness of the disc. The discs are thickest in the lumbar region and thinnest in the thoracic region where the range of movement is necessarily limited because of the compression of the anterior end of the ribs which would inevitably follow any considerable amount of flexion of the thoracic vertebral column. The intervertebral discs are supported by anterior and posterior longitudinal ligaments.

The **anterior longitudinal ligament** is a tough glistening band that stretches from the atlas vertebra to the first piece of the sacrum. It is firmly attached to the anterior surfaces of the intervertebral discs and the adjacent margins of the vertebral bodies. Its lateral margin is difficult to define as it fades into the periosteum [FIG. 77].

The **posterior longitudinal ligament** is much narrower than the anterior longitudinal ligament. It lies on the posterior surfaces of the vertebral bodies within the vertebral canal [FIG. 81]. The margins of the ligament are scalloped, for it is wide where it is attached to the intervertebral discs and the adjacent margins of the vertebral bodies, and narrow opposite the vertebral bodies. Here it is separated from the vertebral bodies by the **basivertebral veins** which emerge anterior to it and pass backwards round its lateral margins to join the internal vertebral venous plexus [FIG. 180].

The intervertebral discs not only allow movements to take place between the vertebrae, but they also absorb shocks applied to the vertebral column and resist the compression forces due to contraction of the powerful erector spinae group of muscles. These forces are considerable, *e.g.*, when an 80 kg. man jumps from a height and lands on his feet, or when he lifts a 50 kg. sack. It is, therefore, not uncommon to find that the nucleus pulposus has been extruded either through the posterior part of the disc, or into the adjacent vertebral body. This herniation of the nucleus pulposus

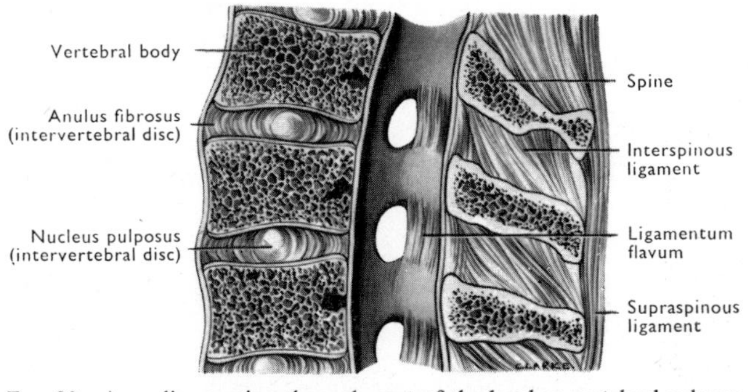

FIG. 80 A median section through part of the lumbar vertebral column.

markedly interferes with the function of the intervertebral disc owing to the loss of pressure in it and the consequent narrowing of the disc. Progressive narrowing of the discs from this and other causes is seen with increasing age, but herniation of the nucleus pulposus may occur at any age and is one cause of pain in the back. If the herniation passes posteriorly through the thinnest part of the anulus fibrosus, it may press on the spinal medulla or on the spinal nerve, which at its exit is posterior to the disc.

The **vertebral arches** are held together by strong, yellow, elastic ligaments (**ligamenta flava**) between the laminae. In the thoracic region these are relatively narrow and arise from the upper margins of the laminae medial to the superior articular facets, and are inserted into the anterior surfaces of the laminae above, medial to the inferior articular facets. With the laminae they form a smooth posterior surface to the vertebral canal. In the median plane, between the two halves of each ligament, there is a slight gap which is filled with areolar tissue and transmits small blood vessels [FIG. 82].

The **spines** of the vertebrae are united by strong **supraspinous ligaments** which course over their posterior extremities, and by thinner **interspinous ligaments** that unite the adjacent margins of the spines and lie between the supraspinous ligaments and the ligamenta flava. All these ligaments are sufficiently elastic to allow the separation of the laminae

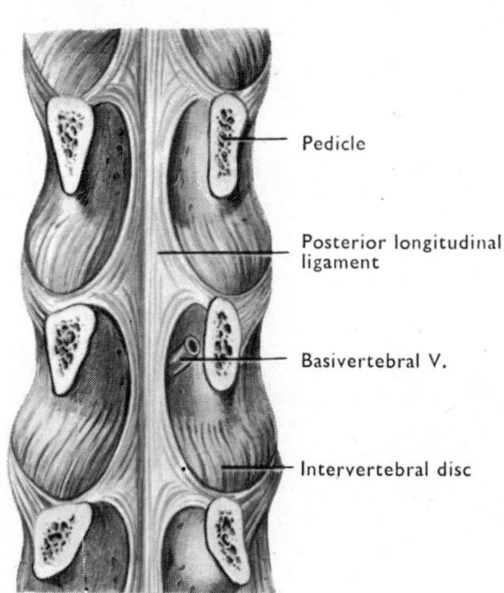

FIG. 81 The posterior longitudinal ligament of the vertebral column. The vertebral arches have been removed.

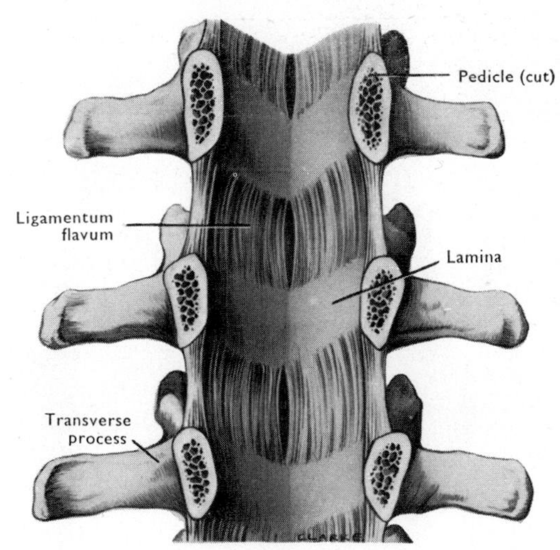

FIG. 82 The lumbar vertebral arches and ligamenta flava seen from in front after removal of the vertebral bodies.

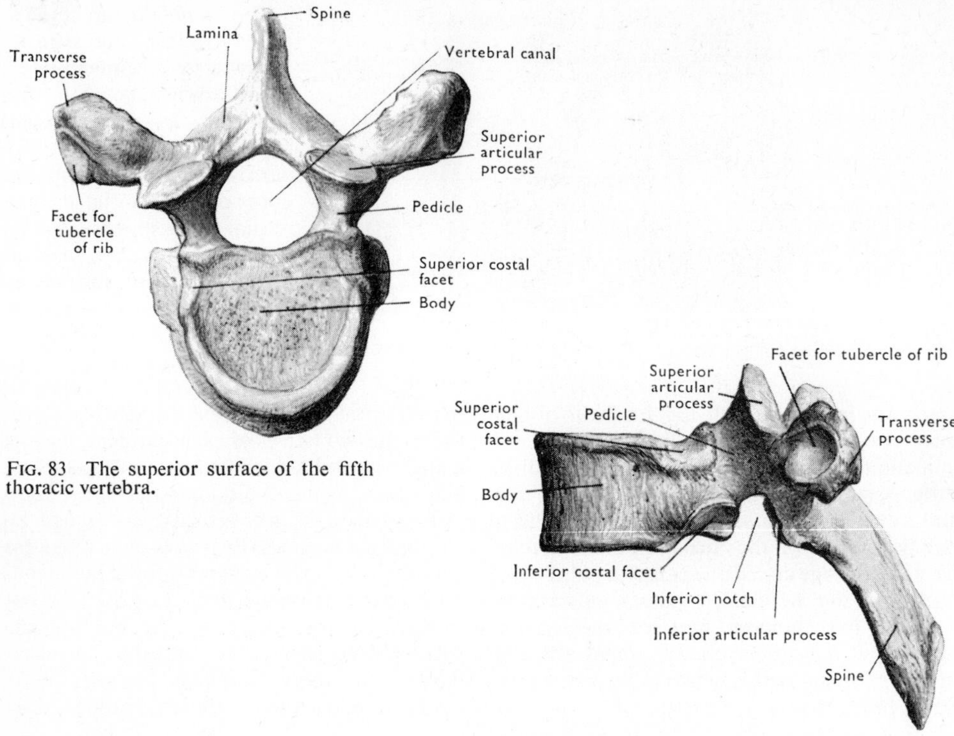

FIG. 83 The superior surface of the fifth thoracic vertebra.

FIG. 84 The lateral surface of the fifth thoracic vertebra.

FIG. 85 The superior surface of the third lumbar vertebra.

FIG. 86 The lateral surface of the third lumbar vertebra.

and spines which occurs on flexion of the vertebral column, and they help to return the vertebral column to its resting position when flexion ceases.

DISSECTION. If the spinal medulla has been removed, proceed to cut out a length of the thoracic vertebral column, and then split it with a saw in the median plane. Identify the parts of the intervertebral discs and note their relation to the vertebral canal and intervertebral foramina.

Examine macerated specimens of vertebrae from the various regions of the vertebral column, and confirm the attachments of the ligaments by the rough areas and lines which they leave on the bone.

Articular Facets. Compare these structures in the cervical, thoracic, and lumbar regions. In the thoracic region [Fig. 83], the plane of these synovial joints is approximately on the arc of a circle with its centre in the nucleus pulposus, thus indicating that rotation is possible in this region though restricted by the thin intervertebral discs. By contrast, in the lumbar region, the inferior articular facets [Figs. 85, 86] fit between the superior articular facets in such a manner that rotation around the body is not possible unless they are first separated to a considerable degree by flexion. Though not so obvious, the same limitation applies in the cervical region for here the two superior facets lie parallel to each other in an oblique coronal plane sloping upwards and forwards. They are relatively further apart than in the other regions, and thus effectively prevent rotation except for a small amount which can occur either after flexion, or in lateral flexion. In the latter case the elevated inferior facet slides anteriorly on the sloping superior facet below, the opposite movement taking place on the other side where the inferior facet, passing downwards, is displaced posteriorly on the sloping superior facet below.

The maximum range of movement is in the lumbar region and consists of flexion, extension, and lateral flexion. The minimum range is in the thoracic region and consists principally of rotation. The movements in the cervical region (ignoring the movements between the first two cervical vertebrae and between the first cervical vertebra and the skull) are intermediate in range, and their direction is the same as in the lumbar region. However a greater degree of extension is normally possible in the cervical region because the spines are smaller than in the lumbar region, and do not overlap as in the thoracic region [Fig. 79].

THE ABDOMEN

POSITION

Before any dissection is begun, it is important to appreciate the position of the abdomen in relation to the other parts of the body. This is best achieved by examining the bony points in a living individual while relating these to the bones of a mounted skeleton. In the abdomen, as elsewhere, it is rarely possible to obtain satisfactory information from the embalmed cadaver unless it is very thin and the bony points are readily visible.

In the following section the relative positions of certain structures are described, but these are approximations only, since there are considerable variations between individuals, and in one individual at different ages and in different positions. Thus the distance between the iliac crest and the costal margin is greater in infants and children (where the ribs are more horizontally placed) than it is in adults, and is still further reduced in old age both because of the progressive narrowing of the intervertebral discs and the tendency to stoop. The same distance is less in the standing position (because of the lower position taken up by the ribs) than it is when lying supine, and it is greater in inspiration than in expiration.

In the median plane anteriorly, the abdominal wall extends from the xiphoid process (at the level of the ninth thoracic vertebra) to the pubic symphysis, the superior border of which is in the same horizontal plane as the coccyx. Elsewhere the abdominal wall is in great measure replaced by the thoracic cage (with the contained pleura and lungs) and the gluteal region of the lower limb, both of which overlap the abdominal contents posteriorly and laterally. Thus in an adult of average build, the costal margin extends inferiorly to the level of the third lumbar vertebra in the mid-axillary line (usually the lowest point is formed by the eleventh costal cartilage) and is less than 4 cm. from the iliac crest. The iliac crest marks the superior limit of the gluteal region and its highest part reaches the level of the fourth lumbar vertebra. Thus penetrating wounds of the lower thorax or buttock may well involve the abdominal contents.

The abdominal contents fill the concavity of the diaphragm, and thus extend into the thorax to the level of the eighth thoracic vertebra, or in the case of the right dome of the diaphragm to the level of the fifth rib in the mid-clavicular line, in full expiration. Yet the pleural sac crosses the tenth rib in the mid-axillary line and the twelfth rib in the paravertebral line. Hence the upper abdominal contents are overlapped by the pleural cavities and lungs, though separated from them by the diaphragm [Fig. 20].

Since the mobile diaphragm forms the superior limit of the abdominal cavity, the abdominal contents move up and down with respiration, a fact that is made use of in clinical examination because certain organs (*e.g.* liver or enlarged spleen) may be exposed to palpation inferior to the costal margin on deep inspiration, though hidden by the thoracic cage in quiet respiration.

SURFACE ANATOMY

Find the **xiphoid process** where the costal margins meet at the **infrasternal angle.** Trace the **costal margin** inferolaterally and note its relation to the iliac crest, the curved bony ridge which is set in a furrow between the abdominal wall and the gluteal region. Posterior to its most inferior point, the costal margin ascends to the **twelfth rib** which may only just be palpable lateral to the paravertebral mass of muscle (erector spinae) or may extend some distance beyond this. In the angle between the costal margin and erector spinae the abdominal wall lies immediately posterior to the lower part of the kidney [FIG. 167].

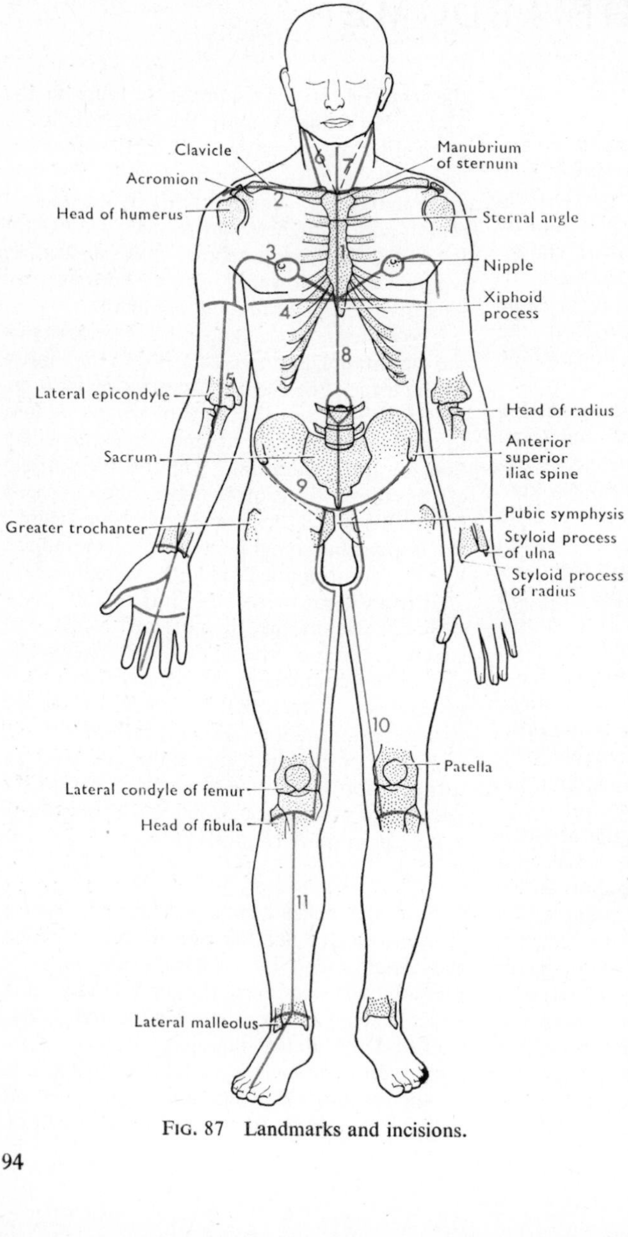

Trace the **iliac crest** anteriorly and posteriorly. Its highest point lies at the level of the fourth lumbar vertebra (slightly inferior to the normal level of the umbilicus), while the rounded knob of bone at its anterior extremity (**anterior superior iliac spine**) lies on the same horizontal plane as the sacral promontory, though its actual position is altered markedly by changing the tilt of the pelvis. Thus it is lowered relatively by increasing the lumbar curvature (lordosis) and raised by bending forwards. Since the level of a horizontal plane passing through the anterior superior iliac spines is approximately that of the sacral promontory, the part of the anterior abdominal wall between this plane and the pubic symphysis lies opposite the superior aperture of the pelvis [FIG. 112].

Posteriorly the iliac crest ends in the **posterior superior iliac spine.** This bony point is difficult to palpate because of the dense fascia which covers erector spinae and is attached to the posterior part of the iliac crest, but it may be felt in a dimple opposite the second sacral spine approximately 4 cm. from the median plane.

Five to seven centimetres posterior to the anterior superior iliac spine, the outer margin of the iliac crest protrudes to form the **tubercle of the crest,** which lies in the same horizontal (intertubercular) plane as the fifth lumbar vertebra.

The groove in which the iliac crest lies is produced by the attachment of the fasciae of the abdominal wall and gluteal region to the crest. A similar groove passes inferomedially

FIG. 87 Landmarks and incisions.

from the anterior superior iliac spine and then transversely in the fold of the groin to the pubis. It marks the line of attachment of the fascia of the anterior abdominal wall to the fascia of the thigh (**fascia lata**), and it lies inferior to a tendinous band (inguinal ligament) which stretches from the anterior superior iliac spine to the pubic tubercle. The **inguinal ligament** is convex inferiorly, and is the inrolled inferior margin of the aponeurosis of the most superficial muscle of the abdominal wall (the external oblique). The **mid-inguinal point** lies on the inguinal ligament half way between the **pubic symphysis** and the **anterior superior iliac spine,** and marks the point where the external iliac artery escapes from the abdomen into the lower limb, posterior to the inguinal ligament, to become the femoral artery.

Palpate the inguinal ligament and feel the pulsations of the **femoral artery** at the mid-inguinal point. Run a finger laterally from the pubic symphysis along the superior surface of the pubis (**pubic crest**) to a small prominence where the inguinal ligament is attached, the **pubic tubercle.** In the male the pubic tubercle is partly covered by a soft rounded cord (**spermatic cord**) which descends to the scrotum from a triangular aperture (**superficial inguinal ring,** FIG. 90) in the aponeurosis of the external oblique immediately superior and lateral to the tubercle. The margins of the ring are readily felt in the male by placing the tip of the little finger on the loose skin of the upper part of the scrotum over the spermatic cord and invaginating it upwards along the line of the cord. Where the cord disappears, the sharp margins of the ring will be felt by pressing posteriorly. Pick up the spermatic cord between finger and thumb; note the firm cord buried deep in its posterior part. This is the duct of the testis, the **ductus deferens.**

In the female the ring is smaller, transmits only the **round ligament of the uterus,** and is more difficult to palpate. It may be felt by invaginating the skin in the same position as in the male, but the greater amount of subcutaneous fat in the female in this region makes palpation difficult.

Superior to the pubic symphysis a slight median groove passes upwards to the xiphoid process. Deep to this lies the **linea alba** where the aponeuroses of the three flat muscles on each side of the abdominal wall meet and fuse after ensheathing the muscle **(rectus abdominis)** which runs longitudinally on each side of the midline [FIG. 93]. The **umbilicus** lies in the linea alba, nearer the pubis than the xiphoid, and is the puckered scar formed by the remnants of the root of the umbilical cord through which the foetus *in utero* is attached to the placenta.

The linea alba and umbilical scar are formed entirely of white fibrous tissue and are relatively avascular. Incisions into the abdominal cavity may be made through the linea alba without injury to nerves or blood vessels of any size, but its avascularity is associated with poor healing properties, so that wounds in it are slow to heal and liable to break down.

The lateral edge of each rectus abdominis muscle is marked by a slight groove (**linea semilunaris**) which is readily visible only in a slim or muscular person, and is most obvious in the superior two-thirds of the abdomen. The linea semilunaris crosses the costal margin at the **ninth costal cartilage,** the surface marking of the **fundus of the gall-bladder** on the right, and three transverse grooves may be seen connecting the median groove to the linea semilunaris. One such groove lies at the level of the umbilicus and two between it and the xiphoid process. They are formed by the tendinous intersections which cross the rectus abdominis muscles and are fused to the aponeuroses on the anterior surfaces of these muscles.

DISSECTION. Make incisions 8 and 9 [Fig. 87] through the skin, and carry 8 round both sides of the umbilicus and 9 posteriorly along the iliac crest. If the thorax has not been dissected, make incision 4 also, and carry it posteriorly at least to the mid-axillary line. Reflect the large flap of skin so defined, but take care to leave the superficial fascia on the abdominal wall.

Superficial Fascia

This is similar to the superficial fascia elsewhere but the amount of fat is extremely variable and is usually greatest over the inferior half of the abdomen. Here the fascia is divisible into a superficial fatty and a deep membranous, elastic layer. The latter represents the thick, elastic suspensory layer of quadrupeds but is poorly developed in Man. Inferiorly the lateral parts of the **membranous layer** pass over the inguinal ligaments to fuse with the fasciae latae of the thighs a short distance distal to the ligaments, while the intermediate portion passes downwards over the front of the pubis as a flattened, funnel-shaped extension into the perineum. This part is attached laterally to the pubic tubercle, the body of the pubis, and the sides of the pubic arch. It encloses the spermatic cords and forms a membranous layer covering the perineum. In the median plane it is thickened to form the **suspensory ligament of the penis** or **clitoris**, and in the male is continuous with the fascial

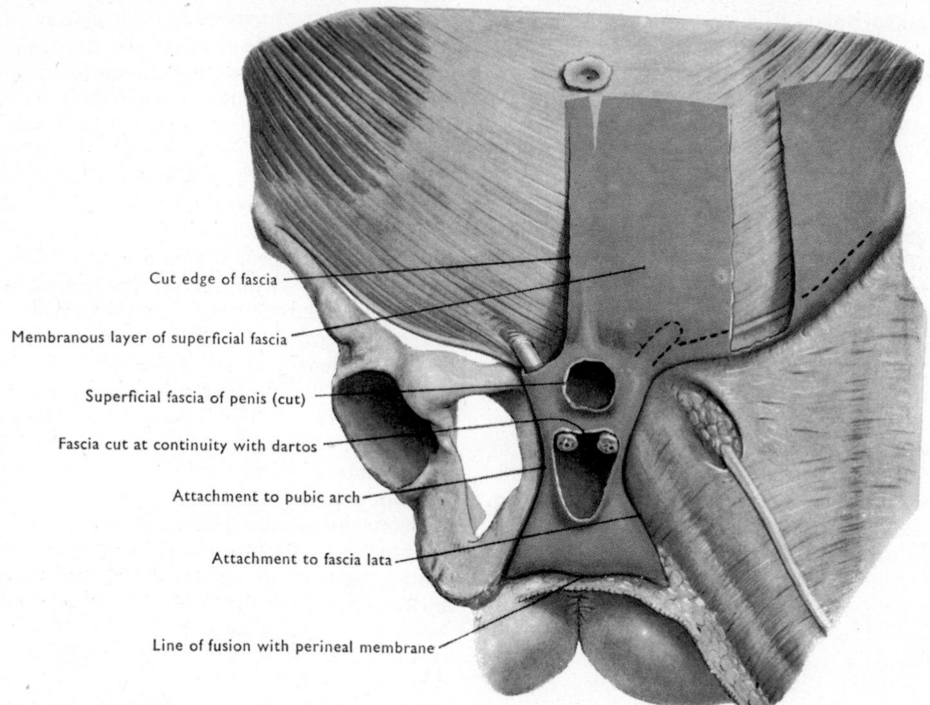

FIG. 88 A diagram to show the membranous layer of the superficial fascia of the abdomen and its extension into the perineum in the male.

sheath of the penis and the fascial layer of the scrotum which contains much smooth muscle, the **dartos muscle.** In the female the lateral attachments are the same, but it is split in the median plane by the vulva, and so passes only into each labium majus [FIG. 194].

DISSECTION. Make a transverse incision through the entire thickness of the superficial fascia from the anterior superior iliac spine to the median plane. Raise the lower margin of the cut fascia, identify the two layers, fatty and membranous, and pass the fingers inferiorly deep to the membranous layer. This is readily separated from the aponeurosis of the external oblique muscle which lies deep to it because of the loose areolar tissue connecting them. The fingers may be passed down for a short distance distal to the inguinal ligament, but close to the median plane one finger may be passed along the spermatic cord, anterior to the pubis, into the perineum. Once in this position, the finger can not be carried laterally because of the lateral attachment of the membranous layer of fascia to the pubic bone. Note the anterior cutaneous branch of the iliohypogastric nerve passing through the aponeurosis of the external oblique into the fascia a short distance superior to the superficial inguinal ring.

If the urethra in the male is ruptured in the perineum, urine escapes deep to the membranous layer of fascia and readily extends superiorly into the anterior abdominal wall in front of the pubis, but it cannot pass into the thigh because of the attachment of the membranous layer to the pubic bone and the fascia lata. It can also extend deep to the sheath of the penis and scrotum. The presence of fluid in this fascial pouch causes a characteristic circumscribed swelling of the perineum and inferior anterior abdominal wall [FIG. 88].

Cutaneous Nerves

The muscles and skin of the abdominal wall are almost entirely supplied by the **lower intercostal** and **subcostal nerves,** with the exception of the most inferior part which is supplied by two branches of the first lumbar nerve, the **iliohypogastric** and **ilioinguinal** nerves. All these nerves are arranged on the same plan as the higher intercostal nerves [FIG. 10] with lateral and anterior cutaneous branches in series with them, but the ilioinguinal nerve has only an anterior cutaneous branch that passes through the superficial inguinal ring. This supplies skin on the medial side of the thigh and on the scrotum (or in the female the labium majus which corresponds to the scrotum).

Anterior Cutaneous Branches. These pierce the anterior wall of the sheath of the rectus either close to the median line or a short distance from it. They send minute cutaneous branches medially and laterally, and are arranged in series such that the **tenth thoracic nerve** emerges close to the umbilicus while the **iliohypogastric** (L.1) is above the superficial inguinal ring.

DISSECTION. To expose the anterior cutaneous branches, divide the superficial fascia along the median line and reflect it laterally by blunt dissection.

To find the lateral cutaneous branches, divide the superficial fascia along the posterior axillary line as far inferiorly as the iliac crest. Reflect the fascia forwards by blunt dissection, and find the nerves emerging between the slips of origin of the external oblique muscle.

Lateral Cutaneous Branches. These emerge between the slips of origin of the external oblique muscle. The subcostal and iliohypogastric nerves pierce the external oblique muscle in the same line as the others (the latter immediately superior to the iliac crest), but run downwards over the iliac crest to supply the skin of the upper anterior part of the gluteal region. The lateral cutaneous branches of the lower intercostal nerves give small posterior and large anterior branches, the latter passing forwards to the lateral margin of the rectus abdominis.

Cutaneous Vessels

The small arteries that accompany the lateral cutaneous branches of the nerves are branches of the **posterior intercostal arteries,** while those that accompany the anterior cutaneous branches arise from vessels within the sheath of the rectus abdominis. These are the superior and inferior **epigastric arteries** which arise from the internal thoracic and external iliac arteries respectively, and they enter the rectus sheath at its superior and inferior ends.

The skin and superficial fascia below the level of the umbilicus are supplied by three small branches of the femoral artery in the groin (Vol. 1, Fig. 93). The **superficial external pudendal** runs medially to supply the skin of the scrotum (or labium majus) and penis. The **superficial circumflex iliac** passes towards the anterior superior iliac spine. The **superficial epigastric** runs superomedially, across the inguinal ligament, as far as the umbilicus.

Superficial Veins

Below the umbilicus these drain with the superficial arteries to the **great saphenous vein** in the groin, and thus eventually to the inferior vena cava. Above the umbilicus they pass to the axilla and so to the superior vena cava. Both groups anastomose with each other and with small veins which pass to the umbilicus from the liver along the line of the obliterated umbilical vein. In obstruction of the superior or inferior vena cava these veins may be distended to form an alternative route for venous return. Also if the venous drainage through the liver is blocked, distended veins from the liver may enter this system at the umbilicus and drain in both directions on each side. Such distended veins radiating from the umbilicus are known as a 'caput medusae'.

MUSCLES OF ANTERIOR ABDOMINAL WALL

These muscles are arranged in three layers. All are muscular posterolaterally but become thin, sheet-like tendons (aponeuroses) anteromedially. These aponeuroses partially surround a paramedian longitudinal muscle (rectus abdominis) and fuse with each other and those of the opposite side in the median **linea alba**. The muscle fibres of the three layers run in different directions, and thus strengthen the abdominal wall to resist the tendency of the abdominal contents to bulge through it when under pressure. The nerves and vessels run between the inner and middle layers as in the thoracic wall.

DISSECTION. Clean the fascia from the superficial layer of muscle (external oblique) and from its aponeurosis. Take special care superiorly where the aponeurosis is thin and easily removed, and inferiorly where it is pierced by the spermatic cord (in the male) or the round ligament of the uterus (in the female) at the inferior margin 4–5 cm. from the median plane.

External Oblique Muscle [Fig. 89]

This muscle arises from the outer surfaces of the lower eight ribs by slips which interdigitate with those of serratus anterior and latissimus dorsi. The fibres fan out from this curved origin; the postero-inferior pass vertically downwards to the anterior half of the iliac crest, are muscular throughout, and form a free border to the muscle posteriorly. The middle (oblique) and upper (transverse) fibres pass into the aponeurosis. This is wider below than above and its fibres continue the oblique inferomedial direction of the muscle fibres.

Medially the **aponeurosis** passes anterior to the rectus abdominis and interlocks with its fellow in the linea alba [Fig. 95] between the xiphoid process and the anterior surface of the symphysis pubis. Superiorly the aponeurosis gives attachment to the lower fibres of pectoralis major, while inferiorly it has a free margin between the anterior superior iliac spine and the pubic tubercle. This margin is rolled posteriorly on itself to form the **inguinal ligament,** which lies at the junction of the abdominal wall with the thigh. The deep fascia of the thigh (**fascia lata**) is attached inferiorly to the inguinal ligament, and the tension of this fascia makes the ligament convex inferiorly.

Superficial Inguinal Ring [Figs. 89, 90]. This is a triangular aperture in the aponeurosis of the external oblique, immediately superior to the pubic tubercle and the medial part of the inguinal ligament. Here the fibres of the aponeurosis diverge to form the inferolateral and superomedial margins (**lateral** and **medial crura**) of the ring. The ring transmits the spermatic cord in the male or the round ligament of the uterus in the female, and each of these is covered by a sleeve of **external spermatic fascia** derived from the margins of the ring.

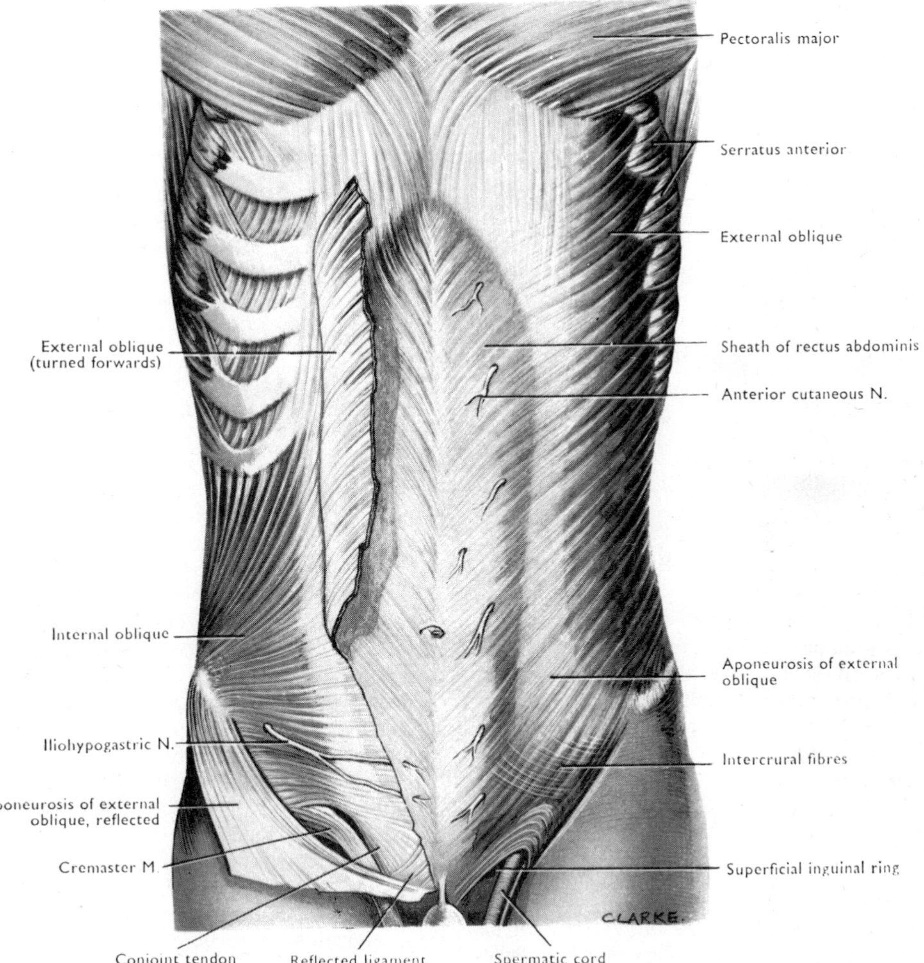

FIG. 89 A dissection of the anterior abdominal wall. The external oblique has been reflected on the right side.

This fascia rapidly fuses with the round ligament, but forms a complete investment for the testis and spermatic cord produced by the testis as it descends through the abdominal wall to the scrotum from its origin in the abdomen.

DISSECTION. Separate the external spermatic fascia from the margins of the ring and define its borders by blunt dissection.

The **lateral crus** of the ring curves inferomedially below the spermatic cord to the pubic tubercle, while the **medial crus** runs obliquely downwards over the front of the body of the pubis to meet its fellow. At the superolateral angle of the ring the crura are bound together by a number of **intercrural fibres** [FIG. 90].

The size of the superficial inguinal ring is very variable. It is much larger in the male

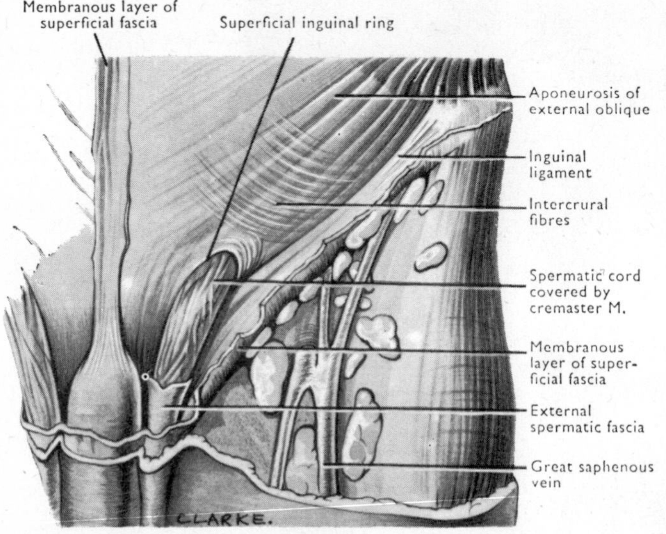

FIG. 90 A superficial dissection of the inguinal region.

than the female, but still scarcely admits the tip of a finger unless stretched.

The **round ligament** of the uterus spreads out into the fascia of the labium majus (the homologue of the scrotum), and is the remnant of part of a fibrous cord (**gubernaculum testis**) which guides the testis to the scrotum in the male, but which is represented in the female by a ligament that joins the ovary to the uterus and the uterus to the labium majus (see below).

DISSECTION. Detach the upper six digitations of the external oblique and cut vertically through the muscle to the iliac crest, leaving the posterior two digitations of the muscle in situ. Separate the anterior part of the external oblique from the iliac crest, avoiding injury to the lateral cutaneous nerves which pierce it close to the iliac crest.

Turn the superior part of the external oblique forwards and clean the internal oblique and its aponeurosis to the line along which it fuses with the aponeurosis of the external oblique, anterior to rectus abdominis. Beginning superiorly, divide the external oblique aponeurosis lateral to the line of fusion, and reflect it inferiorly to expose the remainder of the internal oblique. Carry this line of division medial to the superficial inguinal ring as far as the pubis. Fold the external oblique downwards on the inguinal ligament, and examine the superior surface of the ligament and the deep surface of the external oblique aponeurosis. Medially the superior surface of the inguinal ligament can be seen by lifting the spermatic cord or round ligament from it, but laterally it is hidden by the internal oblique and transversus abdominis muscles which are attached to it.

Inguinal Ligament [FIGS. 90–94]. This inrolled, free margin of the external oblique aponeurosis extends from the anterior superior iliac spine to the pubic tubercle. At the medial attachment, the deeper, inrolled fibres curve horizontally backwards to a linear attachment from the pubic tubercle along the pecten pubis. This part is the curved **lacunar ligament** [FIG. 96], which is continued laterally as a strong ridge of fibrous tissue (**the pectineal ligament**) on the pecten pubis as far as the iliopubic eminence. The medial part of the inguinal ligament, the lacunar ligament, and the pectineal ligament surround the anterior, medial, and posterior surfaces, respectively, of the neck of the **femoral sheath,** a fibrous funnel through which the external iliac vessels pass into the thigh to become the femoral vessels. Clean the lacunar ligament by blunt dissection, and note that its sharp lateral edge abuts on the medial edge of the femoral sheath.

The **spermatic cord** (or round ligament) lies on the superior surfaces of the medial part of the inguinal ligament and of the lacunar ligament as the cord turns forwards through the superficial inguinal ring.

The **reflected ligament** is of no great importance. It consists of the lowest fibres of the aponeurosis of the external oblique which pass through the linea alba. These are inserted into the opposite pubis deep to the aponeurosis of that side.

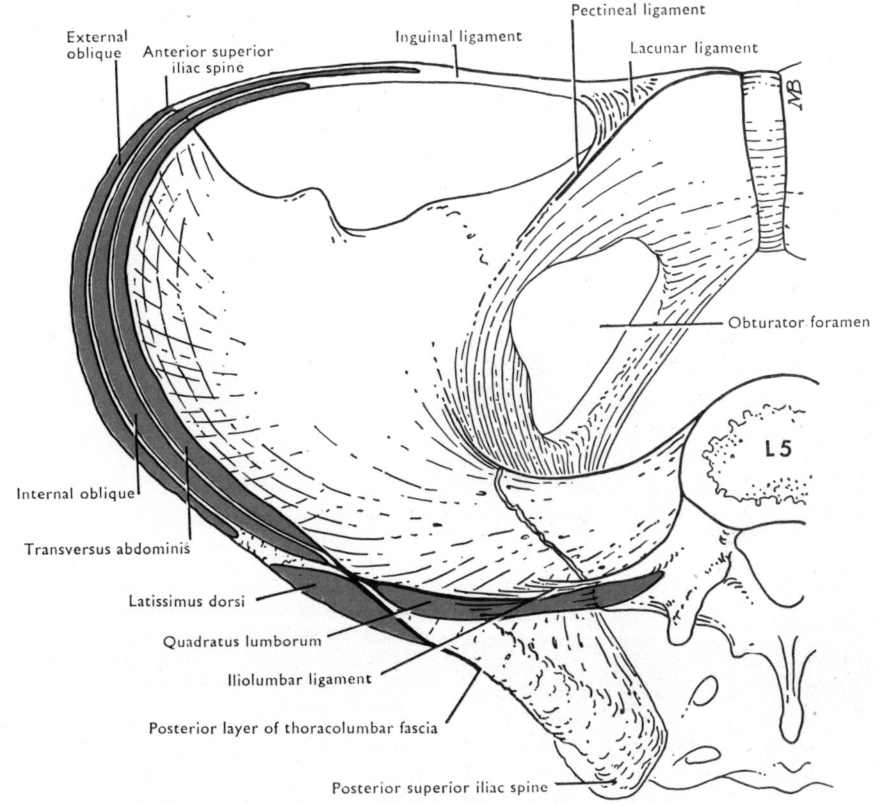

FIG. 91 The bony pelvis and fifth lumbar vertebra seen from above.

DISSECTION. Clean the surface of internal oblique. Retain the branches of the nerves which pierce it superior to the anterior part of the iliac crest and the lateral part of the inguinal ligament. Define the inferior border of the muscle and note its relation to the spermatic cord or round ligament, particularly the muscle bundles (cremaster muscle) passing on to the spermatic cord from the medial edge of the muscle.

Internal Oblique Muscle [FIG. 89]

The muscle arises from the lateral two-thirds of the inguinal ligament, the anterior two-thirds of the iliac crest [FIG. 91], and the lumbar fascia [FIG. 110]. The fibres run upwards and forwards from these origins; the most posterior pass to the cartilages of the lower three ribs, while the remainder form a wide aponeurosis. Most of this splits to enclose the rectus abdominis and passes into the linea alba. The superior part turns upwards to the costal margin formed by the ninth to seventh costal cartilages and to the xiphoid process, while the most inferior part turns downwards to the pubis as part of the conjoint tendon (see transversus abdominis for details of the attachments of the aponeurosis).

Cremaster Muscle. The fibres of the inferomedial edge of the internal oblique are carried downwards by the descending testis which traverses the deeper parts of the abdominal wall 1 cm. above the inguinal ligament at the mid-inguinal point. These muscle fibres form a number of separate loops (cremaster muscle)

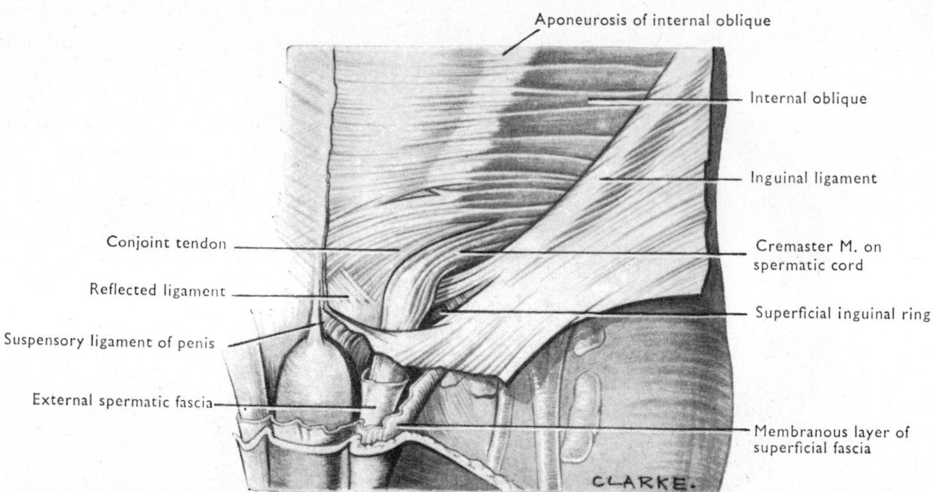

FIG. 92 A dissection of the inguinal region. The external oblique is turned down to show the spermatic cord in the inguinal canal.

which pass over the anterior surface of the spermatic cord for a variable distance, and turning on to its medial and deep surfaces, ascend to be inserted with the other inferior fibres of internal oblique into the pubic crest and tubercle. Only a few of the muscle loops reach the testis, and some end in the fascial layer (**cremasteric fascia**) which accompanies them and forms a complete sheath for the testis and spermatic cord. This is derived from the internal oblique muscle, and lies deep to the external spermatic fascia.

Nerve supply: the genital branch of the genitofemoral nerve (L. 1 and 2). Action: it raises the testis to the superficial inguinal ring, thereby shortening the length of the ductus deferens, the contraction of which is responsible for the discharge of spermatozoa. If the skin of the medial side of the upper thigh is stroked firmly, cremaster contracts reflexly provided the sensory nerve supply to that skin (L. 1–2), the spinal medulla segments (L. 1 and 2), and the genitofemoral nerve are all intact (**cremasteric reflex**).

DISSECTION. Cut through the attachments of the internal oblique to the inguinal ligament, iliac crest, and costal margin. Take care not to cut too deeply as the nerves lie immediately deep to this muscle on transversus abdominis and are easily damaged. Cut vertically through the internal oblique from the twelfth costal cartilage to the iliac crest, and strip the muscle forwards from the transversus and the nerves. This is difficult superiorly owing to the dense fascia between these muscles, and is often impossible inferiorly. The superior part of the internal oblique and its aponeurosis should be freed as far as the lateral edge of the rectus abdominis. Here the aponeurosis will be seen to pass partly anterior and partly posterior to rectus abdominis.

Clean the surface of transversus abdominis and the nerves and vessels which lie on it, including the cutaneous nerves which have been seen piercing the internal and external oblique muscles. Follow the aponeurosis of the transversus abdominis posterior to the rectus abdominis to fuse with the posterior layer of the internal oblique aponeurosis down to the arcuate line [Fig. 93].

NERVES OF ANTERIOR ABDOMINAL WALL

These are the ventral rami of the lower six thoracic nerves (intercostal and subcostal nerves) and the first lumbar nerve (iliohypogastric and ilioinguinal nerves).

The lower five **intercostal nerves** leave the intercostal spaces between the slips of transversus abdominis attached to the internal surfaces of the costal cartilages, and pass between that muscle and the internal oblique either directly (11th) or deep to the upturned ends of the costal cartilages. They run antero-inferiorly to enter the rectus sheath, pierce and supply rectus, and emerge through the anterior wall of the sheath as the **anterior cutaneous branches.** These nerves, with the subcostal, iliohypogastric and ilioinguinal nerves, supply the muscles of the abdominal wall. The last three enter the same layer as the others by piercing the transversus abdominis posteriorly, but they differ from the others in that: (1) The lateral cutaneous branches of the **subcostal** and **iliohypogastric nerves** pierce both oblique muscles close to the iliac crest and descend over it to the gluteal skin. (2) The iliohypogastric pierces the internal oblique 2–3 cm. anterior to the anterior superior iliac spine, and the external oblique 2–3 cm. superior to the superficial inguinal ring to become cutaneous. (3) The **ilioinguinal nerve** has no lateral

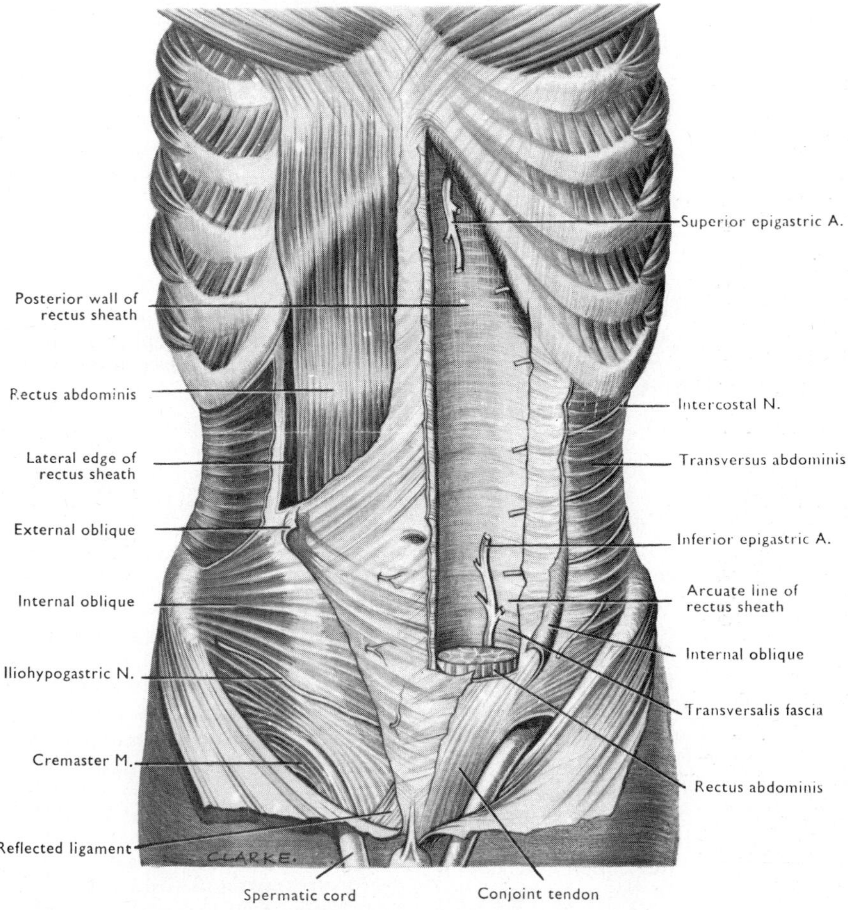

FIG. 93 A deep dissection of the anterior abdominal wall. On the left side the external and internal obliques, the anterior wall of the rectus sheath, and the greater part of the rectus abdominis have been removed. On the right side the external oblique and upper parts of the internal oblique and anterior wall of the rectus sheath have been removed.

cutaneous branch, but pierces the internal oblique above the lateral part of the inguinal ligament, and runs with the spermatic cord or round ligament through the superficial inguinal ring. It is cutaneous to the upper part of the front of the thigh and the anterior parts of the external genitalia.

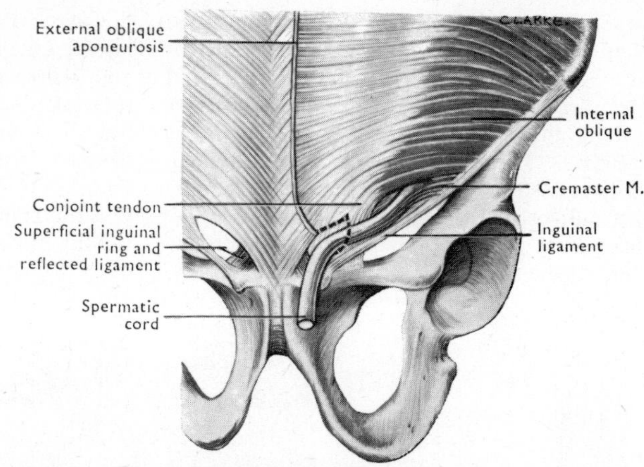

FIG. 94 A diagram of the inguinal canal to show the conjoint tendon and internal oblique. Note that the latter arches over the spermatic cord and gives fibres (cremaster muscle) on to it.

Transversus Abdominis Muscle [FIGS. 91, 93, 97]

This muscle arises from the lateral third of the inguinal ligament, the anterior two-thirds of the iliac crest, the lumbar fascia [FIG. 110], and from the internal surfaces of the lower six costal cartilages by slips that interdigitate with the slips of origin of the diaphragm. The horizontally directed muscle fibres form a broad aponeurosis which fuses with that of the internal oblique. Superior to a horizontal line half way between the pubis and the umbilicus, the aponeurosis fuses with the posterior layer of the internal oblique aponeurosis to form the **posterior wall of the rectus sheath.** The anterior layer of the aponeurosis of internal oblique passes anterior to rectus abdominis to fuse with that of the external oblique and form the **anterior wall of the rectus sheath** [FIG. 95]. Inferior to the horizontal line, the aponeuroses of all three muscles pass anterior to the rectus abdominis, and the posterior wall of the sheath ends in a curved margin, the **arcuate line** [FIG. 93]. Of the three aponeuroses anterior to the lower quarter of rectus abdominis, that of the external oblique is relatively separate from the other two which are completely fused, and their lowest fibres arch inferiorly to be inserted into the **pubic crest** and the medial part of the **pecten pubis** as the conjoint tendon [FIG. 97].

Conjoint Tendon. The conjoint tendon is formed from the fused lowest parts of the aponeuroses of transversus abdominis and internal oblique. It arches downwards, posterior to the inferomedial part of the aponeurosis of the external oblique and the superficial inguinal ring, to reach the pubic crest and the pecten pubis. The conjoint tendon therefore strengthens the abdominal wall deep to the superficial inguinal ring. It passes to the pecten pubis at right angles to the horizontal lacunar ligament, which has the spermatic cord or round ligament lying on its superior surface, anterior to the conjoint tendon. Here the spermatic cord turns forwards through the superficial inguinal ring.

Medial to the rectus abdominis, the aponeuroses of all three muscles fuse with each other and with the corresponding aponeuroses of the opposite side in the **linea alba,** and this tendinous raphe separates the two rectus muscles.

The most superior muscle fibres of transversus abdominis lie posterior to the rectus abdominis, and form a continuous sheet with the transversus thoracis in the thorax.

DISSECTION. Open the rectus sheath by a vertical incision along the middle of the muscle. Reflect the anterior layer of the sheath medially and laterally, cutting its attachments to the tendinous intersections of the rectus muscle. Raise the medial and lateral margins of the rectus and note in its upper three-quarters that the sheath is closed medially by the fusion of its walls in the linea alba, and laterally by the splitting of the aponeur-

osis of the internal oblique. Find the intercostal and subcostal nerves entering the sheath and piercing rectus.

Clean the lowest part of rectus and identify the pyramidalis muscle if present. This small, triangular muscle arises from the front of the pubis and the pubic symphysis, and passes anterior to rectus to be inserted into the lowest part of the linea alba. A small branch of the subcostal nerve leaves rectus to supply it.

Divide the rectus transversely at its middle, and cutting the nerves which enter it, define its attachments and expose the posterior wall of the rectus sheath by turning its parts superiorly and inferiorly. Identify and clean the superior and inferior epigastric arteries passing longitudinally deep to the muscle. Note that the posterior wall of the rectus sheath is not adherent to the muscle, and that it ends inferiorly in a more or less sharp line (arcuate line) half way between the umbilicus and the pubis where the aponeuroses of the internal oblique and transversus pass anterior to the rectus. The arcuate line may be defined by blunt dissection.

Rectus Abdominis

This muscle arises from the superior surface of the pubis and the pubic crest posterior to the conjoint tendon. It passes superiorly, widening rapidly, to a horizontal attachment on the anterior surfaces of the fifth to seventh costal cartilages. Horizontal **tendinous intersections** partially divide the muscle at the level of the umbilicus, at the tip of the xiphoid process, and midway between these, with a fourth occasionally present between the umbilicus and pubis. The anterior layer of the rectus sheath is fused with the tendinous intersections, but the posterior layer is not, for they do not extend through the thickness of the muscle.

Rectus Sheath. This has already been described, but its major parts are: (1) in the superior three-quarters the anterior and posterior walls are formed by the aponeuroses of the external oblique and transversus abdominis respectively, each with one half of the split aponeurosis of the internal oblique fused with it; (2) superior to the costal margin, the posterior wall is formed by the fifth to seventh costal cartilages, and the anterior wall solely by the external oblique; and (3) in the inferior quarter, where the posterior wall is missing, the rectus abdominis lies on the fascial layer deep to transversus abdominis (transversalis fascia), since the aponeuroses of all three muscles pass anterior to rectus [FIG. 95].

The rectus sheath also contains the superior and inferior epigastric arteries and the terminal parts of the lower eight thoracic ventral rami.

Nerve Supply of Abdominal Muscles. The two obliques, transversus, and rectus are supplied by the lower five or six intercostal and the subcostal nerves. In addition the oblique and transverse muscles receive twigs from the iliohypogastric and ilioinguinal nerves.

Actions of Abdominal Muscles. Contraction of these muscles when the vertebral column, diaphragm, and ribs are fixed, turns the

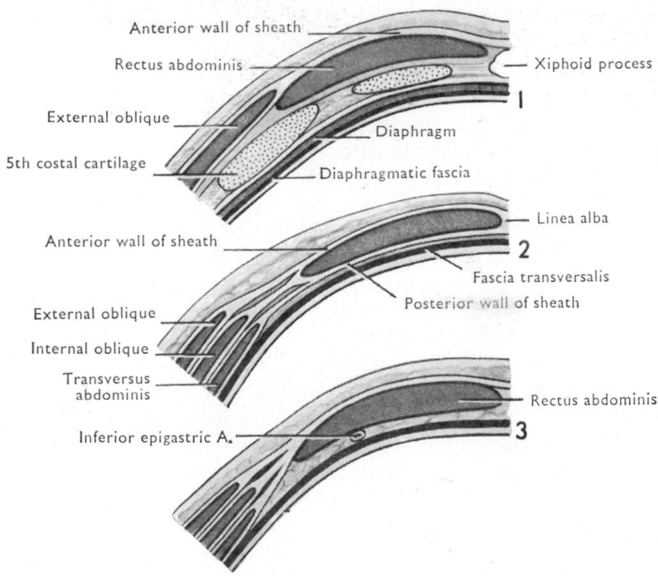

FIG. 95 Transverse sections of the anterior abdominal wall to show the varying formation of the rectus sheath. 1. Above the costal margin. 2. Upper three-quarters of the abdominal wall. 3. The lower quarter of the wall.

abdominal wall into a rigid structure which can withstand heavy blows or form a rigid base on which the upper limbs can work effectively. The rectus is a powerful flexor of the vertebral column when the ribs are fixed by contraction of the expiratory muscles against a closed glottis, which prevents the escape of air from the lungs. This action is particularly obvious when lifting the head and shoulders or pelvis off the ground from the supine position. If the ribs are not fixed, it draws them down and assists expiration, a function in which the oblique muscles also take part.

Contraction of the abdominal muscles as a whole increases intra-abdominal pressure, and this is used to force the abdominal contents and diaphragm upwards into the thorax to assist expiration and to cause violent expulsion of air in sneezing or coughing. The increased intra-abdominal pressure also impels blood from the abdomen into the thorax, assists micturition, defaecation, and parturition, and is the force used to cause vomiting.

The level of intra-abdominal pressure reached in coughing and straining is considerable, and may lead to the abdominal contents being forced through weak parts in the abdominal wall (*e.g.*, the inguinal canal, the femoral sheath, or the oesophageal hiatus in the diaphragm) thus producing a rupture or hernia. It may also cause discharge of urine through a weakened sphincter (stress incontinence). Thus the presence of a chronic cough, the lifting of heavy weights, or straining to pass urine through a partially obstructed urethra may aggravate or cause a hernia.

Linea Alba. This fibrous strip extends from the xiphoid process to the pubic symphysis and contains the umbilicus a little inferior to its middle. It consists of the interlacing fibres of the aponeuroses of the oblique and transverse muscles of the two sides, and having this structure (raphe) is capable of being stretched longitudinally to some extent without damage. It is narrower below than above the umbilicus, and is widest at the umbilicus because of the inclusion of the dense umbilical scar in which collagen fibres run in all directions and give added strength to this region.

Incisions to open the abdominal cavity are sometimes made through the linea alba because of its relative avascularity, but this factor is also responsible for a slower rate of healing. It is also possible to open the abdomen by splitting the muscle layers successively along the direction of their fibres. This has the advantage of producing a valve-like aperture which is closed by the very muscle contraction that raises the intra-abdominal pressure, and would stress any wound in the aponeuroses or linea alba.

Transversalis Fascia. This layer of fascia covers the internal surface of transversus abdominis, but it is part of a much more extensive layer which lines the abdominal and pelvic walls, and is variously named according to the structures on which its parts lie. Thus it is continuous superiorly with the fascia on the inferior surface of the diaphragm (**diaphragmatic fascia**), posteriorly with the fascia which surrounds the kidneys, suprarenal glands (**renal fascia**), and the great vessels of the posterior abdominal wall. Inferiorly it covers the iliacus (**iliac fascia**) and psoas muscles in the greater pelvis, and descends into the lesser pelvis as **pelvic fascia.**

The transversalis and iliac fasciae meet at and are fused to the internal lip of the iliac crest and the lateral half of the inguinal ligament. Medial to this the transversalis fascia is fused to the inguinal ligament, but is separated from the iliac fascia by the external iliac vessels which descend into the thigh as femoral vessels posterior to the inguinal ligament. These vessels carry with them a sheath (**femoral sheath**) of this abdominal fascia formed by the transversalis fascia anteriorly and the iliac fascia posteriorly.

Medial to the femoral sheath, the transversalis fascia passes deep to the conjoint tendon and is attached to the pubis deep to rectus abdominis. Inferior to this it is continuous with the pelvic fascia over the postero-superior surface of the pubis.

One centimetre superior to the mid-inguinal point, the transversalis fascia extends outwards as a sleeve (**internal spermatic fascia**) over the spermatic cord or round ligament,

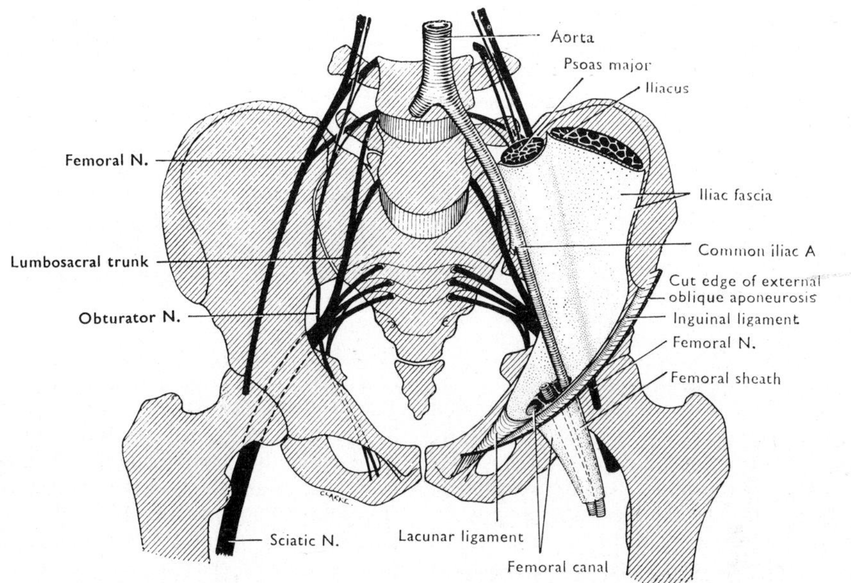

FIG. 96 A diagram to show the structures in the inguinal region and the nerves of the lower limb related to the pelvis.

and the opening thus produced in it is the **deep inguinal ring.** In the male, the internal spermatic fascia, like the cremasteric and external spermatic fasciae which subsequently surround it, forms a continuous sheath for the spermatic cord and testis, while it rapidly fuses with the round ligament in the female.

Immediately medial to the deep inguinal ring, the inferior epigastric artery ascends in the abdominal wall deep to the transversalis fascia. Medial to this the transversalis fascia is thickened where it fills the gap between the free inferior border of the transversus abdominis muscle and the inguinal ligament. Here it is separated from the aponeurosis of the external oblique muscle by the spermatic cord or round ligament running inferomedially on the inguinal ligament and by the most medial part of the internal oblique muscle.

DISSECTION. Divide the remaining ribs in the mid-axillary line. Turn down the sternum, costal cartilages, and the anterior parts of the ribs, and clean the exposed part of the superior surface of the diaphragm. Note the slips by which it arises from the xiphoid process and the costal cartilages, and identify: (1) the musculophrenic artery; (2) the slips of origin of transversus abdominis; and (3) the continuity of transversus abdominis with transversus thoracis superiorly. Divide these slips of the diaphragm in front of the mid-axillary line, and cut vertically through the transversus abdominis in the mid-axillary line to the iliac crest, avoiding injury to the peritoneum deep to the transversalis fascia. Turn down the remnants of the anterior abdominal wall with the sternum, costal cartilages, and ribs, and attempt to strip the peritoneum from the transversalis fascia for a short distance. This is usually possible if the extraperitoneal fatty tissue is plentiful. Having identified the peritoneum, divide and reflect it with the abdominal wall, cutting the fold of peritoneum which passes from the median part of the supra-umbilical anterior abdominal wall to the liver (falciform ligament, Fig. 127) together with the ligamentum teres (obliterated umbilical vein, Fig. 126) which ascends from the umbilicus to the liver in the free posterior border of the falciform ligament.

When the anterior abdominal wall has been turned down, examine its posterior surface, and identify five ill-defined folds (two on each side and one median) passing upwards towards the umbilicus. These are the lateral, medial, and median umbilical folds, and they

cover respectively the inferior epigastric vessels, the lateral umbilical ligaments (obliterated umbilical arteries which ascend posterior to the conjoint tendons, and which carry blood to the placenta in the foetus), and the median umbilical ligament (the remnant of the intra-abdominal part of the allantois—urachus, Fig. 209—which is attached inferiorly to the apex of the bladder). Strip the peritoneum from the infra-umbilical part of the anterior abdominal wall to expose these structures and the attachments of the transversus abdominis and the conjoint tendon. Before removing the transversalis fascia from the inguinal ligament, pull on the spermatic cord or round ligament from the anterior surface, and confirm the continuity of that fascia over these structures as internal spermatic fascia.

INGUINAL CANAL

This is the passage between the deep and superficial inguinal rings which passes obliquely through the anterior abdominal wall superior to the inguinal ligament. It is approximately 4 cm. long, transmits the spermatic cord and is much larger in the male than in the female where it only transmits the round ligament. Since it lies where the posterior and anterior abdominal walls meet inferiorly, it is subjected to most of the weight of the abdominal viscera when the body is erect, and is, therefore, a common site for the development of herniae. The canal is valvular in nature because of its oblique course through the layers of the abdominal wall. Thus an increase in intra-abdominal pressure forces the walls together and obliterates the passage, minimizing the chance of hernia so long as the strength of the walls is maintained.

The walls of the inguinal canal have been described already, but they should be confirmed from the external and internal aspects. The *floor* (inferior wall) is formed throughout by the inguinal ligament, with the addition of the lacunar ligament medially. The *anterior wall* is the aponeurosis of the external oblique, strengthened in the lateral half by the most anterior fleshy fibres of the internal oblique muscle. The latter arch over the canal and its

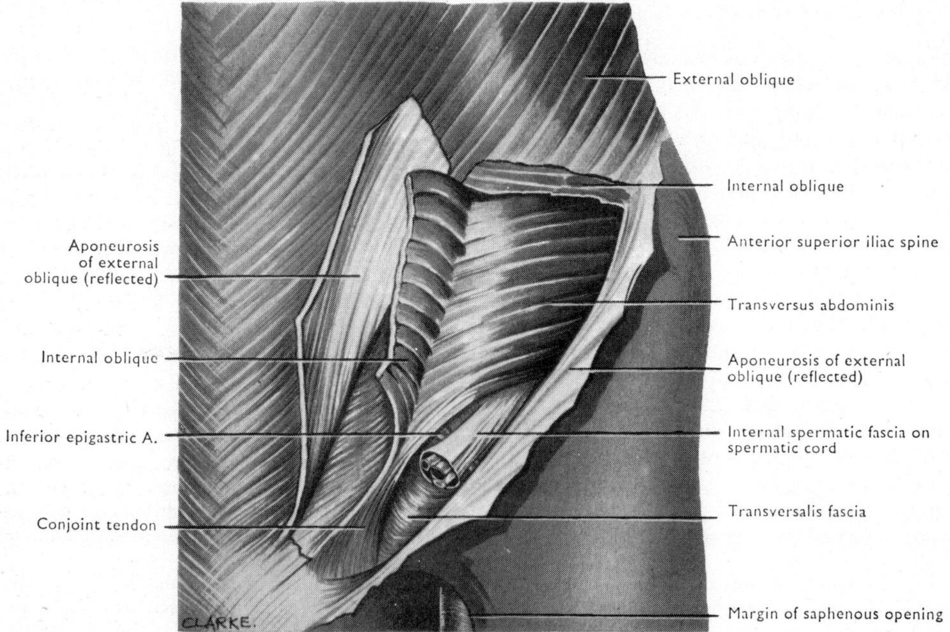

FIG. 97 A deep dissection of the inguinal region. Parts of the internal and external obliques have been reflected. The spermatic cord and internal spermatic fascia are cut across.

contents to the conjoint tendon, thus forming the *roof*. The *posterior wall* consists of transversalis fascia, but its real strength lies in the conjoint tendon, which is posterior to the superficial inguinal ring and the medial half of the canal [Fig. 98].

The **inguinal triangle** is the area bounded by the inferior epigastric artery, the lateral border of rectus abdominis, and the inguinal ligament.

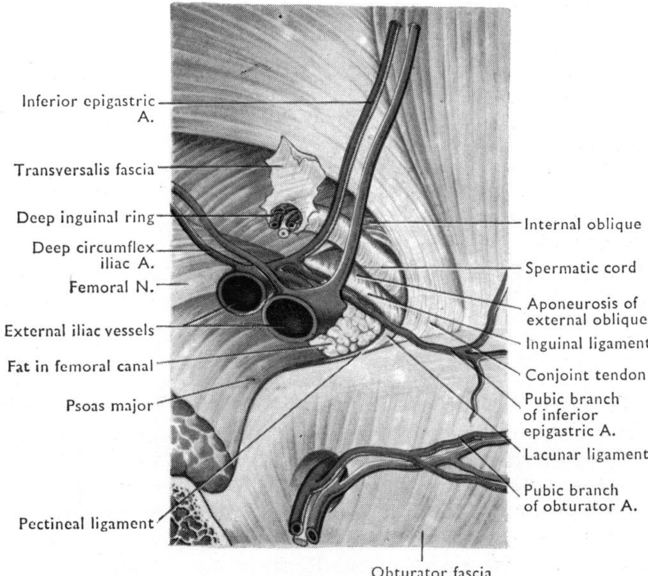

Fig. 98 A dissection of the posterior surface of the anterior abdominal wall in the inguinal region. Note the pubic branches of the obturator and inferior epigastric arteries which anastomose. They may replace the proximal part of the obturator artery (abnormal obturator artery).

Hernia

Hernia is the term applied to the abnormal protrusion of any of the abdominal contents (usually a loop of small intestine or a part of the greater omentum) through the abdominal wall. It tends to occur at points where the abdominal wall is weak, more especially in its inferior part which is subjected to continuous pressure from the abdominal viscera in the erect position. The potential sites of weakness are the inguinal canal, the femoral sheath, and the umbilicus.

At the inguinal canal and umbilicus, the abdominal wall is traversed during development by a tube of peritoneum, and at both there may be a small pocket of peritoneum internally which represents the proximal part of the obliterated peritoneal sleeve. This may form the beginning of a peritoneal pouch which can be pushed through a weakened abdominal wall by the pressure of the intra-abdominal contents assisted by any force tending to increase that pressure, *e.g.*, coughing or straining, etc. The persistence of a peritoneal channel either in the inguinal canal (processus vaginalis, Fig. 101) or traversing the umbilicus presents a ready made hernial track for a *congenital* inguinal or umbilical hernia, but in all other cases the peritoneum is carried in front of the herniating abdominal contents to form a new hernial sac. The proximal part of the sac is known as the *neck*. Each hernial sac receives a covering from the structures through which it pushes its way, in a manner similar to the descending processus vaginalis and testis.

Femoral Hernia. The space which leads into the thigh between the inguinal ligament and the hip bone is closed laterally by the fusion of the transversalis and iliac fasciae, but medially these fasciae are carried out as a sleeve (**femoral sheath**) over the external iliac vessels. The medial part of this sleeve (**femoral canal**) lies between the external iliac vein laterally, the lacunar ligament medially, and the inguinal ligament anteriorly. It is filled with fat which contains an occasional lymph node and some lymph vessels. The peritoneum which overlies the abdominal end of the canal may be forced along it, more especially in women where the space is wider than in men because of the greater over-all width of the pelvis. Also when the abdominal wall is distended it pulls a weakened inguinal ligament anteriorly, thus increasing the space between the ligament and the hip bone. Such a femoral hernia extends along the femoral sheath into the thigh, and tends to turn forwards through the thin cribriform fascia which lies anterior to it and through which the great saphenous vein passes posteriorly to join the femoral vein. It thus presents as a swelling on the anterior surface of the upper thigh, inferior to the inguinal ligament, and may be confused with a distended great saphenous vein beside which it lies [FIG. 99].

The hernial sac and its contents enter the thigh through a constricting ring formed by the **inguinal** and **lacunar ligaments,** and the pressure on the contents at this point may be sufficient either to obstruct a loop of the small intestine in the sac, or even to cut off its blood supply so that it becomes gangrenous, and rupturing, infects the sac. Both conditions are acute surgical emergencies. Relief of the constriction is most easily achieved by division of the lacunar ligament, but this may injure an abnormal obturator artery [p. 111] with severe haemorrhage if care is not taken.

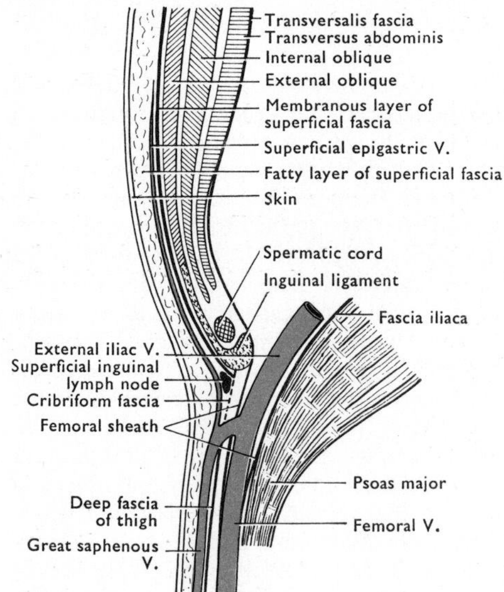

FIG. 99 A diagram of a sagittal section along the external iliac and femoral veins, to show the fasciae and muscles of the inguinal region.

Inguinal Hernia. Between the deep inguinal ring and the lateral margin of the conjoint tendon, only transversalis fascia and peritoneum separate the abdominal contents from the inguinal canal. Here a pouch of peritoneum may be forced through the posterior wall of the canal, and passing along its medial part, appear at the superficial inguinal ring. The neck of such a sac lies superior to the inguinal ligament, *medial to the inferior epigastric artery*, and lateral to the lateral umbilical ligament. In cases where the abdominal wall is considerably weakened, the conjoint tendon may be stretched and a direct hernia occur through it to the superficial inguinal ring which lies anterior to it. Both these types of hernia are known as *direct inguinal herniae* and they occur in the elderly, especially males where the superficial inguinal ring and the inguinal canal are larger than in the female.

Oblique inguinal hernia is the production of a hernial sac which passes through the inguinal canal from the deep ring to the superficial ring, and often extends into the scrotum or labium majus. This type of hernia is commonest in the male because of the greater size of the inguinal canal, and more rarely because of the persistence of the processus vaginalis in whole or in part. It may also occur in both sexes by the production of an entirely new hernial sac starting at the deep inguinal ring and following the inguinal canal throughout its length. Where there is persistence of the entire processus vaginalis, the hernia enters the tunica vaginalis (which surrounds the testis; see below), but more usually the sac is separate from it. The oblique inguinal hernia differs from the direct hernia in having the neck of the sac at the deep inguinal ring, *lateral to the inferior epigastric artery.*

Umbilical hernia can occur either through a persistent peritoneal channel perforating the fibrous umbilical scar, or as a result of the progressive weakening and stretching of the scar which may follow repeated pregnancies or gross abdominal distension with fat. It is often associated with weak rectus abdominis muscles which become separated owing to stretching of the linea alba.

ARTERIES OF ANTERIOR ABDOMINAL WALL

Inferior Epigastric Artery. This arises from the external iliac artery immediately superior to the inguinal ligament and inferior to the deep inguinal ring. It passes round the medial margin of the deep inguinal ring, and running superomedially to the lateral edge of rectus abdominis, pierces the transversalis fascia and courses over the deep surface of the rectus, supplying it and sending branches through it to the skin. It anastomoses with the superior epigastric artery within the rectus sheath.

As the artery curves round the deep inguinal ring, it is inferior and then medial to the spermatic cord or round ligament, and it gives a small branch (**cremasteric artery**) on to the spermatic cord to supply the cremaster muscle and anastomose with the testicular artery at or near the testis. The corresponding artery in the female is the smaller **artery of the round ligament.**

On the deep surface of the inguinal ligament, the inferior epigastric artery gives off a small **pubic branch.** This passes inferomedially on the inguinal ligament, and crossing the superior surface of the lacunar ligament, anastomoses with the pubic branch of the obturator artery on the posterosuperior surface of the body of the pubis. Occasionally this anastomosis replaces the proximal part of the **obturator artery,** in which case the pubic branch of the inferior epigastric artery is of considerable size [Fig. 98].

Deep Circumflex Iliac Artery. This artery arises from the external iliac artery close to the inferior epigastric. It runs postero-inferior to the inguinal ligament, and reaches the anterior superior iliac spine. In this part of its course it gives an **ascending branch** into the lower anterior abdominal wall between the transversus abdominis and internal oblique muscles. From the anterior superior iliac spine it runs posteriorly, close to the iliac crest, pierces the transversus abdominis about the middle of the crest, and ramifies in the abdominal wall between that muscle and the internal oblique.

Superior Epigastric Artery. This terminal branch of the internal thoracic artery enters the rectus sheath posterior to the seventh costal cartilage. It ramifies on the deep surface of the rectus abdominis, supplies it, sends branches to the overlying skin, and anastomoses with the corresponding inferior epigastric artery. The right superior epigastric artery sends a few slender branches through the falciform ligament to anastomose with the hepatic arteries at the liver. These branches run with the small veins that connect the veins of the anterior abdominal wall to the portal vein at its entry to the liver [p. 98].

Musculophrenic Artery. This artery runs along the upper surface of the costal origin of the diaphragm as far as the eighth intercostal space. It gives branches to the diaphragm and the anterior abdominal wall.

DISSECTION. Clean the transversalis fascia from the posterior surface of the rectus sheath. Identify the arcuate line, and note that transversalis fascia is the only structure separating the rectus abdominis from the extraperitoneal tissue inferior to the arcuate line.

Dissectors of the female abdomen should now dissect the loin.

THE MALE EXTERNAL GENITAL ORGANS

These are the penis, the scrotum and its contents, and the spermatic cords.

SCROTUM

This pendulous sac of dark coloured, rugose skin contains the testes, their associated ducts, and the lower parts of the spermatic cords, all in their coverings. In the median plane there is a ridge or raphe which indicates the embryological line of fusion of the two halves of the scrotum.

The **superficial fascia** is totally devoid of fat

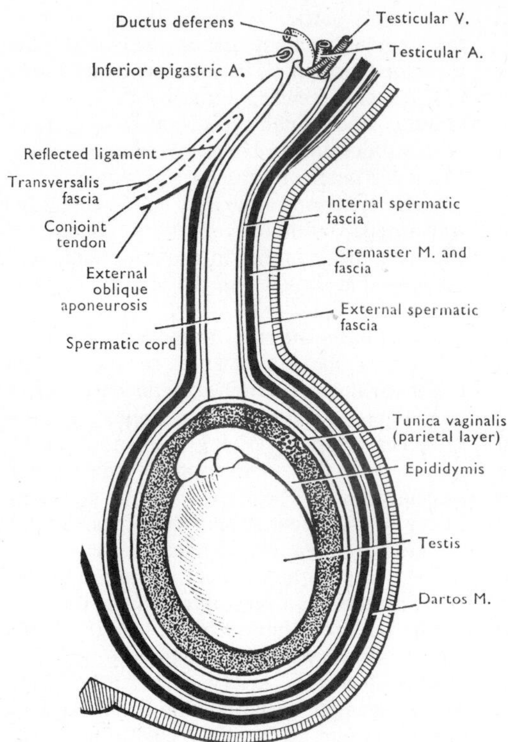

FIG. 100 A diagram of a coronal section through the spermatic cord and scrotum.

and is reddish in colour because of a layer of involuntary muscle (**dartos**). It decreases the surface area of the scrotum by its contraction, thus helping to regulate the loss of heat through the thin, fat free skin and so control the temperature of the testes; a factor which is essential for normal spermatogenesis. The dartos layer passes inwards from the raphe as an incomplete septum between the testes, each of which is separately covered by the same layers that surround the spermatic cord (external spermatic fascia, cremasteric fascia and muscle, and internal spermatic fascia, which are here fused together and difficult to differentiate). In addition each testis is invaginated into the posterior wall of a serous sac (**tunica vaginalis testis**). In the foetus this is the distal end of a tubular extension of the peritoneal cavity (**processus vaginalis**; FIG. 101) which passes through the inguinal canal into the corresponding half of the scrotum.

The processus vaginalis precedes the descending testis, which enters the scrotum approximately at birth, and at this time or subsequently, the cavity of the part of the processus within the spermatic cord is obliterated, and the processus reduced to a fibrous thread. This remnant of the processus vaginalis is usually only present in the proximal part of the spermatic cord, but occasionally it may persist throughout the spermatic cord, or even remain patent in part or all of its length. Thus there may be isolated cavities derived from the processus which can become swollen with fluid and form hydroceles of the spermatic cord.

The precise mechanism of descent of the processus vaginalis and testis is unknown. However, the caudal pole of the testis is attached to the rudiment of the scrotum by a fibromuscular band (**gubernaculum testis**) which extends from the caudal pole of the developing testis down the posterior abdominal wall immediately posterior to the peritoneum, and passes through the inguinal canal. As the gubernaculum shortens relative to the growing foetus, the testis is drawn down the posterior abdominal wall, and is preceded through the inguinal canal to the scrotum by the peritoneum applied to the anterior aspect of the gubernaculum.

The descent of the testis may be arrested at any stage, *e.g.*, in the abdomen, the inguinal canal, or the groin. Such undescended testes usually do not produce spermatozoa and are more commonly the site of tumour formation than the normally placed testis.

DISSECTION. Make an incision through the skin of the anterolateral aspect of the scrotum from the superficial inguinal ring inferiorly. Carefully reflect the skin from the dartos which is attached to it. Reflect the dartos layer from the layer of loose areolar tissue (external spermatic fascia) deep to it. Towards the median plane, the dartos layer extends superiorly be-

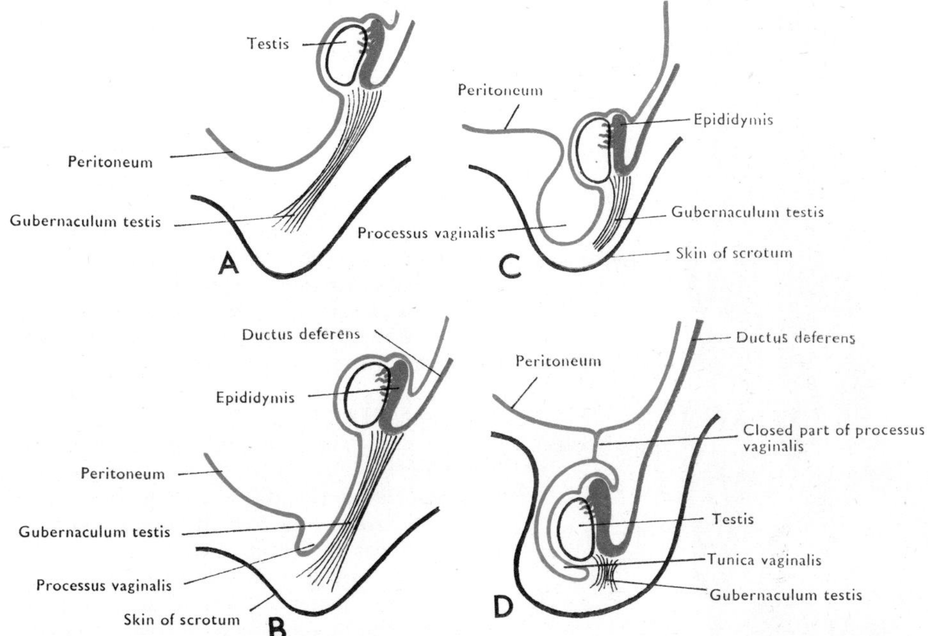

FIG. 101 Diagrams to illustrate the descent of the testis and the formation of the tunica vaginalis.

tween the testes [Fig. 100]. Complete the separation of the layer of areolar tissue from the deep surface of the dartos, stripping it superiorly to the superficial inguinal ring. Lift the testis and spermatic cord from the scrotum.

Carefully lift the peritoneum away from the extraperitoneal tissue at the deep inguinal ring by blunt dissection. A fine thread may be seen passing from the peritoneum into the beginning of the spermatic cord. This is the vestige of the processus vaginalis.

SPERMATIC CORD

This bundle of structures which passes to and from the testis, is wrapped in three concentric layers of fascia derived from the layers of the anterior abdominal wall [p. 107]. It begins at the deep inguinal ring and ends at the superior pole of the testis.

Structures in Spermatic Cord

1. The ductus deferens, the duct of the testis.

2. Blood vessels { Arteries { Artery of the ductus deferens; Testicular }; Veins: Pampiniform plexus }

3. Lymph vessels which drain the testis and the immediately associated structures, but not the scrotal wall.

4. Nerves. Sympathetic filaments on the arteries and pelvic autonomic fibres on the ductus deferens.

DISSECTION. Cut through the spermatic cord at the superficial inguinal ring and remove it together with the testis to a tray on which it may be pinned out under water. Incise and reflect the three coverings in turn, external spermatic fascia, cremaster muscle, and internal spermatic fascia. Begin superiorly for the layers become progressively less distinct inferiorly. When the coverings have been removed, separate the various structures in the spermatic cord. It is possible to identify the ductus deferens and the blood vessels, but

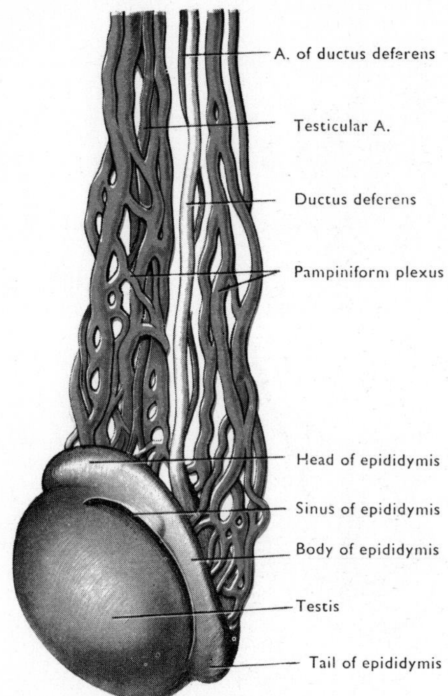

FIG. 102 A dissection of the left spermatic cord.

the nerves and lymphatics are not visible as separate structures.

Ductus Deferens. This is the thick-walled, muscular part of the duct system of the testis through which spermatozoa are transported to the urethra. It is firm and readily palpable in the living, and its muscular wall is responsible for the sudden discharge of the mature spermatozoa which are stored in it. It begins in continuity with the lower pole of the epididymis [FIG. 106] and its first part is convoluted. It ascends along the medial aspect of the epididymis, posterior to the testis, and runs in the posterior part of the spermatic cord to the deep inguinal ring. Here it hooks round the lateral side of the inferior epigastric artery, and leaving the other structures of the spermatic cord, arches inferomedially into the pelvis. It is accompanied throughout by the artery of the ductus deferens (a slender branch of the inferior vesical artery) which anastomoses with the testicular artery.

Testicular Artery. This vessel arises from the front of the abdominal aorta at the level of the second lumbar vertebra (the level of origin of the testis) and descends on the posterior abdominal wall to the deep inguinal ring. Here it enters the spermatic cord and runs through it to the posterior border of the testis. Small branches enter the posterior border of the testis, while the larger branches pass forwards on both sides of the testis, between it and the dense layer of fibrous tissue (tunica albuginea) which encloses it. They form a vascular layer on the surface of the testis stroma [FIG. 103].

Veins. Numerous veins leave the posterior border of the testis to form the extensive **pampiniform plexus** [FIG. 105] which makes up a large part of the bulk of the spermatic cord. At or near the deep inguinal ring, the testicular vein is formed from the plexus and ascends over the posterior abdominal wall to end either in the renal vein (left side) or the inferior vena cava (right side) at the same level. The function of the pampiniform plexus is not known, but it is probably concerned with maintaining the temperature of the structures in the spermatic cord at a level similar to that of the testis. The venous channels forming the plexus may be greatly distended to produce a varicocele of the spermatic cord.

Lymph Vessels. The testicular lymph vessels ascend through the spermatic cord, and passing over the posterior abdominal wall, end in the lumbar lymph nodes at the side of the aorta from its bifurcation to the level of the renal veins [FIG. 176].

Nerves. The sympathetic nerves run with the testicular artery from the renal or aortic sympathetic plexuses, and occasional small ganglia are found along the artery. The nerve fibres on the ductus deferens (deferential plexus) are derived from the inferior hypogastric plexus in the pelvis.

DISSECTION. With a hypodermic syringe and needle or a blowpipe, force some air or water into the tunica vaginalis of the testis through the anterior wall. This demonstrates the extent of the cavity which passes

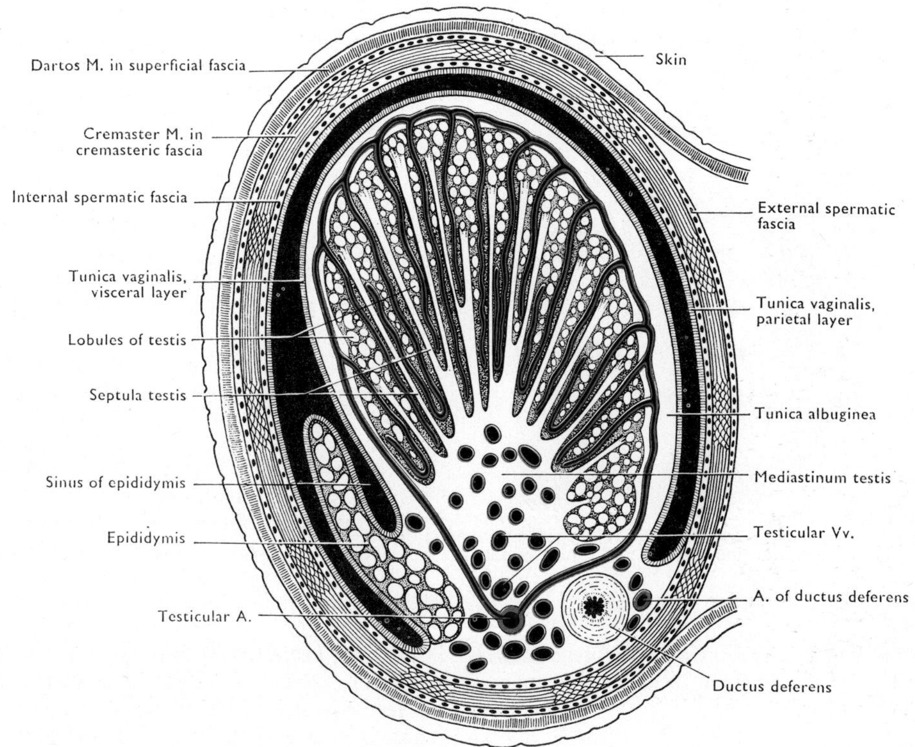

FIG. 103 A diagrammatic horizontal section through the left half of the scrotum and left testis. The cavity of the tunica vaginalis (black) is distended to make it obvious.

upwards on to the front of the spermatic cord for a short distance [Fig. 104]. Open the anterior surface of the cavity.

Tunica Vaginalis Testis

This is a closed serous sac which has the testis and epididymis invaginated into its posterior wall. It consists of a parietal layer which lines the internal spermatic fascia, and a visceral layer which covers the front and sides of the testis and epididymis and is continuous with the parietal layer near the posterior border of the testis. Normally there is only a thin film of fluid between the two layers, but in certain pathological conditions the space may be distended with fluid to form a hydrocele. On the lateral side, the visceral layer is tucked between the testis and epididymis to form the slit-like **sinus of the epididymis** [FIGS. 102, 103].

TESTIS

This oval body is variable in size, but is approximately 4 cm. long, 2·5 cm. antero-posteriorly, and 2 cm. transversely. It is enclosed in a thick, dense layer of white fibrous tissue, the **tunica albuginea,** and this is covered by the visceral layer of the tunica vaginalis except where it is directly in contact with the epididymis superiorly and posteriorly. The **appendix testis** is a small, sessile body attached to the upper part of the anterior border of the testis. It is thought to be a remnant of the proximal end of the embryonic paramesonephric duct, which forms the fimbriated extremity of the uterine tube in the female.

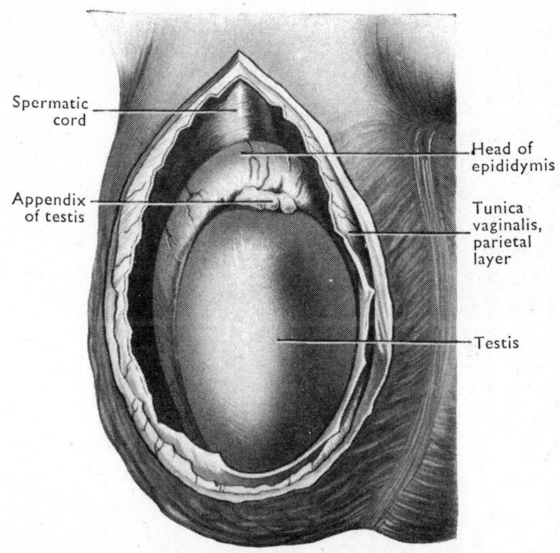

FIG. 104 The right testis and epididymis exposed by remova of the anterior wall of the scrotum and tunica vaginalis.

Structure of Testis. The testis is enclosed in the thick, fibrous tunica albuginea, and this forms a longitudinal thickened ridge (the **mediastinum testis**) which projects forwards into the posterior border of the testis. The mediastinum is traversed by the blood and lymph vessels of the testis, and by a network of seminal channels, the **rete testis** [FIG. 103].

Fibrous strands pass radially from the mediastinum towards the other surfaces of the testis. These are the incomplete **septula** which divide the testis into two or three hundred lobules. These contain the convoluted seminiferous tubules, which are lined with thick, multi-layered germinal epithelium that produces immature spermatozoa. The **convoluted tubules** appear as fine, highly plicated, thread-like loops which join each other and become straighter (**straight seminiferous tubules**) as they pass towards the mediastinum. The straight seminiferous tubules do not produce spermatozoa, but discharge into the spaces of the rete testis which are lined by cubical epithelium. Every lobule contains two to four convoluted tubules, which measure approximately 60 cm. in length, and thus the over-all length of seminiferous tubules is approximately 500 m. Groups of interstitial cells which are responsible for secreting male sex hormone lie in delicate areolar tissue between the convoluted tubules.

DISSECTION. Attempt to unravel some of the tubules on the cut surface of the testis by drawing them out with a fine probe under water. Only a general idea of the arrangement can be obtained by this method. With the aid of a stream of water and gentle agitation of the probe, remove the tubules from part of the testis and uncover the fibrous septula.

At the superior pole of the testis, divide the tunica vaginalis which joins it to the head of the epididymis. Gently separate the testis and epididymis, and with gentle blunt dissection attempt to demonstrate the efferent ductules passing from the rete to the head of the epididymis.

Structure of Epididymis. Fifteen to twenty delicate **efferent ductules** pass from the rete testis to the epididymis. In this structure they

The **appendix of the epididymis,** a small, pedunculated structure on the superior pole of the epididymis, represents the degenerated remains of the cephalic tubules of the mesonephros of the embryo.

Epididymis

This comma-shaped structure overlies the superior and posterolateral surfaces of the testis. The superior and inferior extremities are the **head** and **tail** respectively, while the intermediate part, which is partly separated from the testis by the sinus of the epididymis, is the **body.** The ductus deferens arises from the tail of the epididymis, and ascends on the posterior border of the testis medial to the body and head of the epididymis [FIG. 105].

The epididymis consists almost entirely of a single, complexly convoluted tube (the **duct of the epididymis**) which is 6–7 m. in length, and in which the spermatozoa undergo maturation as they pass towards the ductus deferens for discharge.

DISSECTION. Trace the blood vessels into the testis, and then free the tail and body of the epididymis from it. Make a transverse cut through the testis, and examine its structure with a hand lens.

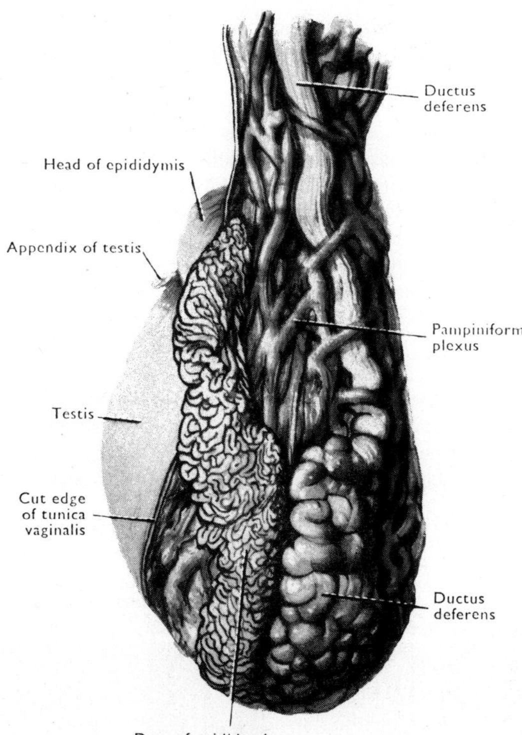

FIG. 105 The left testis, epididymis, and lower part of spermatic cord seen from behind.

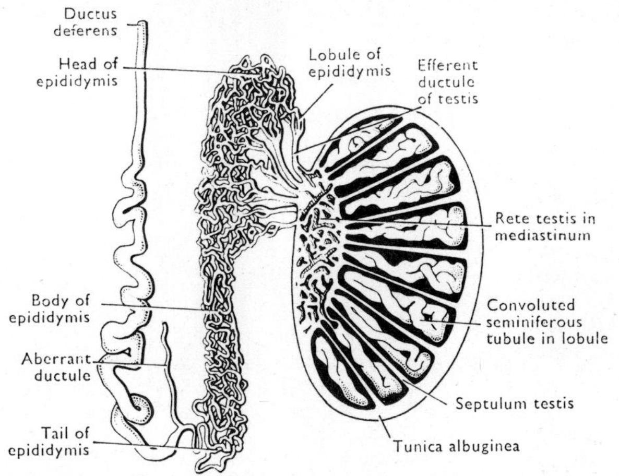

FIG. 106 A diagram of a sagittal section of the testis, epididymis, and ductus deferens.

become spirally coiled to form the conical **lobules of the epididymis.** These unite in the head to form the convoluted **duct of the epididymis** which extends to the inferior pole of the testis where it joins the ductus deferens. The extent of the convolution of the duct of the epididymis can be gauged by the fact that its over-all length is approximately 6–7 m.

One or more small **aberrant ductules** may enter the ductus at the tail of the epididymis. These represent persistent tubules of the mesonephros of the embryo of which the efferent ductules of the testis are the only functional members.

An attempt should be made to unravel at least part of the duct of the epididymis. This duct is lined by tall columnar epithelial cells which have large, non-motile processes (stereocilia). The spermatozoa go through part of their maturation in this duct.

PENIS

[FIGS. 107–109]

The penis consists of three parallel, cylindrical bodies. (1) The two dorsally placed **corpora cavernosa** which are fused together in the body of the penis, but diverge in the perineum to form the **crura of the penis** which are attached to the sides of the pubic arch. (2) The **corpus spongiosum** lies on the ventral surface between the corpora cavernosa. It transmits the urethra and enlarges proximally to form the **bulb of the penis** where it is attached between the crura to the perineal membrane. Distally it expands to form the **glans penis** into which the tapered distal ends of the corpora cavernosa are inserted, and through the extremity of which the **external urethral orifice** opens as a vertical slit. The glans penis is conical in shape and is much more extensive on the dorsal than the ventral surface. The projecting margin of its base is the **corona glandis.**

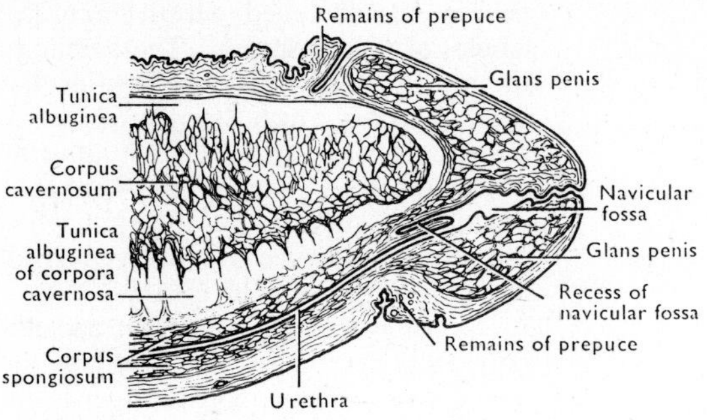

FIG. 107 A median section through the terminal part of a circumcised penis.

The skin of the penis is delicate, elastic, and hairless except at the base. It is freely moveable over the surface of the penis, and distally forms a tubular fold (the **prepuce,** FIGS. 107, 208) which extends over the glans for a variable distance. The skin at the distal end of the prepuce turns in to line its deep surface and become continuous, just proximal to the corona, with the skin which passes distally over the glans and is firmly bound to its surface. In the midline ventrally, a narrow, free fold of skin (the **frenulum of the prepuce**) passes from the inferior margin of the external urethral orifice to the deep surface of the prepuce. The greater part of the prepuce is removed in the operation of circumcision [FIG. 107].

The superficial fascia of the penis is composed of loose areolar tissue devoid of fat. The deep fascia forms a close-fitting sheath around the corpora.

DISSECTION. Cut through and reflect the skin along the dorsum of the penis from the symphysis pubis to the end of the prepuce. Find the suspensory ligament of the penis passing from the pubic symphysis to the superficial fascia of the penis. Clean the superficial dorsal vein of the penis and trace it proximally. Clean the deep fascia, dividing it in the same line as the skin. Uncover and clean the dorsal vein with the dorsal arteries and nerves on each side of it [Fig. 108].

The **suspensory ligament** is a fibro-elastic structure which spreads out from the anterior surface of the pubic symphysis to fuse with the deep fascia on the dorsum and sides of the body of the penis, the dorsal vessels and nerves passing deep to it.

Dorsal Vessels and Nerves of Penis. The superficial and dorsal veins are both median structures. The superficial vein lies in the superficial fascia and divides proximally into right and left branches which pass to the external pudendal veins of the corresponding thigh. The dorsal vein lies deep to the deep fascia, and enters the pelvis proximally by passing below the pubic symphysis. It ends in the prostatic plexus of veins.

The two dorsal arteries and nerves are the terminal branches of the internal pudendal arteries and the pudendal nerves respectively. The nerves lie lateral to the arteries, and both supply the skin and glans of the penis.

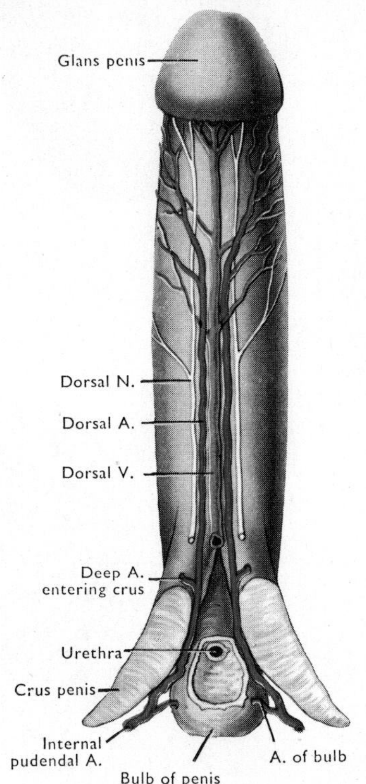

FIG. 108 A dissection of the dorsal surface of the penis.

DISSECTION. Make a transverse section through the body of the penis, but leave the two parts connected by the skin on the inferior surface. Examine the cut surface [Fig. 109].

Structure of Penis. The **corpora cavernosa** are a pair of cylindrical bodies consisting of a mass of cavernous erectile tissue enclosed in a dense sheath of white fibrous tissue, the **tunica albuginea.** Medially the tunicae albugineae fuse to form an incomplete median **septum** through which the cavernous tissue of the two corpora is continuous. In the centre of each corpus cavernosum the **deep artery of the penis** may be seen. When this artery is dilated, blood fills the cavernous spaces under pressure, and thus makes the corpora cavernosa rigid inside the dense tunicae albugineae.

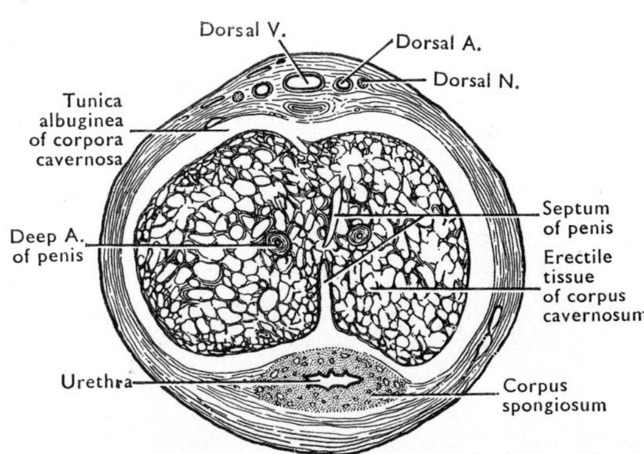

FIG. 109 A transverse section through the body of the penis.

The **corpus spongiosum** has a finer meshwork of erectile tissue surrounding the urethra and a more delicate fibrous capsule (tunica albuginea). It therefore does not prevent the distension of the urethra when the cavernous tissue is filled with blood. The **arteries of the bulb** traverse the corpus spongiosum longitudinally, inferior to the urethra. Thus the parts of the penis each have their separate blood supply.

THE DISSECTION OF THE LOIN

Provided the whole extent of latissimus dorsi has been cleaned, the body should be placed in the prone position and the posterior parts of the muscles of the abdominal wall should be cleaned, together with the serratus posterior inferior and the thoracolumbar fascia.

DISSECTION. Clean the free posterior border of the external oblique muscle and the inferior part of latissimus dorsi to the iliac crest, and note the interval (lumbar triangle) which is usually present between them immediately superior to the iliac crest. Reflect the remains of latissimus dorsi inferiorly and the external oblique anteriorly, thus exposing the posterior part of the internal oblique and the thoracolumbar fascia to which it is attached.

Thoracolumbar Fascia [FIG. 110]

This layer of fascia extends from the sacrum to the neck. It binds the long muscle of the back (erector spinae) to the posterolateral surfaces of the vertebrae. In the *thoracic region* it is a thin transparent lamina which extends from the spines of the vertebrae to the angles of the ribs. In the upper thoracic region it passes deep to **serratus posterior superior** and enters the neck. At the junction of the thoracic and lumbar regions it lies deep to **serratus posterior inferior** which extends superolaterally from the thoracolumbar fascia to the last three or four ribs. In the *sacral region* it stretches between the sacral spines and the ilium and sacrotuberous ligament, and is attached inferiorly to the back of the sacrum and coccyx.

It is very strong in the *lumbar region* (lumbar fascia) and consists of three layers. These enclose the erector spinae and quadratus lumborum muscles between them, and unite laterally to give origin to the internal oblique and transversus abdominis muscles [FIG. 110].

DISSECTION. Clean the posterior layer of the thoracolumbar fascia by removing the remains of latissimus dorsi and dividing serratus posterior inferior transversely. Remove the part of that muscle attached to the fascia.

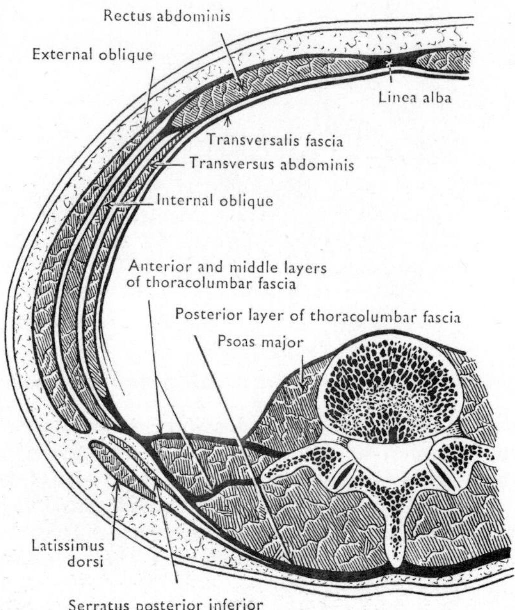

FIG. 110 A horizontal section through the abdominal walls at the level of the second lumbar vertebra, to show the thoracolumbar fascia.

The **posterior layer** of the thoracolumbar fascia, now exposed, is the strongest of the three layers. It passes from the lumbar spines over the erector spinae to fuse with the middle layer lateral to that muscle.

DISSECTION. Divide the posterior layer vertically from the level of the last rib to the iliac crest, and making horizontal cuts at the upper and lower ends, reflect the posterior layer. Pull erector spinae medially and trace the attachments of the middle layer anterior to it.

The **middle layer** separates erector spinae from quadratus lumborum. Medially it is attached to the tips of the lumbar transverse processes, and extends from the twelfth rib superiorly to the iliolumbar ligament and iliac crest inferiorly. Laterally it fuses first with the posterior layer at the lateral edge of erector spinae, and then with the anterior layer at the lateral edge of quadratus lumborum. The internal oblique arises lateral to the first fusion, the transversus abdominis lateral to the second.

DISSECTION. Divide the middle layer along its superior, medial, and inferior attachments, and reflect it laterally. Push quadratus lumborum medially and run a finger over the posterior surface of the anterior layer in front of the muscle. Note the attachments of the anterior layer.

The **anterior layer** of the thoracolumbar fascia is thin but strong. It lies anterior to quadratus lumborum, is attached medially to the anterior surfaces of the lumbar transverse processes, and inferiorly to the iliolumbar ligament and the iliac crest. Superiorly it is attached to the twelfth rib, and is thickened to form a transverse tendinous strip (**lateral arcuate ligament**) which gives attachment to the muscle fibres of the diaphragm anterior to quadratus lumborum. The **subcostal vessels and nerve** pass into the abdomen from the thorax posterior to the lateral arcuate ligament. Since the middle and anterior layers are attached to the **twelfth rib** superiorly and the **iliolumbar ligament** and the iliac crest inferiorly, only the posterior layer of the lumbar part of the thoracolumbar fascia extends into the thoracic and sacral regions.

DISSECTION. Divide the anterior layer of the thoracolumbar fascia longitudinally. Scrape away the exposed fat and uncover the posterior surface of the kidney with the subcostal, iliohypogastric, and ilio-inguinal nerves crossing it [Figs. 167, 179]. At the lateral margin of the kidney is part of the colon, and superior to this the liver on the right and the spleen on the left. The structures posterior to the kidney will be seen later from the abdominal aspect.

THE ABDOMINAL CAVITY

The abdominal cavity is enclosed by the abdominal walls and is completely filled by the abdominal viscera. These consist of the stomach and intestines, their associated glands (liver and pancreas with their ducts), blood and lymph vessels and the spleen, together with the kidneys and suprarenal glands. The kidneys and suprarenal glands lie on the posterior abdominal wall enclosed in the fascial lining of the abdominal cavity [p. 106], while anterior to these are the other structures surrounded to a greater or lesser extent by the peritoneal cavity.

The **peritoneum** consists of a tough layer of elastic areolar tissue lined with simple squamous epithelium. It forms the largest of the three serous sacs of the body, and is similar to the pleura and pericardium in consisting of parietal and visceral layers which are separated from each other by a thin film of fluid. This lubricates their smooth surfaces and facilitates the movements of those parts of the abdominal viscera which are ensheathed by the visceral layer. The most mobile parts of the intra-abdominal gut tube are surrounded by the visceral peritoneum except where (like a cloth draped over a tube) it passes from the gut tube to the posterior abdominal wall as two parallel layers (suspensory fold of peritoneum, **mesentery**, or ligament). These layers are separated by a variable amount of extraperitoneal fatty areolar tissue in which the blood and lymphatic vessels and nerves run to and from the gut tube. Where the layers meet the fascial lining of the posterior abdominal wall, they become continuous with the parietal peritoneum, while the areolar tissue between them is continuous with the extraperitoneal fatty areolar tissue that separates the parietal peritoneum from the fascial lining of the abdominal walls.

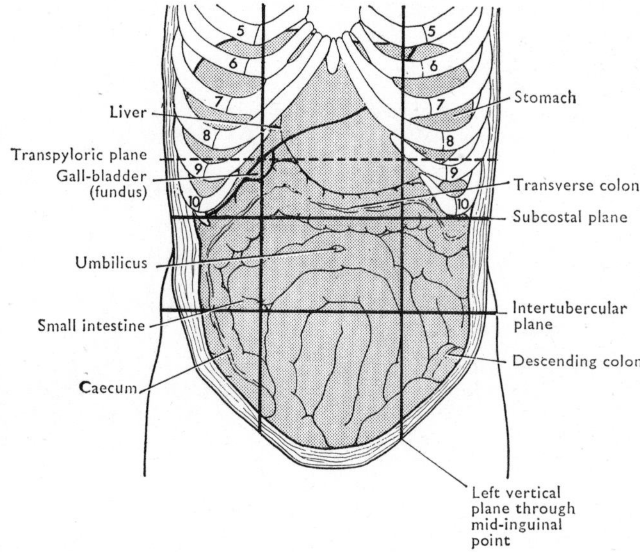

FIG. 111 The abdominal viscera after removal of the anterior abdominal wall and greater omentum. Note that the eighth costal cartilage reaches the sternum in this case.

DISSECTION. In the preliminary examination of the abdominal cavity, it is important to avoid any dissection, as otherwise important relations of the organs may be disturbed and parts of the peritoneum torn before their full significance is appreciated.

The **parietal peritoneum** forms a relatively simple layer on the internal surface of the fascial lining of the abdominal walls, but the **visceral peritoneum,** which passes as mesenteries to surround the intricately folded and tightly packed gut tube, liver and spleen, is a complex layer, the various parts of which are applied to and move on each other in addition to sliding on the parietal peritoneum.

The **peritoneal cavity** is the slit-like interval between the parietal and visceral layers of the peritoneum. It also extends between the parts of the visceral peritoneum surrounding the structures mentioned above, and forming the mesenteries. The cavity has a very small volume because of the tight packing of the abdominal viscera, but it may be extended as far as the abdominal walls will allow by the introduction of fluid or air.

In the embryo, all parts of the gut tube have a mesentery, but during development certain parts (duodenum, ascending and descending colon, and pancreas) are applied to and fused with the peritoneum on the posterior abdominal wall in such a manner that the parietal peritoneum runs directly over their anterior surfaces and they have no mesenteries.

There are, therefore, four distinct layers of structures making up the abdomen from behind forwards, and each layer contains its own blood and lymphatic vessels and nerves.

1. The **posterior abdominal wall.** This consists of the vertebral column and the muscles attached to it [FIG. 110].

2. The **fascial lining of the abdominal walls.** This encloses (a) the kidneys (and their ducts the ureters) and the suprarenal glands, on each side of the vertebral column, and (b) the great vessels (abdominal aorta and inferior vena cava) on the anterior surface of the vertebral column [FIGS. 124, 175].

3. The viscera (**duodenum, pancreas, ascending and descending colon**) which are attached to the posterior wall of the peritoneal cavity.

4. The viscera which appear to be invaginated into the peritoneal cavity, and which are supported by mesenteries that attach them to the parietal peritoneum on the posterior abdominal wall (**dorsal mesenteries**).

All the parts of the gut tube forming layer 4 have dorsal mesenteries, but the stomach and the proximal 2–3 cm. of the duodenum have, in addition, a **ventral mesentery** that attaches them to the anterior abdominal wall. This is divided into two parts by the presence of the liver between its layers, so that it consists of a part which joins the stomach and proximal duodenum to the liver (**lesser omentum**) and a part passing from the liver to the anterior abdominal wall (**falciform ligament**).

Thus, when the anterior abdominal wall is removed it is only attached to the abdominal viscera (liver) by the falciform ligament, and the only parts of the viscera immediately visible are those which comprise layer 4 and the ascending and descending parts of the colon.

The **cavity of the lesser pelvis** extends posteriorly and then inferiorly from the postero-inferior part of the abdominal cavity [FIG. 112]. Its antero-inferior wall is short and consists of the pubic symphysis, while the roof and posterior wall are formed by the sacrum and coccyx. The floor is the **perineum,** a fibromuscular diaphragm pierced by the rectum, urethra, and the vagina in the female. The lateral walls are the hip bones covered by the obturator internus muscles. The peritoneal

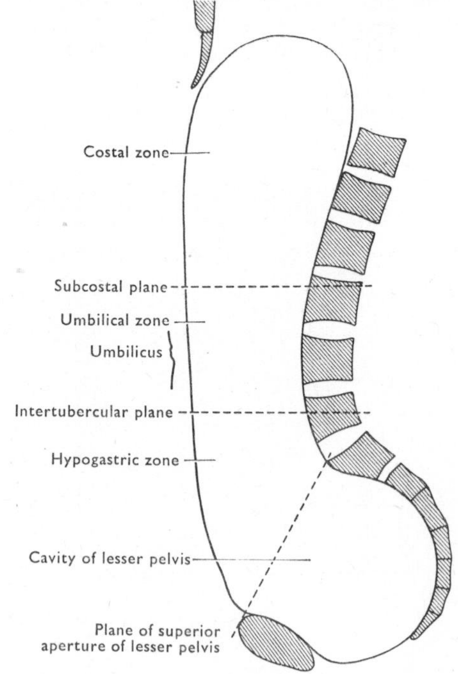

FIG. 112 An outline of the abdominal and pelvic cavities as seen in median section.

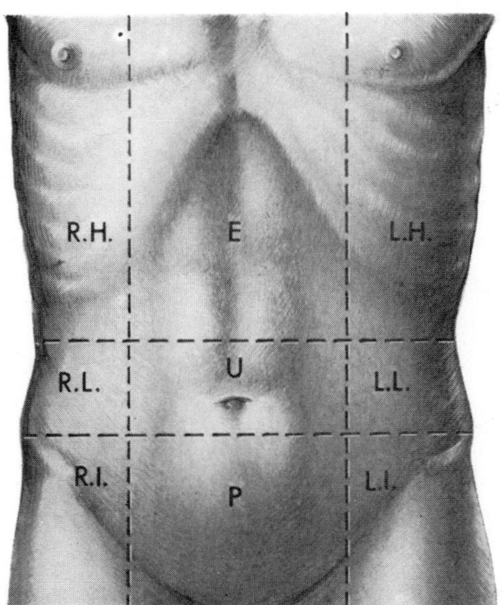

FIG. 113 The planes of subdivision of the abdominal cavity.

R.H. and L.H. Right and left hypochondriac regions.
E. Epigastric region.
R.L. and L.L. Right and left lateral regions.
U. Umbilical region.
R.I. and L.I. Right and left inguinal regions.
P. Pubic region.

cavity extends into the superior part of the pelvis above the bladder (or bladder and uterus in the female) and anterior to the rectum. In the male it is a closed sac, but in the female the uterine tubes open into it and there is a direct channel to the exterior through those tubes, the uterus and the vagina.

For the purposes of description the abdomen is artificially divided into a number of regions by imaginary horizontal and vertical planes [FIGS. 111, 113]. The horizontal planes are: (1) the **subcostal plane,** situated at the level (third lumbar vertebra) of the lowest part of the costal margin as seen from the front (10th costal cartilage), and (2) the **intertubercular plane**, which passes through the tubercles of the iliac crests (the highest parts of these crests seen from in front) and the fifth lumbar vertebra. In addition there is a third horizontal plane, the **transpyloric plane,** which lies at a level half way between the pubic symphysis and the jugular notch of the sternum (approximately half way between the umbilicus and the xiphoid process). It passes through the first lumbar vertebra and the ninth costal cartilage where the linea semilunaris crosses the costal margin (the position of the fundus of the gall-bladder on the right). Though known as the transpyloric plane, it seldom passes through the pylorus which is usually at a lower level.

The **vertical planes** pass through the mid-inguinal points on both sides. The nine regions thus marked out are shown in FIGURE 113.

Shape of Abdominal Cavity [FIGS. 112, 115, 116, 118, 123]

In transverse section the abdominal cavity is kidney shaped because of the protrusion of the vertebral column into it in the midline posteriorly. There is, therefore, a deep paravertebral groove on each side which is separated from its thoracic counterpart by the diaphragm. The groove lodges the kidney and suprarenal gland and ascending (right) or descending (left) part of the colon. Because of the anterior convexity of the lumbar vertebral column, the upper vertebrae lie further posteriorly than the lower vertebrae. The anteroposterior extent of the abdominal cavity is therefore much greater in the superior than the inferior parts, especially in the midline, though it is reduced in the uppermost part where the diaphragm arches forwards anterior to the pleural cavity, above the first lumbar vertebra [FIG. 116]. Thus the anterior abdominal wall may be no more than 5 cm. from the great vessels on the anterior surface of the lower lumbar vertebral column in the supine position, and from this level the paravertebral grooves slope posterosuperiorly.

Boundaries of Abdominal Cavity

The roof is the diaphragm which also forms the upper parts of the lateral and posterior walls. The anterior wall is formed by the muscles and aponeuroses, while the remainder of each lateral wall is formed by the abdominal

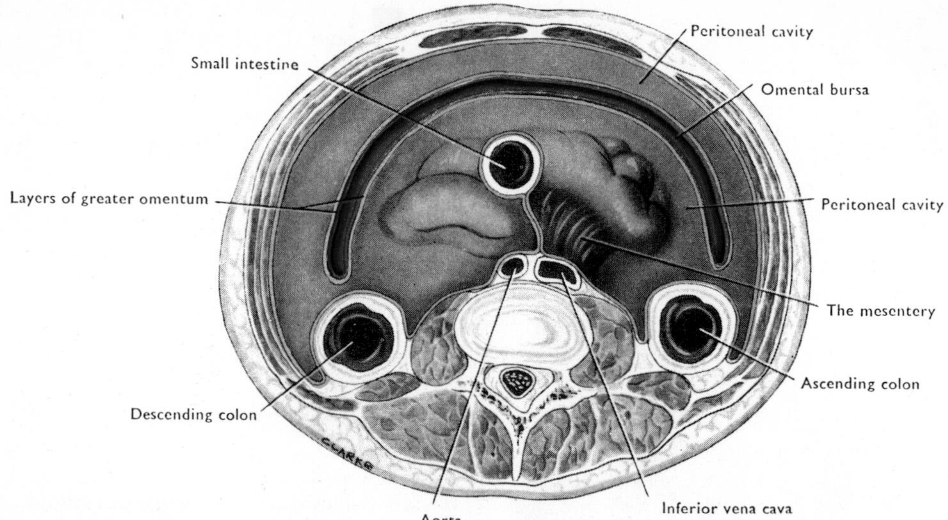

FIG. 114 A diagrammatic horizontal section through the abdomen at the level of the fourth lumbar vertebra. The peritoneal cavity is shown distended. Blue: peritoneal cavity. Red: omental bursa of peritoneal cavity.

muscles and below that by the ilium covered internally by the iliacus muscle. The posterior wall is formed by the vertebral column, the muscles attached to it (especially psoas and quadratus lumborum) and the thoracolumbar fascia, and inferiorly by the posterior part of the ilium and iliacus.

Divisions of Peritoneal Cavity

When the anterior abdominal wall is removed the greater part of the peritoneal cavity is opened, but there is a smaller extension of the main cavity which passes posterior to the stomach and forms a considerable bursa between it and the posterior abdominal wall [FIGS. 115, 116, 123, 125]. This **omental bursa** is produced in the embryo by an extension of the peritoneal cavity into the right side of the dorsal mesentery of the stomach. The small sac thus formed in the mesentery balloons out the left wall of the mesentery to the left and inferiorly, and is at first posterior to the stomach, but later extends beyond it [FIG. 121]. Superiorly the wall of the sac is carried to the left against the diaphragm, and the spleen develops on its left wall. Thus the spleen is held in position against the diaphragm by this part of the dorsal mesentery of the stomach, the anterior part of which passes between the stomach and the spleen (**gastrosplenic ligament**), while the posterior portion connects the spleen to the posterior abdominal wall in the region of the kidney, the **lienorenal ligament** [FIG. 115]. The term ligament applied to certain parts of the mesenteries does not mean that they are specially strengthened or ligamentous. Of the two layers of peritoneum forming these ligaments, that on the right forms the left wall of the omental bursa, while the left layers of both meet the spleen (lien) close together at its hilus and then diverge to enclose the spleen. Superior to the spleen, the dorsal mesentery passes directly from the superior part (fundus) of the stomach to the diaphragm (**gastrophrenic ligament**).

The part of the dorsal mesentery of the stomach which is carried inferiorly by the expanding omental bursa, passes as a double fold of peritoneum (the **greater omentum**) between the anterior surface of the abdominal viscera inferior to the stomach and the parietal

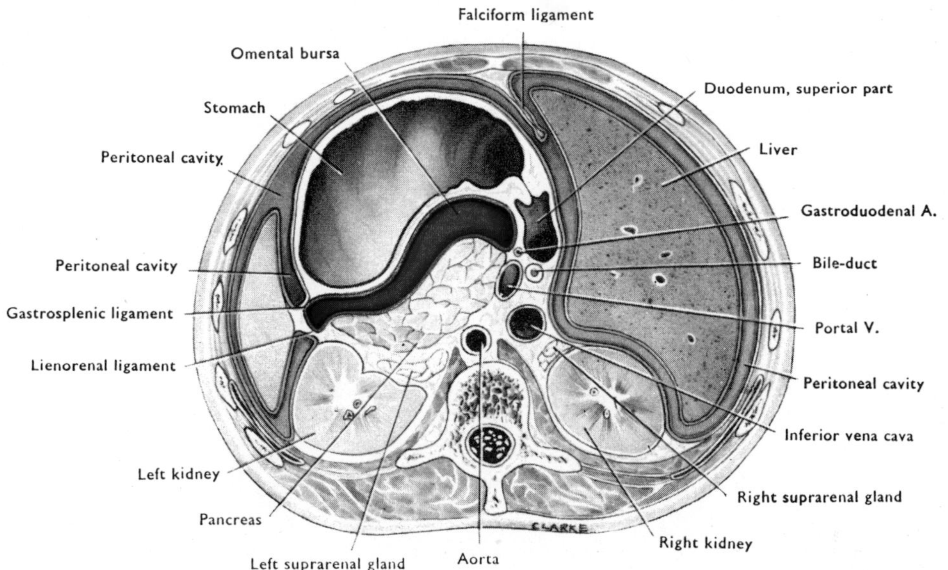

FIG. 115 A horizontal section through the abdomen at the level of the pylorus. Blue : peritoneal cavity. Red : omental bursa.

peritoneum on the posterior surface of the anterior abdominal wall [FIG. 122]. Initially the greater omentum contains part of the cavity of the omental bursa, but the walls fuse and convert it to a simple flap of peritoneum which often contains a considerable quantity of fat in its extraperitoneal areolar tissue. The greater omentum overlies part of the large intestine (transverse colon), and this, together with its mesentery, fuses with the posterior surface of the greater omentum. This compound flap partially divides the peritoneal cavity into anterosuperior and postero-inferior compartments which are frequently known as the *supracolic* and *infracolic compartments* because of the presence of the transverse colon fused to the greater omentum [FIG. 123].

DISSECTION. Identify and lift up the greater omentum, and note the transverse colon fused with its posterior surface a short distance inferior to the stomach.

The **supracolic compartment** of the peritoneal cavity surrounds the liver, stomach, spleen, and the superior part of the duodenum, and lies anterior to parts of the pancreas, duodenum, kidneys, and suprarenal glands. The following brief description gives only the general arrangement of the abdominal viscera which may be examined without dissection. *It is important to confirm the various points on the specimen without damaging the structures which will be dissected later.* The positions given for the various structures are only approximate since all abdominal viscera move to a greater or lesser extent with respiration, and change their position in relation to the age and bodily habitus of the individual. The relative position of organs is also changed by distension and movement of the hollow viscera, particularly those which are free to move on a mesentery.

The **liver** fills the greater part of the right hypochondrium, and is mainly under cover of the diaphragm and ribs. Most of its surface is covered with peritoneum, and it is divided into large right and small left **lobes** by the **falciform**

ligament which is attached on its anterior surface to the right of the median plane. The sharp inferior edge of the right lobe lies approximately along the costal margin as far anteriorly as the tip of the ninth costal cartilage. Close to this the rounded **fundus of the gall-**

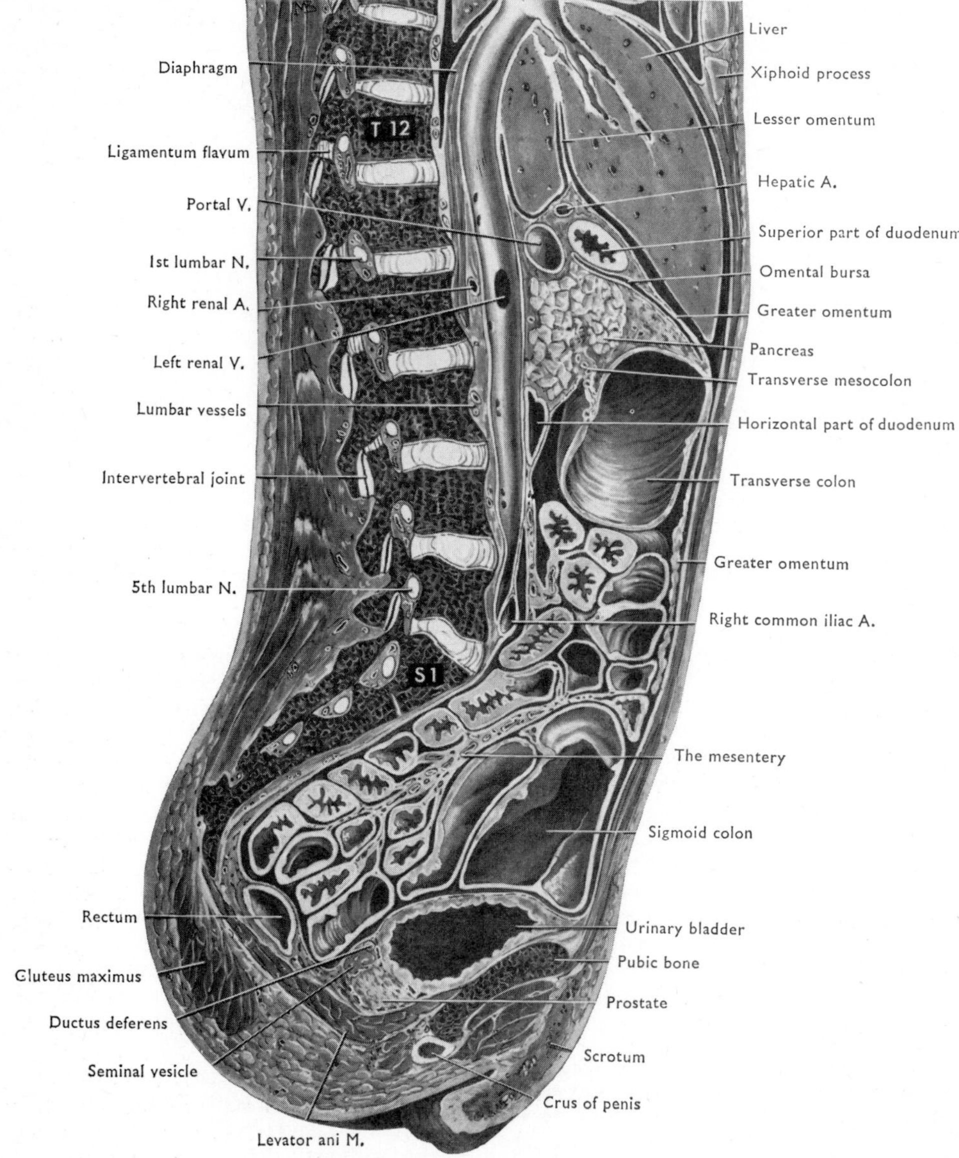

FIG. 116 A sagittal section through the abdomen and pelvis along the inferior vena cava.

bladder protrudes below the inferior edge of the liver. The right lobe then appears from behind the costal cartilages and almost immediately joins the left lobe between the right and left costal margins. The inferior edge of the left lobe then continues in the same direction, and near the left costal margin turns more steeply upwards to end by meeting the superior surface, posterior to the fifth left costal cartilage, close to the fifth rib [FIG. 111]. The superior surface of the right lobe fits into the right dome of the diaphragm, and so reaches the level of the upper border of the fifth rib in the mid-clavicular line, while posteriorly it lies on the superior part of the right kidney, the right suprarenal gland, and the posterior part of the diaphragm [FIG. 125].

The **stomach** lies obliquely across the supracolic compartment from upper left to lower right in a J or Ɔ-shaped curve. The greater part is hidden by the liver, diaphragm, and ribs, but part of its anterior surface is in contact with the anterior abdominal wall inferior

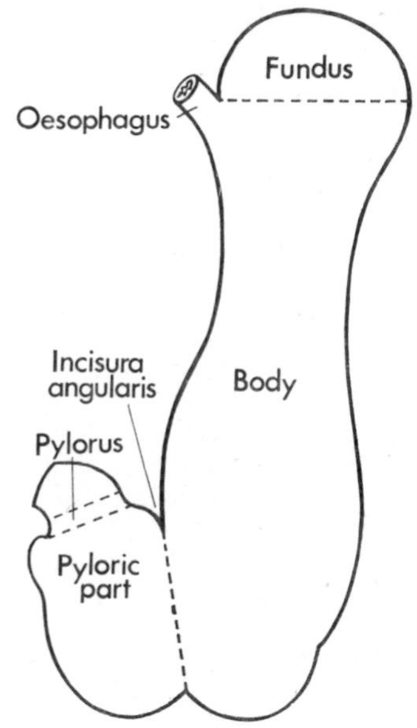

FIG. 117 A diagram of the anterior surface of the stomach to show its parts.

to the left lobe of the liver. Pass a hand upwards over the anterior surface of the stomach and identify its superior, rounded **fundus,** and the **oesophagus** entering the right border below the fundus, immediately posterior to the liver. Lift up the inferior margin of the liver and trace the right, concave border of the stomach (**lesser curvature**) from the entry of the oesophagus downwards and to the right till a thickening (the **pylorus**) is felt in the wall of the stomach where it meets the small intestine (superior part of the **duodenum**). Note a sharp angulation (**incisura angularis**) of the lesser curvature nearer the pylorus than the oesophagus. It marks the junction of the body of the stomach with the pyloric part.

Identify the sheet of peritoneum that passes from the lesser curvature of the stomach to the liver (**lesser omentum**). Superiorly it is narrow where the abdominal part of the oesophagus lies against the liver, but traced inferiorly and to the right it becomes wider and ends in a free edge on the superior part of the duodenum. Pick up the free edge and note that the peritoneum surrounds certain structures in it. These are the **portal vein, hepatic artery,** and **bile-duct,** all of which run between the superior part of the duodenum and a small area on the liver, the **porta hepatis.**

Pass a finger to the left, posterior to the free edge of the lesser omentum. The finger passes through the **epiploic foramen** into the omental bursa posterior to the stomach and lesser omentum. If the tip of the finger is directed upwards after passing through the foramen, it enters a narrow extension of the omental bursa (the **superior recess,** FIG. 124) between the liver and the diaphragm. A finger in the thorax pushed inferiorly between the diaphragm and the descending aorta lies immediately posterior to the finger in the superior recess, but is separated from it by the diaphragm.

Trace the left, convex border of the stomach (**greater curvature**) from the fundus to the pylorus, and note the sheet of peritoneum that passes from it. Superiorly this sheet runs from the fundus to the diaphragm (**gastrophrenic ligament**), while inferior to that it extends first to the spleen (**gastrosplenic ligament**), and more inferiorly forms the **greater omentum** which ends where the superior part of the duodenum becomes adherent to the posterior abdominal wall.

Pull the upper part of the greater curvature to the right and expose the **spleen** deep in the left hypochondrium, posterior to the stomach and anterior to the upper part of the left kidney. Laterally the spleen lies against the diaphragm which separates it from the pleural cavity. Confirm this with a finger in the pleural sac, and note that the spleen lies parallel to the tenth rib, between the ninth and eleventh ribs, posterior to the mid-axillary line. The spleen is covered with peritoneum except for a small area (**hilus**) on the anteromedial surface to which the gastrosplenic and lienorenal ligaments are attached. Thus if the right hand is passed between the spleen and the diaphragm, the fingers can be flexed round its postero-inferior (renal) surface without passing through the peritoneum.

Follow the superior part of the **duodenum**

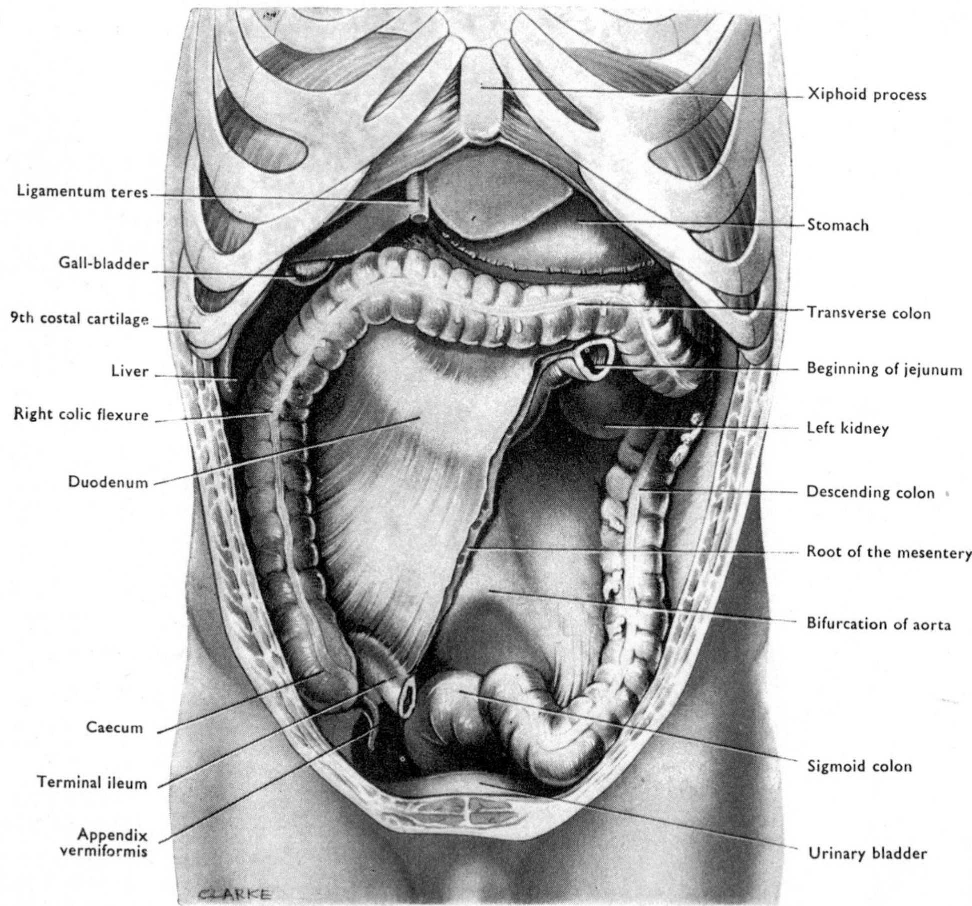

FIG. 118 The abdominal viscera after removal of the jejunum, ileum, and greater omentum.

posterosuperiorly till it turns abruptly downwards as the **descending part.** This part is adherent to the abdominal wall anterior to the medial part of the right kidney. It connects the supracolic part of the gut tube with the infracolic part by passing posterior to the attachment of the mesentery of the transverse colon, to the right of its fusion with the greater omentum [FIG. 124]. The head of the pancreas lies medial to this part of the duodenum.

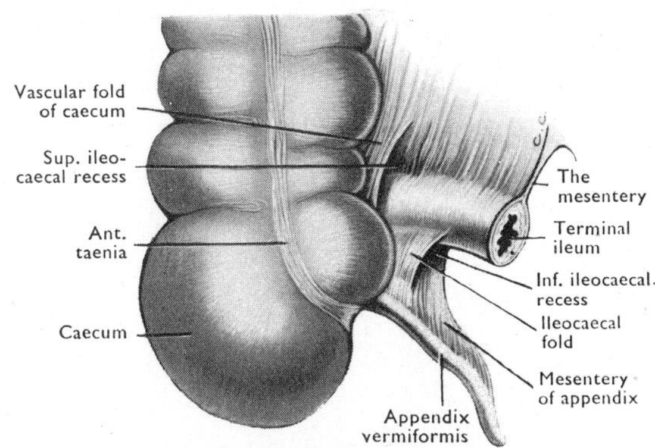

FIG. 119 The anterior surface of the ileocaecal region.

Turn the greater omentum upwards and find the **transverse colon** adherent to its posterior surface. The colon differs from the small intestine in having a wall which (1) is sacculated between the three narrow, straight bands of thickened longitudinal muscle (**taeniae coli**) which pass along it, and (2) has small, projecting sacs of peritoneum filled with fat (**appendices epiploicae**). Trace the transverse colon and its mesentery (mainly fused with the greater omentum and attached with it to the lower part of the body of the pancreas) in both directions, and note that the transverse colon is continuous through the right and left flexures respectively with the **ascending** and **descending colon,** both of which are adherent to the posterior abdominal wall. They lie in the paravertebral gutters which form a route of communication between the supracolic and infracolic parts of the peritoneal cavity, lateral to the ascending and descending parts of the colon (paracolic gutters). Fluid in these gutters gravitates upwards in the recumbent position because of the greater depth of the upper abdomen. Hence infected material (*e.g.*, from a ruptured appendix) may extend into the upper abdomen and form a subphrenic abscess between the liver and either the diaphragm or the upper pole of the right kidney.

The **right colic flexure** lies close to the inferior margin of the liver, anterior to the inferior part of the right kidney, while the **left colic flexure** lies at a much higher level in contact with the anterior (colic) surface of the spleen [FIG. 147].

In the right iliac fossa the inferior part of the ascending colon expands into the blind-ended **caecum** with the retrocaecal recess of the peritoneal cavity posterior to it. Note the relation of the terminal part of the ileum and the **appendix vermiformis** to each other and to the medial surface of caecum [FIG. 119]. Follow the taeniae coli over the surface of the caecum to the base of the appendix where they fuse with its longitudinal muscle coat which is of uniform thickness.

At the brim of the lesser pelvis, the descending colon is continuous with the **sigmoid colon** which loops postero-inferiorly into the lesser pelvis to become continuous with the rectum

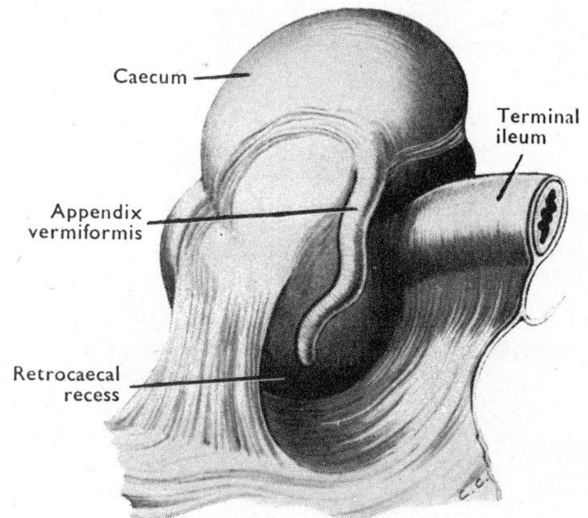

FIG. 120 The inferior surface of the ileocaecal region. The caecum has been turned forwards to open the retrocaecal recess in which the appendix vermiformis commonly lies.

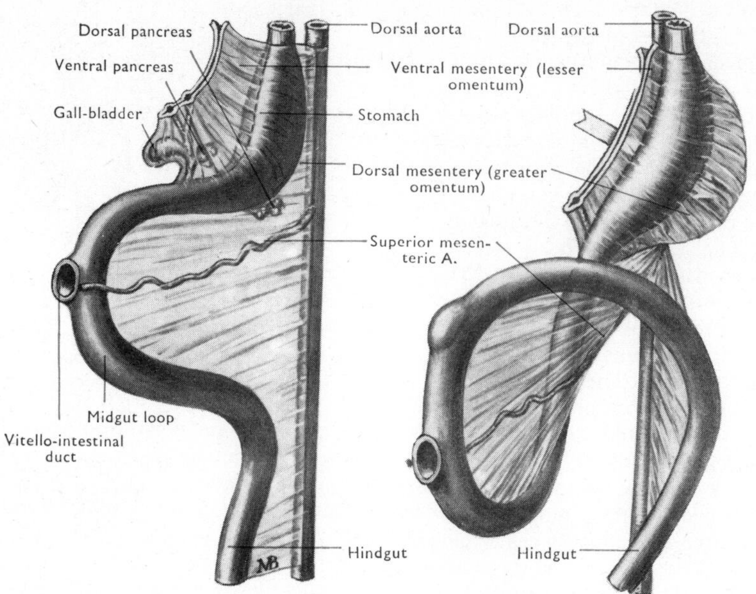

FIG. 121 A diagram to show two early stages in the development of the abdominal part of the gut tube and its mesenteries. Note the rotation of the midgut loop and the ballooning of the dorsal mesentery of the stomach to the left by the extension of the omental bursa (indicated by the arrow) into that mesentery.

on the pelvic surface of the third piece of the sacrum. The sigmoid colon has a short mesentery attached across the margin of the superior aperture of the lesser pelvis [FIG. 124], and where it joins the rectum, the taeniae coli spread out into the longitudinal muscle layer of the rectum.

The infracolic part of the small intestine consists of the inferior half of the duodenum, the jejunum, and the ileum. It is centrally placed within the frame formed by the caecum and colon. This margin is incomplete inferiorly between the caecum and the sigmoid colon, and here coils of small intestine descend into the lesser pelvis. The infracolic part of the **duodenum** completes this C-shaped structure. It comprises the remainder of the descending part, the **horizontal part** which crosses the vertebral column immediately anterior to the aorta on the third lumbar vertebra, and the short **ascending part** which ends by joining the jejunum to the left of the median plane beside the second lumbar vertebra. The **jejunum** and **ileum** lie in the free edge of *the* mesentery which runs obliquely across the central region between the duodenojejunal and ileocaecal junctions, thus partly dividing this part of the peritoneal cavity into right superior and left inferior regions, both of which are filled with coils of small intestine. Note that the appendix vermiformis lies at the right extremity of the left inferior region where it is directly continuous with the pelvic peritoneal cavity.

Pick up *the* **mesentery** and note that its short attachment to the posterior abdominal wall is out of proportion to its long free margin which is complexly folded to accommodate the jejunum and ileum. These two parts of the small intestine cannot be differentiated clearly, but there is less fat in the jejunal mesentery, and thus the vessels are readily visible between its layers and have clear spaces like windows between them. It is usual to reckon the jejunum

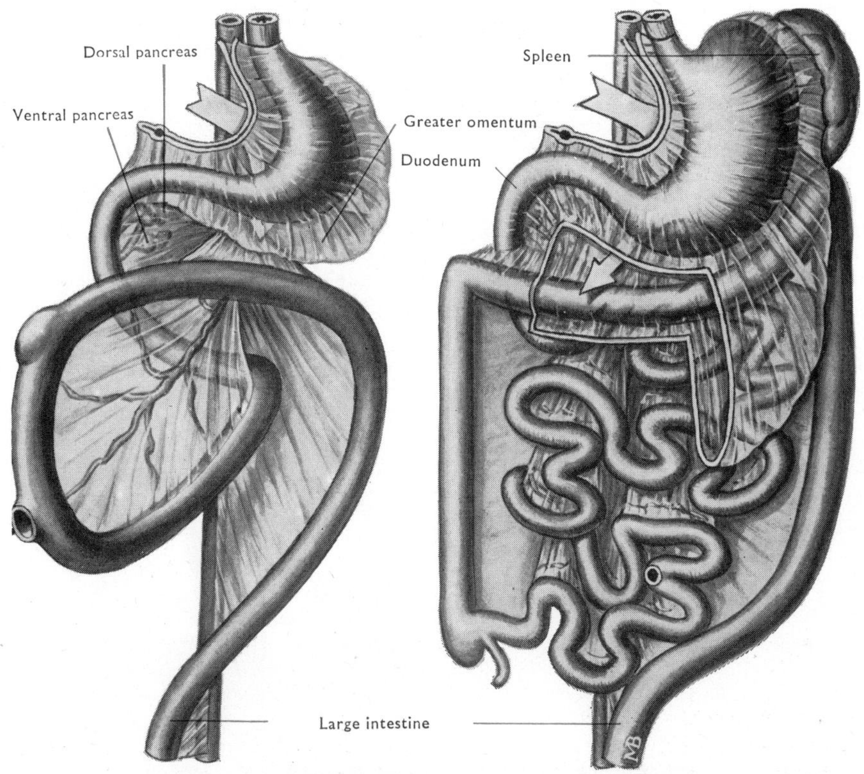

FIG. 122 A diagram of two later stages in the development of the abdominal part of the gut tube and its mesenteries. Note the changes in position of the various parts of the gut tube and the extension of the omental bursa with consequent formation of the greater omentum and the ligaments of the spleen from the dorsal mesentery of the stomach. The duodenum and the ascending and descending parts of the colon become fused to the posterior abdominal wall while the other parts of the gut tube retain their mesenteries. Cf. FIG. 121.

as two-fifths of the 6 m. which this part of the intestine is said to measure. The length is very variable in life, and certain methods of measurement give readings as low as 2·5 m.

A number of accessory but variable peritoneal folds are found, especially in relation to the ascending part of the duodenum and the caecum [FIGS. 119, 120]. Each of these is associated with a **peritoneal recess** within which a loop of small intestine may become lodged and obstructed, thus forming an internal hernia. These folds and recesses should be noted as they are exposed.

The apparently complex arrangement of the viscera described above is readily appreciated from its development. The midgut, which lies between the descending part of the duodenum and the left colic flexure, initially forms a simple loop which extends through the umbilical orifice. This loop rotates 180 degrees anticlockwise (as seen from the anterior surface) on itself so that the ends of the loop, the terminal part of the duodenum, and the future left end of the transverse colon take up reversed positions; the duodenal part lying inferior to the colonic part and to the right of the hindgut and its mesentery [FIGS. 121, 122]. The twist also imparts to the duodenum its final C shape. When the midgut loop returns to the abdominal cavity, the small intestine falls into the central part, while the caecum and midgut parts of the colon lie across the abdomen (anterior to the descending part of the duodenum) superior and to the right of the small intestine. The centrally placed small intestine increases in length and displaces the surrounding parts of the large intestine outwards, the caecum and ascending colon to the right, the hindgut (descending colon) to the left, and the transverse colon (which lies anterior to the small intestine) upwards and forwards against the greater omentum. The mesenteries of all three parts of the colon fuse with the peritoneum to which they are applied, the first two with the posterior abdominal wall, and the third with the greater omentum. The small intestine retains its portion of the midgut mesentery between the parts at either end of it which are fused with the posterior abdominal wall, *i.e.*, the duodenum and the caecum.

Ligaments of Liver

The **falciform ligament** is the part of the ventral mesentery which is attached anteriorly to the diaphragm and supra-umbilical anterior abdominal wall close to the median plane [FIG. 124]. The upper part passes to the right to be attached to the liver, while the inferior part has a free posterior border in which lies the **round ligament of the liver** (obliterated umbilical vein).

Trace the falciform ligament superiorly. Above the liver, its right and left layers of peritoneum diverge and are reflected separately from the superior surface of the liver on to the diaphragm to form the margins of an area on the posterosuperior surface of the liver **(bare area of the liver)** where it is directly in contact with the diaphragm without the intervention of peritoneum [FIG. 158]. The right layer becomes the **superior layer of the coronary ligament** which can be followed to the right and posteriorly to end in a sharp margin (the **right triangular ligament**) where it meets the inferior layer of the coronary ligament. This may be felt by pressing the fingers upwards posterior to the right lobe of the liver and anterior to the right kidney. It will be seen to form the inferior margin of the bare area when the liver is removed. The left layer of the falciform ligament passes to the left as the anterior layer of the **left triangular ligament,** and this also ends in a sharp, left margin where it becomes

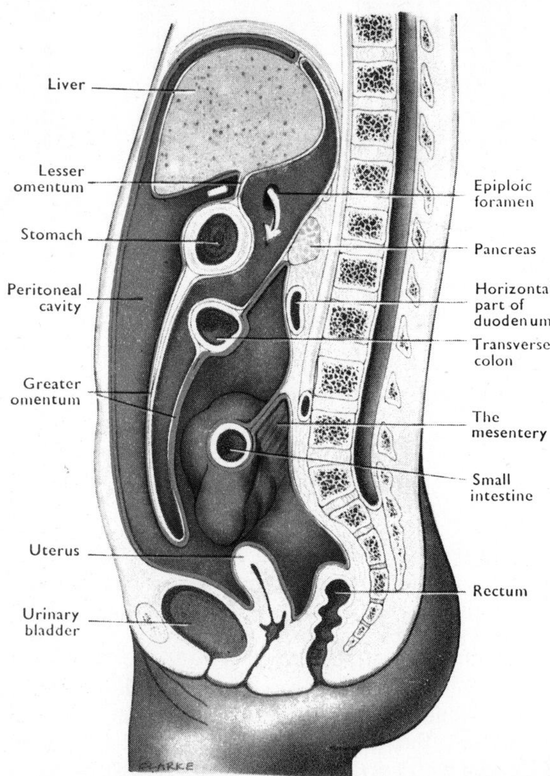

FIG. 123 A diagrammatic median section of the abdomen and pelvis to show the arrangement of the peritoneum. Normally the abdominal viscera completely fill the abdominal cavity and the peritoneal cavity is reduced to a slit. In the diagram the cavity has been distended to make it obvious. Blue : peritoneal cavity. Red : omental bursa of peritoneal cavity. The arrow traverses the epiploic foramen.

continuous with the posterior layer [FIG. 124].

The **round ligament** of the liver leaves the falciform ligament at the inferior border of the liver. It then continues in a fissure on the postero-inferior (visceral) surface of the liver to the left extremity of the porta hepatis. Here it fuses with the left branch of the portal vein [FIG. 156].

DISSECTION. Identify the arterial arcade (gastro-epiploic arteries) in the root of the greater omentum, 2–3 cm. from its junction with the greater curvature of the stomach. Cut through the anterior layers of the greater omentum 2–3 cm. inferior to the vessels, and open the bursa omentalis sufficiently to admit a hand. Explore the bursa.

Omental Bursa

At its right extremity the omental bursa is continuous with the general peritoneal cavity through the **epiploic foramen.** This foramen is posterior to the free edge of the lesser omentum and its contents (the portal vein, hepatic artery, and bile-duct) and anterior to the inferior

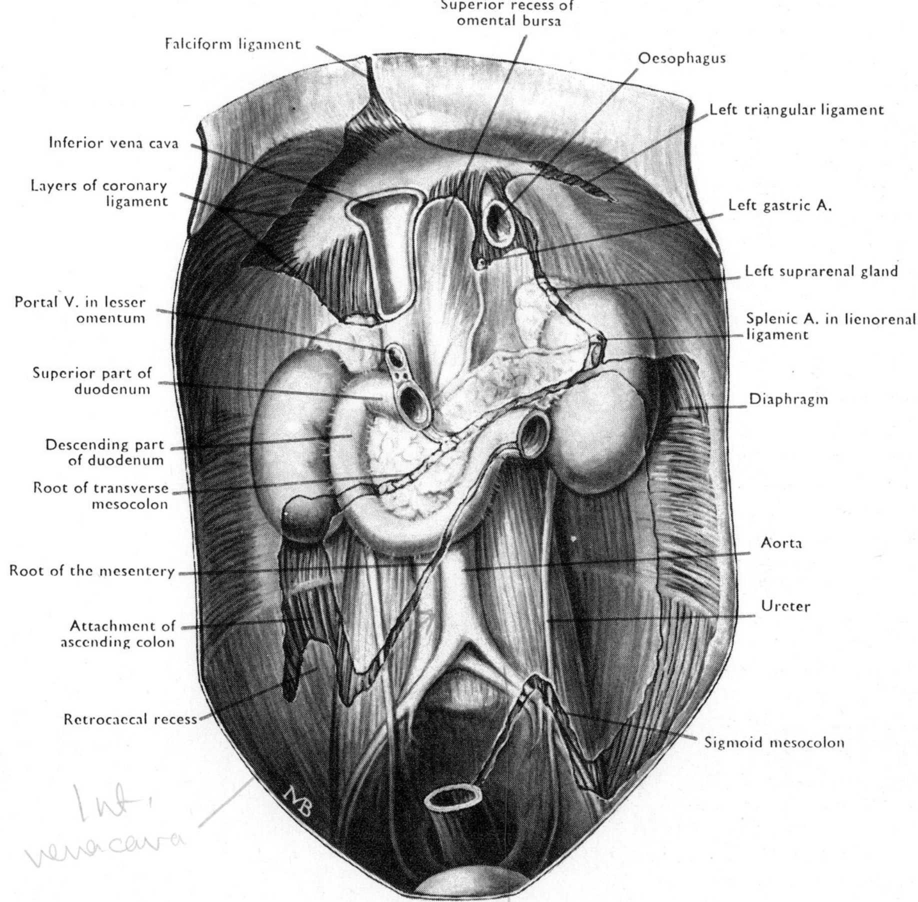

FIG. 124 A dissection of the posterior abdominal wall to show the attachments of the mesenteries and peritoneal ligaments. The oesophagus, duodenum, and rectum are the only parts of the gut tube left *in situ.*

vena cava which is covered anteriorly with peritoneum and lies on the right crus of the diaphragm. Superiorly both portal vein and inferior vena cava enter the liver, and the narrow strip of liver between them (caudate process, FIG. 156) forms the superior limit of the foramen. The inferior wall is formed by the portal vein and bile-duct passing posterior to the superior part of the duodenum.

The epiploic foramen leads into the **vestibule** of the bursa. This is a narrow chamber between the epiploic foramen and the **gastropancreatic peritoneal folds,** which are produced by the left gastric and common hepatic arteries passing anteriorly towards the oesophageal and pyloric ends of the lesser curvature of the stomach.

The **superior recess** of the omental bursa passes superiorly from the vestibule, on the left of the inferior vena cava, and posterior to the caudate lobe of the liver [FIG. 156]. The recess is anterior to the thoracic aorta, but separated from it by the diaphragm.

Between the gastropancreatic folds the vestibule opens into the main body of the bursa, which lies posterior to the lesser omentum and stomach. It passes for a variable distance into the greater omentum **(inferior recess),** extends on the left to the hilus of the spleen and the gastrosplenic and lienorenal ligaments **(splenic recess),** and separates the stomach from the structures on the posterior abdominal wall (the stomach bed).

The omental bursa gives added freedom of movement to the stomach, allowing it to expand after a large meal and to slide on the surrounding tissues during contraction.

DISSECTION. Pull the liver superiorly and tilt its inferior margin anteriorly to expose the lesser omentum. If this gives insufficient exposure, remove the left lobe of the liver by cutting through it to the left of the falciform ligament, the fissure for the round ligament (ligamentum teres), and the attachment of the lesser omentum.

Lesser Omentum

This double layer of peritoneum passes from the abdominal oesophagus, the lesser curva-

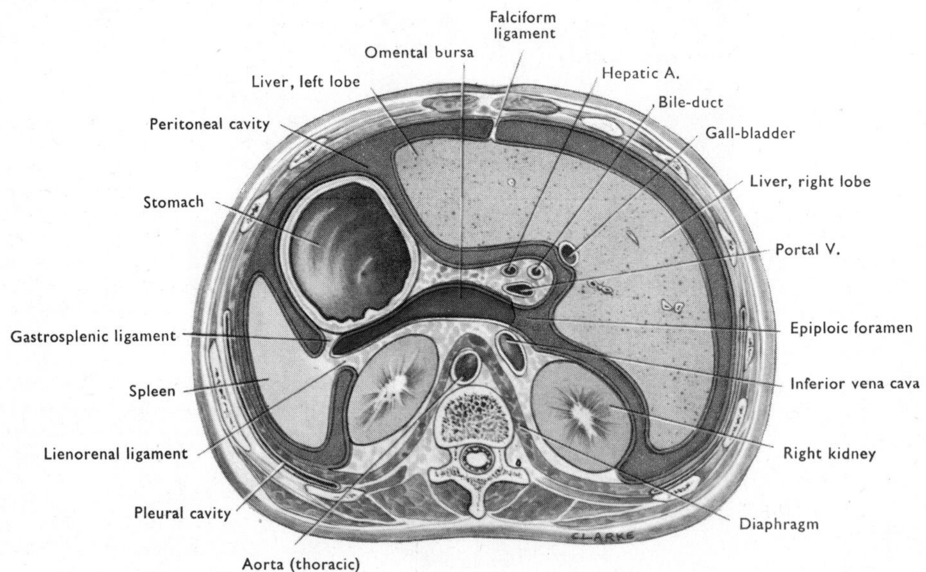

FIG. 125 A horizontal section through the abdomen at the level of the epiploic foramen. Blue: peritoneal cavity. Red: omental bursa.

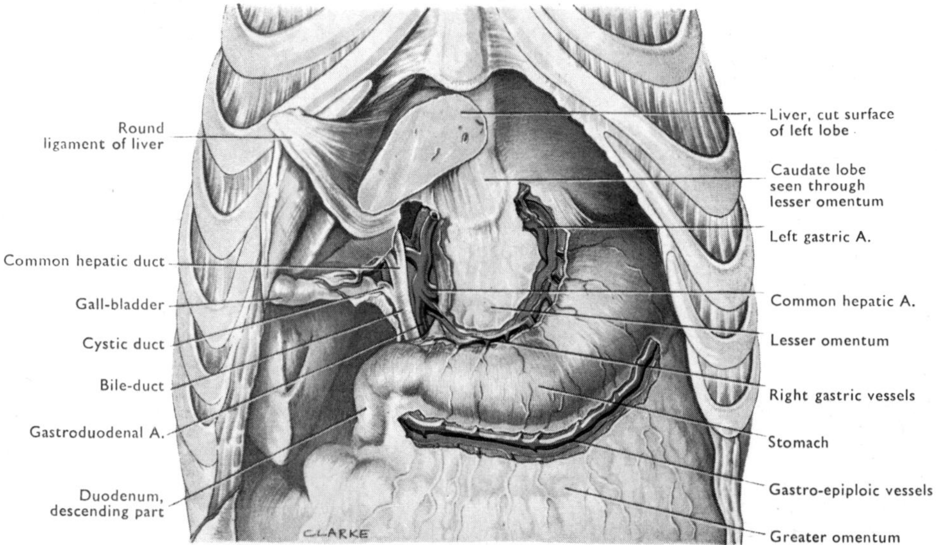

FIG. 126 The interior of the abdomen after removal of part of the left lobe of the liver and dissection of the vessels of the lesser and greater omenta.

ture of the stomach, and the first 2 cm. of the duodenum to be attached to the liver in the depths of the **fissure for the ligamentum venosum** [FIG. 156] and around the margin of the porta hepatis. At the free edge of the omentum, its two layers of peritoneum become continuous with each other around the portal vein, common hepatic artery, and bile-duct. These are accompanied by sympathetic nerves on the artery, parasympathetic branches of the anterior gastric nerve (vagus) passing to the gall-bladder, and by lymph vessels and nodes which drain the liver and the adjacent part of the stomach. Elsewhere the layers are separated by extraperitoneal areolar tissue, and by the right and left **gastric vessels** which run along the lesser curvature of the stomach, supply this part of the stomach, and anastomose with each other. Not uncommonly a branch of the left gastric artery passes between the layers of the omentum to supply part of the left lobe of the liver.

DISSECTION. To expose the structures in the lesser omentum remove the anterior layer of peritoneum. Begin at the middle of the lesser curvature and attempt to trace the left gastric vessels towards the oesophagus till they curve posteriorly around the superior surface of the omental bursa. Trace the oesophageal branch to the oesophagus. Find the anterior vagal trunk on the anterior surface of the oesophagus, and trace its branches on to the stomach.

Trace the right gastric artery to the common hepatic, and the vein to the portal vein. Clean the common hepatic artery and its branches to the porta hepatis. Trace the cystic duct from its union with the neck of the gall-bladder to its junction with the common hepatic duct. Follow the latter to the porta hepatis and note its tributaries, the right and left hepatic ducts. Trace the bile-duct inferiorly till it passes posterior to the duodenum, and displacing the artery and bile-duct, clean the portal vein from the duodenum to the porta hepatis.

Remove the remainder of the lesser omentum, leaving the cleaned structures intact, and examine the abdominal wall posterior to the omentum and omental bursa.

The lesser omentum lies between the left lobe of the liver, anteriorly, and the posterior abdominal wall. Bulging parts of the left lobe of the liver (tuber omentale, FIG. 156) and of the pancreas [FIG. 127] press on its

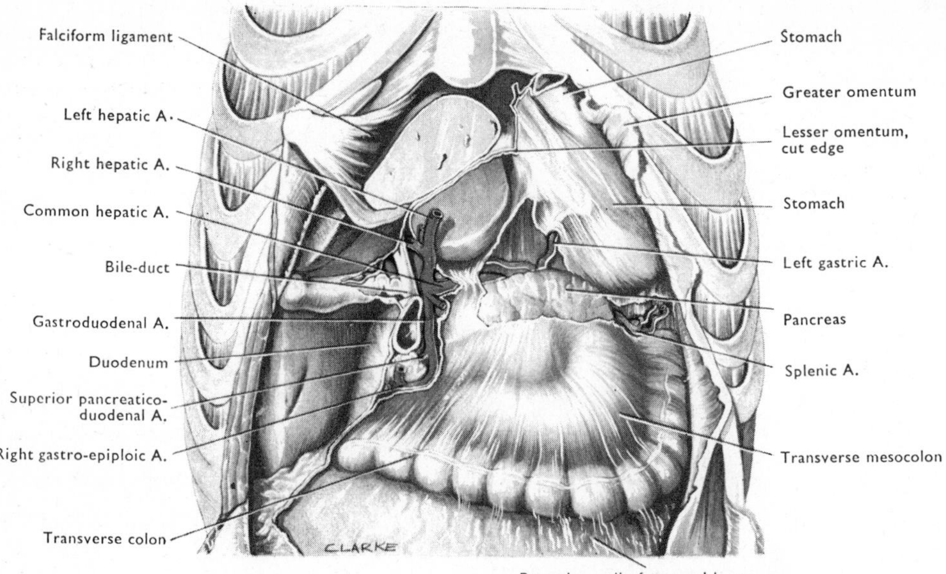

FIG. 127 The posterior wall of the omental bursa. The superior part of the duodenum and the greater part of the lesser omentum are divided and the stomach turned upwards with the anterior layers of the greater omentum.

anterior and posterior surfaces respectively. Immediately superior to the pancreas, the coeliac trunk arises from the aorta which enters the abdomen from the thorax between the two crura of the diaphragm.

Lienorenal and Gastrosplenic Ligaments [FIG. 125]

These have been described already [p. 124], but their position should now be confirmed by placing one hand between the diaphragm and spleen, the other in the omental bursa. Posterior to the spleen, feel the thick lienorenal ligament which contains the tail of the pancreas and the splenic vessels, while anterior to the spleen is the gastrosplenic ligament which contains the branches of the splenic artery passing to the stomach (**short gastric arteries** and the **left gastro-epiploic artery,** both with corresponding veins draining to the splenic vein). Lymph nodes and vessels are also present in both ligaments, and they drain the territories supplied by the blood vessels.

DISSECTION. Identify and clean the vessels in the gastrosplenic ligament to the hilus of the spleen. Confirm the attachment of the ligament to the hilus, and follow the left gastro-epiploic artery through the root of the greater omentum parallel to the greater curvature of the stomach.

SPLEEN

[FIGS. 125, 128, 129, 133, 159]

This is the largest single mass of lymphoid tissue in the body, but it differs from lymph nodes in having a much richer blood supply and in neither receiving afferent lymph vessels nor giving rise to efferent lymph vessels in proportion to its mass. It has a thick **capsule** which contains very little smooth muscle in Man, though there is a considerable quantity in many other mammals where the spleen has more importance as a blood store which can be emptied rapidly, *e.g.*, after haemorrhage.

The spleen lies deep in the left hypochondrium wedged obliquely between the diaphragm, stomach, and left kidney, with the

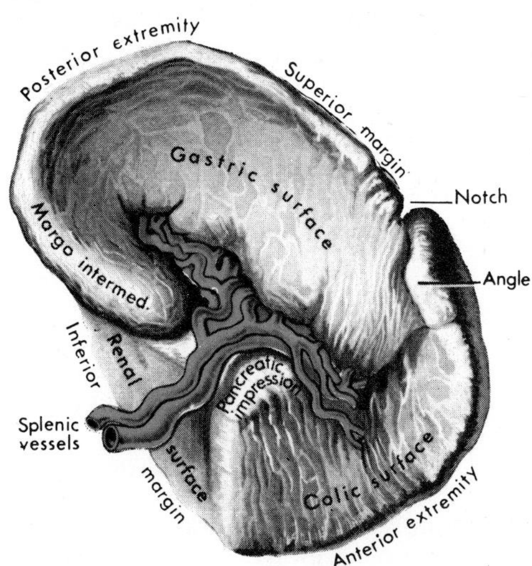

FIG. 128 The visceral surface of the spleen.

left colic flexure applied to its **anterior extremity.** It is almost entirely covered with peritoneum except at the long, linear **hilus** on the medial part of its concave anteromedial **(gastric) surface**. Here the gastrosplenic and lienorenal ligaments are attached, the multiple branches of the splenic artery enter its surface accompanied by the corresponding tributaries of the splenic vein, and the tip of the **tail of the pancreas** may reach it through the lienorenal ligament [FIG. 128].

The convex posterolateral **(diaphragmatic) surface** lies against the diaphragm, parallel and deep to the posterior parts of the ninth to eleventh ribs (the pleural cavity and lung intervening). This surface meets the gastric surface at the relatively sharp **superior margin** which has one or more notches in it near its anterior end. These may be palpated through the anterior abdominal wall when a grossly enlarged spleen extends below the left costal margin along the line of the ribs.

The **renal surface** lies in contact with the lateral part of the upper half of the left kidney. It faces inferomedially and meets the diaphragmatic and gastric surfaces respectively at the blunt **inferior margin** and a low ridge (intermediate margin) close to the hilus.

The spleen develops in the dorsal mesogastrium as a number of separate masses each with its own blood supply. These aggregate but retain their separate circulations, thus blockage of a branch of the splenic artery leads to death (infarction) of a segment of the spleen. Accessory splenic nodules may be found in the gastrosplenic ligament.

Structure and Function. The thick fibroelastic capsule sends a network of **trabeculae** into the pulp of the spleen to join those which arise in the hilus around the entering blood vessels. The pulp is of two kinds, red and white. The **white pulp** consists of lymphatic follicles scattered throughout the spleen, in which active production of lymphocytes takes place. The **red pulp** consists of large numbers of sinusoids separated by reticular fibres intermingled with phagocytic cells of the reticulo-endothelial series and red and white blood cells, some of which may be found within the phagocytes in the process of destruction. The branches of the arteries which leave the trabeculae are ensheathed in lymphocytes, and pass to supply the lymphatic follicles. They then branch into contractile vessels (ellipsoids) which discharge into the sinusoids, the walls of which allow the passage of cells to and from the red pulp. The sinusoids drain into the splenic veins.

The spleen is the major site of destruction of red and white blood cells and platelets, and the products of their destruction are carried through the splenic vein to the portal vein and liver. In common with the rest of the lymphoid tissue in the body it plays a considerable role in the development of immunity; and though not essential to life, its removal tends to increase the susceptibility of the individual to infections.

DISSECTION. Complete the cleaning of the gastro-epiploic vessels in the greater omentum, and follow them as far as possible to the right and left. A plexus of sympathetic nerve fibres and an occasional lymph node may be identified in relation to them.

Cut through the stomach immediately to the left of the pylorus, dividing the right gastric and gastro-epiploic vessels. Turn the stomach to the left to expose the omental bursa, and clean the peritoneum from its

left and posterior walls as far inferiorly as the attachment of the combined greater omentum and transverse mesocolon. Note the lymph nodes (pancreaticosplenic) on the superior border of the pancreas as it is cleaned.

Identify the coeliac trunk and clean its branches. Clean the superior part of the left kidney, the left suprarenal gland and its numerous arteries and single vein, and the adjacent part of the diaphragm (crus) with the inferior phrenic arteries on its abdominal surface. Identify the coeliac ganglia on each side of the coeliac trunk, and trace the splanchnic nerves superiorly from them. Remove the peritoneum from the posterior surface of the stomach and trace the posterior vagal trunk and its gastric branches.

COELIAC TRUNK

This large vessel passes forwards for approximately 1 cm. from the uppermost part of the abdominal aorta. It then divides into common hepatic, splenic, and left gastric branches to supply the gut tube from the lower oesophagus to the descending part of the duodenum, the liver, pancreas, and spleen. It is surrounded by a dense plexus of sympathetic nerves from the coeliac ganglia, and these are distributed with its branches.

Left Gastric Artery [Figs. 124, 129]

This small branch runs on the posterior part of the diaphragm towards the oesophagus. It then arches forwards in the superior gastropancreatic fold to run inferiorly along the lesser curvature of the stomach and anastomose with the right gastric artery. It gives ascending, **oesophageal branches** which anastomose with the oesophageal branches of the aorta in the thorax. The **gastric branches** pass to both surfaces of the stomach adjacent to the lesser curvature.

The **left gastric vein** runs along its artery to the coeliac trunk, and then follows the common hepatic artery to the portal vein. Its tributaries are derived from the territory supplied by the artery, and the most important of these are from the oesophagus for they anastomose with thoracic oesophageal veins which drain into the azygos system of veins. If the portal vein is obstructed in liver disease, these vessels form an alternative venous drainage and are often greatly distended, especially the submucous veins of the lower oesophagus. Such oesophageal varices may be a source of severe haemorrhage [Fig. 152].

Splenic Artery [Figs. 128, 133]

This, the largest branch of the coeliac trunk, runs a sinuous course to the left along the superior border of the pancreas, posterior to the omental bursa. With the pancreas, it runs anterior to the left kidney into the lienorenal ligament, and gives five or six branches into the hilus of the spleen.

Branches. (1) Small twigs pass directly into

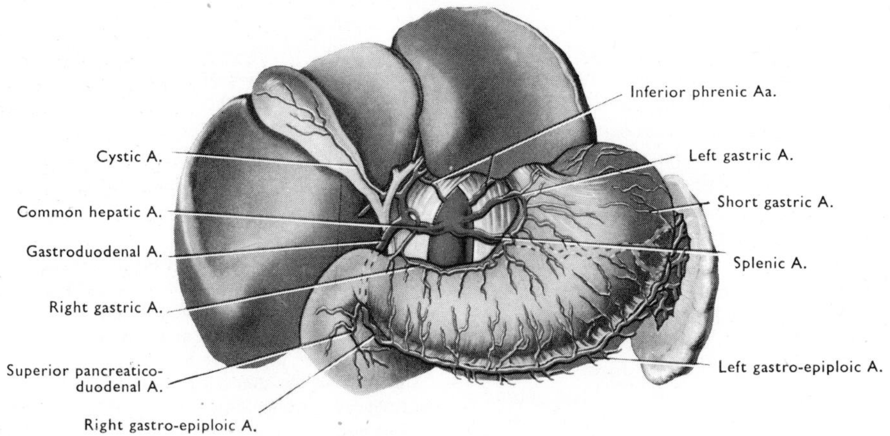

Fig. 129 The coeliac trunk and its branches.

the body and tail of the **pancreas.** (2) Five or six slender, **short gastric arteries** pass through the gastrosplenic ligament from the trunk and splenic branches towards the fundus of the stomach. (3) The **left gastro-epiploic artery** runs through the gastrosplenic ligament, and passes to the right between the layers of the greater omentum parallel to and a short distance from the greater curvature of the stomach. It anastomoses with the right gastro-epiploic artery, supplies both surfaces of the stomach adjacent to the greater curvature, and sends small branches into the greater omentum.

The corresponding **veins** drain into the splenic vein. This lies inferior to the splenic artery, and runs to the right, posterior to the pancreas.

Common Hepatic Artery [FIGS. 127, 129]

This artery passes to the right along the upper border of the pancreas to the superior part of the duodenum. Here the gastroduodenal artery arises, and the common hepatic turns forwards between the duodenum and the epiploic foramen, gives off the right gastric artery, and becoming the **hepatic artery** ascends through the lesser omentum to the porta hepatis, anterior to the portal vein and medial to the bile-duct [FIG. 125]. Inferior to the porta hepatis it divides into right and left hepatic arteries which enter the corresponding lobes of the liver through the porta.

In the lesser omentum, the hepatic artery may give a descending **duodenal branch** to the superior part of the duodenum, while the right hepatic artery sends the **cystic artery** along the cystic duct to supply the gall-bladder. The cystic vein enters the right branch of the portal vein.

Gastroduodenal Artery. This descends anterior to the portal vein, behind the superior part of the duodenum, and divides into the superior pancreaticoduodenal and right gastro-epiploic arteries [FIGS. 127, 129]

The **superior pancreaticoduodenal artery** curves inferiorly between the duodenum and the head of the pancreas, sends branches to both, and anastomoses freely with the inferior pancreaticoduodenal branch of the superior mesenteric artery. The corresponding **vein,** when present, usually drains to the superior mesenteric vein.

The **right gastro-epiploic artery** runs to the left between the layers of the greater omentum near the first 1–2 cm. of the duodenum and the greater curvature of the stomach. It anastomoses with the left gastro-epiploic artery and sends branches to the superior part of the duodenum, the right part of the stomach, and the greater omentum. The corresponding **vein** usually enters the superior mesenteric vein:

Right Gastric Artery. Smaller than the left gastric artery, this branch passes to the left on the first centimetre of the duodenum, the pylorus, and the lesser curvature of the stomach. It gives branches to these, and anastomoses with the left gastric artery. The corresponding **vein** enters the portal vein, and is united to the right gastro-epiploic vein by the **prepyloric vein** which crosses the front of the pylorus and is a landmark for the surgeon.

Variations in the arrangement of the branches of the common hepatic artery are frequent and occasionally the whole artery may arise from the superior mesenteric artery through the anastomosis of the pancreaticoduodenal arteries.

ABDOMINAL PART OF OESOPHAGUS

The oesophagus pierces the muscular part (right crus) of the diaphragm together with the vagal trunks, the oesophageal branches of the left gastric artery, and the corresponding veins. Here it is posterior to the central tendon and grooves the posterior surface of the left lobe of the liver 2–3 cm. to the left of the median plane. Its right surface is directly continuous with the lesser curvature of the stomach, while the left surface meets the fundus of the stomach at an acute angle [FIGS. 134, 136] almost immediately after passing through the diaphragm.

Vagal Trunks

In the inferior part of the posterior mediastinum, the oesophageal plexus reforms into the anterior and posterior vagal trunks. These

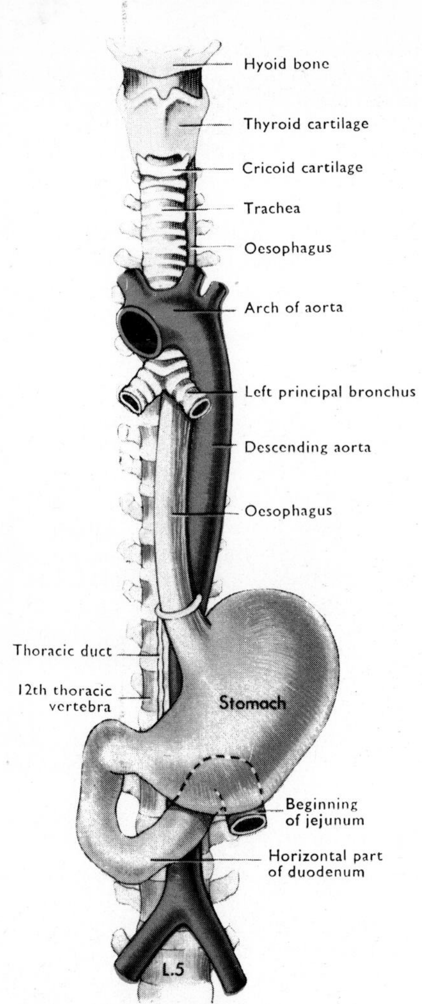

FIG. 130 The oesophagus, stomach, and duodenum.

pass through the diaphragm with the oesophagus and break up into anterior and posterior **gastric branches** respectively. Each vagal trunk consists of nerve fibres from both vagus nerves with the addition of sympathetic nerve fibres from the greater splanchnic nerves [p. 79].

The **anterior gastric branches** supply the stomach and send nerve fibres to the duodenum and pancreas, and to the liver through the lesser omentum.

The **posterior vagal trunk** sends branches to the stomach (posterior gastric) and **coeliac branches** which descend over the diaphragm to the coeliac plexus. Thence the parasympathetic nerve fibres are distributed with the sympathetic fibres that follow the branches of the aorta to the liver, pancreas, kidneys, suprarenal glands, spleen, and intestines.

Replace the stomach and the left lobe of the liver if it has been removed. Then review the shape and position of the stomach.

STOMACH

The stomach is the most distensible organ in the body. Through the oesophagus it receives food mixed with and softened by saliva, and having added a considerable volume of fluid (which contains hydrochloric acid, pepsin, rennin, and lipase), churns the food to a semifluid mass (chyme) by its muscular action. This is discharged slowly through the pylorus into the superior part of the duodenum. It also adds mucus to the food, particularly in the pyloric part through which the chyme passes on its way to the duodenum. This mucus adsorbs and neutralizes a considerable quantity of hydrochloric acid, and not only raises the pH of the chyme passing into the duodenum, but also helps to protect the gastric mucous membrane from digestion.

The stomach curves downwards and to the right across the supracolic compartment of the peritoneal cavity, and tapers from its upper, rounded extremity (the **fundus,** which lies well to the left of the median plane) to the narrow **pylorus** slightly to the right of the median plane. Together with the superior part of the duodenum it forms a U-shaped curve (convex anteriorly) across the anterior surface of the prominent vertebral column; the fundus and superior part of the duodenum lying posteriorly in the paravertebral gutters, while the pyloric part lies anterior to the vertebral bodies and to the structures lying on them.

When empty, the stomach has flattened anterosuperior and postero-inferior surfaces.

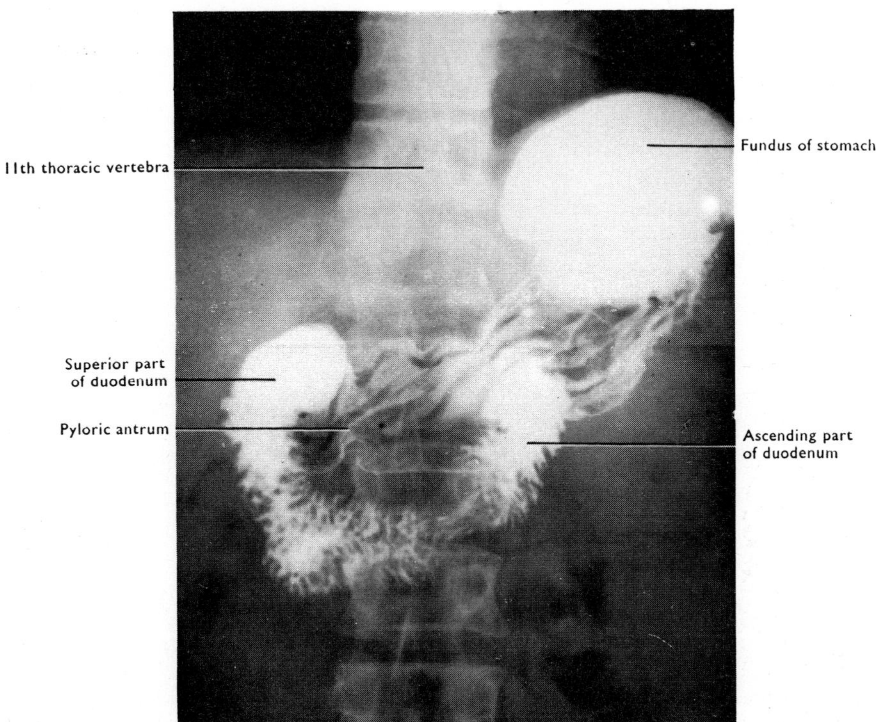

FIG. 131 A radiograph of the transverse type of stomach taken in the recumbent posture. Note that the gas bubble lies in the part of the stomach anterior to the vertebral column and so outlines the folds of gastric mucosa. Heavy contrast medium gravitates into the fundus and superior part of the duodenum which are posterior. Cf. FIG. 132.

Its concave (right) margin [FIG. 134] (the **lesser curvature**) extends from the oesophageal orifice (**cardiac orifice**) to the pylorus, the lesser omentum passing from this margin to the liver. The **incisura angularis** is a notch on this border, nearer the pylorus than the oesophagus. It marks the junction of the superior part of the stomach with the inferior or **pyloric part,** and is sometimes matched by a corresponding groove on the greater curvature.

The right surface of the abdominal oesophagus is directly continuous with the lesser curvature; the left surface meets the right surface of the fundus at an acute angle (**cardiac notch**). A horizontal line drawn through the stomach at the level of the cardiac notch divides the superior part of the stomach into the **fundus** and **body.**

The pyloric part of the stomach is divisible into a dilated proximal portion, the **pyloric antrum,** and a narrow, cylindrical portion (**pyloric canal**) 2–3 cm. long, which is continuous distally with the pylorus. The **pylorus** lies in the thickened portion of the stomach that unites it to the duodenum. The thickening is due to an increase in the amount of circular muscle to form the **pyloric sphincter,** a structure concerned with controlling the rate of discharge of stomach contents into the duodenum. Hence it prevents too much hydrochloric acid passing at one time into the alkaline medium of the duodenum. The pylorus is marked externally by a slight groove and by the prepyloric vein.

On the convex margin of the stomach (**greater curvature**) the layers of peritoneum

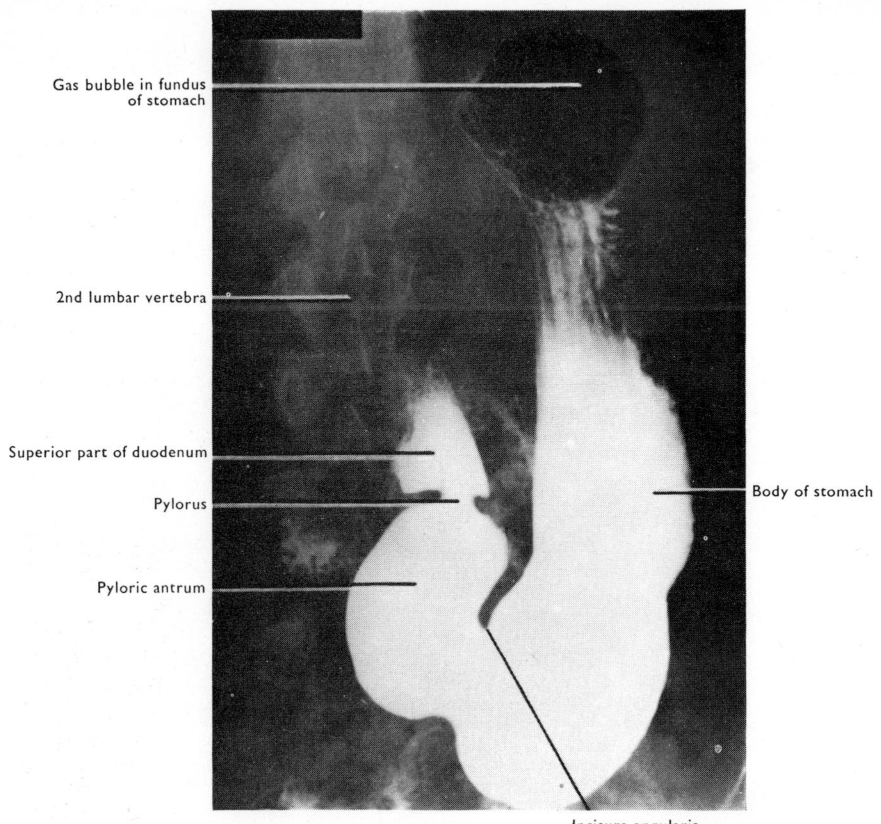

FIG. 132 A radiograph of a J-shaped stomach taken in the erect posture. Note the level of the pylorus and compare this with FIG. 131.

covering its surfaces pass off as a continuous sheet from the cardiac orifice to the pylorus. From the fundus this passes to the diaphragm **(gastrophrenic ligament)** and continues as the **gastrosplenic ligament** from the upper part of the body. The greater omentum is the part which arises from the lower part of the body and the pyloric part of the stomach. Near the oesophagus, the layers of the gastrophrenic ligament separate and the stomach wall adjacent to the cardiac orifice comes directly into contact with the diaphragm—the bare area of the stomach.

The shape of the stomach varies considerably from individual to individual and in the same individual with age, degree of distension, position of the body, and state of contraction of its muscle layers. These differences are partly due to the freedom of movement of the stomach, the greater part of which lies between the omental bursa and the general peritoneal cavity, attached only by the loose omenta. The stomach in thick set individuals and children tends to lie almost transversely across the abdomen, sloping downwards to the duodenum [FIG. 131], though it is more commonly J-shaped [FIG. 132]. In the latter case, the pyloric part lies horizontally or ascends to the superior part of the duodenum, and the lowest part of the greater curvature may even extend into the greater pelvis in the erect posture. Thus the structures in contact with the most mobile parts of the stomach are variable.

The cardiac orifice and fundus are relatively fixed, and only move with the respiratory excursions of the diaphragm.

The **cardiac orifice** lies 10 cm. posterior to the seventh left costal cartilage 2–3 cm. from the median plane, immediately posterior to the liver against the diaphragm.

The **fundus** abuts on the left dome of the diaphragm under cover of the rib cage. It reaches the level of the fifth rib in the midclavicular line anteriorly, and here lies inferior and slightly posterior to the apex of the heart. In the erect posture it is filled with a bubble of swallowed air which moves into the pyloric portion, anterior to the vertebral column, in the supine position [FIGS. 131, 132].

The **pylorus,** supported by the omenta, is highly mobile despite its attachment to the duodenum, most of which is adherent to the posterior abdominal wall. The pylorus may lie anywhere between the first and third lumbar vertebrae 2–3 cm. to the right of the median plane, though it is displaced to the right when the stomach is full. In its higher positions the pylorus is posterior to the right lobe of the liver (quadrate lobe) and lies in front of the pancreas, but is separated from it by the omental bursa.

The part of the anterosuperior surface of the stomach adjacent to the lesser omentum is overlapped by the liver (mainly the left lobe).

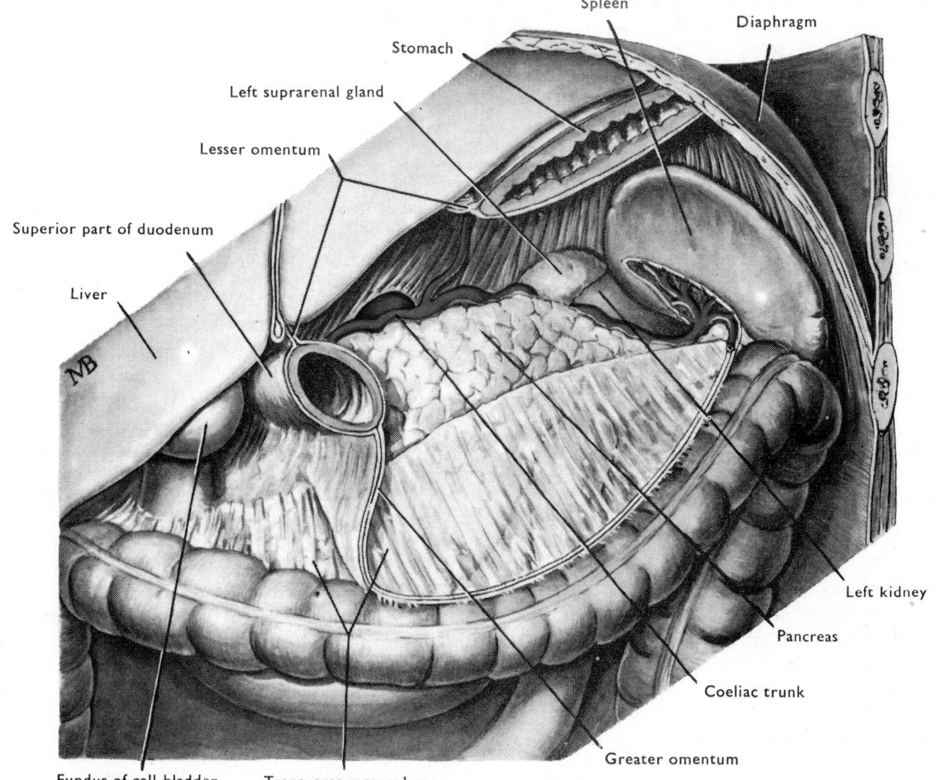

FIG. 133 A dissection to show the structures posterior to the stomach.

The left superior part lies behind the anterior part of the diaphragm and rib cage, and the intermediate part is in contact with the peritoneum on the rectus sheath.

The postero-inferior surface of the stomach lies on the stomach bed, but is *separated from it by the omental bursa.* Superiorly the stomach bed consists of the spleen, upper pole of the left kidney, the left suprarenal gland, and the diaphragm [FIG. 133]. Inferior to these are the upper part of the pancreas [FIG. 115] and associated vessels, with the mesentery of the transverse colon attached to and extending inferiorly from it. In the low type of J-shaped stomach, the transverse colon and even coils of small intestine may be posterior to its inferior part.

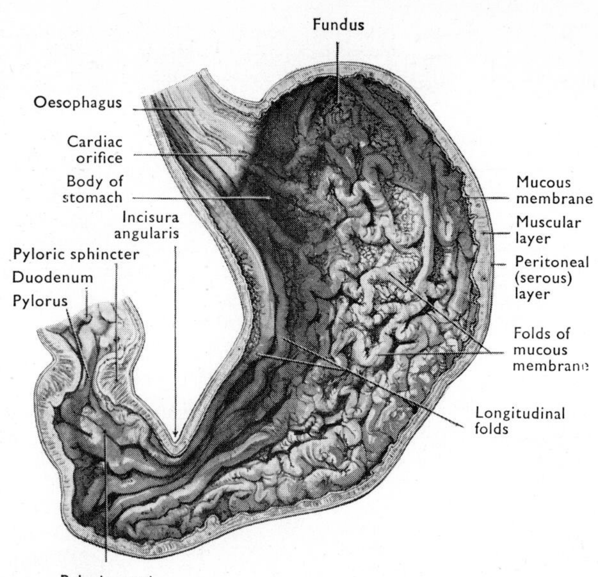

FIG. 134 The posterior wall of the empty, contracted stomach.

Vessels and Nerves. The rich arterial supply is derived from all three branches of the coeliac trunk. The right and left **gastric arteries** anastomose on the lesser curvature, while the right and left **gastro-epiploic arteries** are adjacent to the inferior part of the greater curvature, the superior part of which is supplied by the **short gastric arteries.** Branches of all these arteries run on to both surfaces of the stomach at right angles to its long axis. The supply and anastomoses are sufficiently rich to allow one or more of the major arteries to be tied without ill effects. The **veins** drain with the corresponding arteries.

Parasympathetic and some sympathetic nerve fibres reach the stomach through the anterior and posterior **vagal trunks** and their branches. The majority of the sympathetic fibres arise in the **coeliac plexus** and pass along the branches of the coeliac trunk.

Lymph vessels run with the blood vessels to small lymph nodes on the latter. The main lymph nodes are on the posterior abdominal wall along the pancreas.

DISSECTION. Divide the oesophagus and left gastric vessels close to the diaphragm. Cut through the gastrophrenic and gastrosplenic ligaments and the anterior layers of the greater omentum. Remove the stomach and strip the peritoneum from one of its surfaces to expose the muscle coat. Open the stomach along the greater curvature and examine the mucous membrane with a hand lens.

Mucous Membrane. This is a thick, smooth-surfaced layer which is thrown into longitudinal folds when the stomach is contracted, but is flattened out as it distends. It consists of a layer of tubular glands which open in groups into **pits** [FIG. 135] formed by the surface epithelium, which is a single layer of tall columnar cells that produce a protective surface layer of mucus. In the **body** and **fundus** (the acid secreting part of the stomach) the pits are short and the glands long and tightly packed in a parallel array. They contain several different kinds of cells, including the enzyme secreting types. In the pyloric part of the stomach the pits are deeper, and the glands are coiled, less tightly packed, and entirely of a mucus secreting type. The deepest layer of the mucous membrane is the muscularis mucosae which is thicker in the stomach than else-

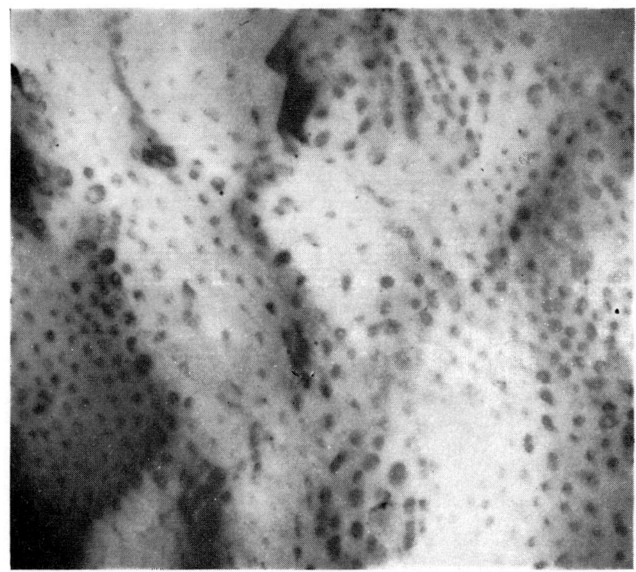

FIG. 135 A photograph of the surface of the human gastric mucosa. Note that it is not quite smooth but has a number of rounded protrusions (mamillae), and that the surface is covered with dark spots of variable size, the gastric pits. A number of simple tubular gastric glands open into the base of each pit.

where, and may have three rather than the two layers found elsewhere.

The submucous layer is formed of loose areolar tissue which allows the mucous membrane to slide on the muscle layers. It contains the blood and lymphatic vessels and the nerves which are distributed to the mucous membrane.

DISSECTION. Divide the stomach along the lesser curvature, and strip the mucous membrane from one half to expose the internal layer of the muscle coat.

Muscle of Stomach. This consists of three layers. The outer two are continuous with the muscle layers of the oesophagus and duodenum, the inner layer is peculiar to the stomach [FIG. 136].

The **outer layer** is of longitudinal muscle and is found principally at the curvatures, but is very thin or absent along the middle of each surface. Some of its fibres turn into the circular layer at the pyloric sphincter, and may help to open the pylorus.

The **middle layer** is a complete circular layer which gradually thickens in the pyloric canal and is accentuated at the pylorus to form the pyloric sphincter. This thickening ceases abruptly at the duodenum [FIG. 137].

The **inner layer** consists of oblique fibres which loop over the cardiac notch. The posterior fibres fan out into the fundus and body of the stomach, but a well developed ridge passes towards the pylorus on each side of the lesser curvature. The contraction of these fibres is believed to approximate the ridges of mucous membrane that lie deep to them and thus cut off a tubular part of the stomach along the lesser curvature through which fluids may pass directly to the pylorus.

DISSECTION. Cut longitudinally through the wall of the superior part of the duodenum close to the pylorus. Open the cut and examine the duodenal aspect of the pylorus. Split the pyloric wall longitudinally.

The **pyloric sphincter** bulges the mucous membrane into the pylorus and narrows the aperture in such a manner that, seen from the duodenal side, it appears as a small opening in the centre of a rounded knob.

DISSECTION. Turn the transverse colon and its mesentery upwards and examine the mesentery of the small intestine. Note its oblique attachment to the posterior abdominal wall in the infracolic compartment.

Pull the small intestine to the left, cut through the peritoneum forming the right layer of the mesentery along the line of attachment to the posterior abdominal wall, and stripping off this layer of the mesentery, expose the superior mesenteric vessels in its root and their branches and tributaries in the mesentery. Note and remove the numerous lymph nodes, and expose the complex mass of fine nerve filaments (superior mesenteric plexus) passing with the vessels.

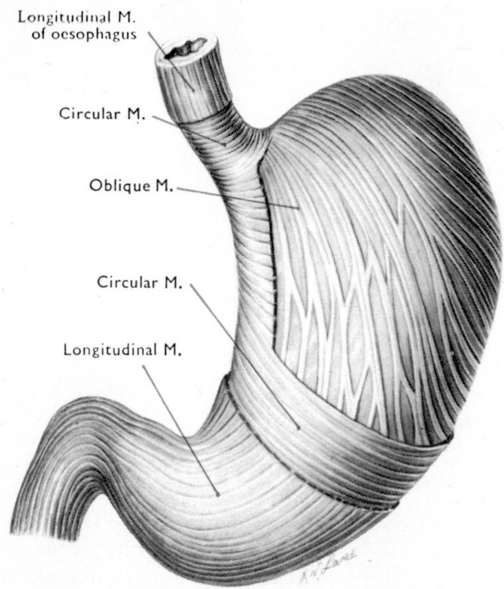

FIG. 136 A dissection of the muscle layers of the stomach.

Remove the peritoneum from the area between the root of the mesentery and the ascending and transverse parts of the colon. Clean the vessels so exposed [Figs. 138, 146] and note the lymph nodes and nerves associated with them.

THE MESENTERY

This is the fold of peritoneum and extraperitoneal tissue by which the jejunum and ileum are attached to the posterior abdominal wall. It is fan-shaped, for although its attachment to the posterior abdominal wall is only 15 cm. long, the free edge is folded to accommodate the whole length of the jejunum and ileum (up to 6 m.). The **attached margin,** with the superior mesenteric vessels in it, runs obliquely from the duodenojejunal flexure to the ileocaecal junction, and crosses the duodenum, the aorta and inferior vena cava, and the right psoas muscle with the testicular or ovarian vessels and ureter on its surface [FIG. 124].

In addition to extraperitoneal tissue and fat, *the* mesentery contains the jejunal and ileal blood vessels, large lacteal lymph vessels passing to the lymph nodes in and at the base of *the* mesentery, and a considerable plexus of sympathetic nerves.

Superior Mesenteric Artery

This large artery arises from the front of the aorta at the level of the first lumbar vertebra, 0·5 cm. inferior to the coeliac trunk, posterior to the body of the pancreas and the splenic vein. It descends anterior to the left renal vein, the uncinate process of the pancreas (q.v.), and the horizontal part of the duodenum, and runs in the root of *the* mesentery to the right iliac fossa. Here it terminates by anastomosing with a branch of the ileocolic artery near the end of the ileum.

Branches. The superior mesenteric artery supplies the intestine from the descending part of the duodenum to the transverse colon by a series of branches which anastomose freely with each other and with branches of the arteries supplying adjacent parts of the gut tube.

The **middle colic artery** [FIG. 138] arises at the lower border of the pancreas, and turning forwards into the transverse mesocolon, divides into right and left branches. These branch and anastomose with each other close to the transverse colon, thus forming part of a **marginal artery** which extends along the ascending,

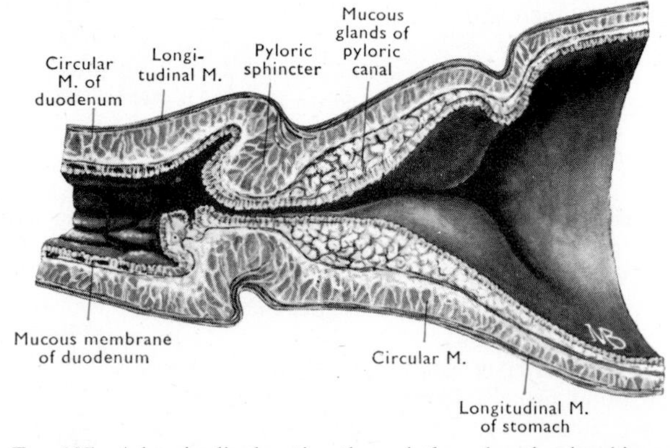

FIG. 137 A longitudinal section through the pyloroduodenal junction. Note the mass of mucous glands in the mucous membrane of the pyloric canal.

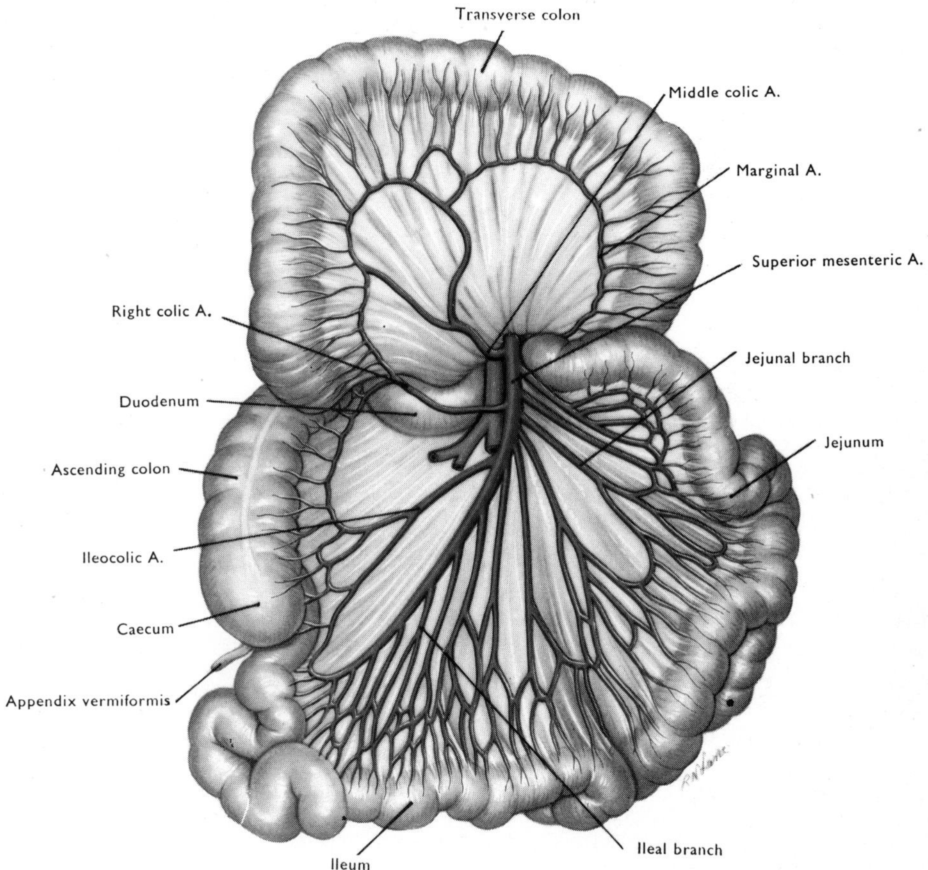

FIG. 138 The superior mesenteric artery and its branches.

transverse, and descending parts of the colon, and receives branches from the other colic arteries. Branches to the colon arise from the marginal artery, and through it the middle colic artery supplies most of the transverse colon.

The **inferior pancreaticoduodenal artery** arises from the superior mesenteric artery as it crosses the duodenum, and passes upwards and to the right between the duodenum and the pancreas. It sends branches to both, and anastomoses with the superior pancreatico-duodenai artery.

The **jejunal** and **ileal branches** enter *the* mesentery, branch and anastomose with each other to form a series of arterial arcades from which further branches form a second, and in the lower part of *the* mesentery, a third and even a fourth tier of arcades. The last arcades send branches to each side of the small intestine within which they branch and anastomose [FIG. 138].

The **right colic artery** passes across the structures on the posterior abdominal wall to join the marginal artery near the superior end of the ascending colon. The ascending branch of the ileocolic artery, which forms the beginning of the marginal artery, is enlarged when the right colic artery is absent.

The **ileocolic artery** arises with the right colic artery, and passing downwards and to the right, sends an ascending branch to the marginal artery, a descending branch which supplies the colon, caecum, appendix vermiformis, and the terminal part of the ileum, and anastomoses with the last ileal branch of the superior mesenteric artery. The **appendicular artery** enters the lowest part of *the* mesentery, and passing posterior to the terminal part of the ileum, enters the mesentery of the appendix [Fig. 143].

Superior Mesenteric Vein

This large vein lies immediately to the right of the superior mesenteric artery, but deviates from it superiorly to join the splenic vein and form the portal vein posterior to the pancreas. It drains blood from the territory of the artery, but receives the right gastro-epiploic vein and, occasionally, the inferior mesenteric and pancreaticoduodenal veins.

Lymph Nodes of the Mesentery

These nodes lie between the layers of *the* mesentery and are very numerous. Close to the intestine they are small (1 mm. or less) but gradually increase in diameter towards the root of *the* mesentery.

The **lymph vessels** of the small intestine are known as **lacteals** because they contain a milky white emulsion of fat (chyle) absorbed from the intestine during life. These vessels converge on and pass successively through the various lymph nodes of *the* mesentery. Those that issue from the large nodes in the root of *the* mesentery unite to form the **intestinal lymph trunk,** which passes to the cisterna chyli [Figs. 75, 176].

DISSECTION. Turn the mesentery and its small intestine to the right. Strip the peritoneum from the posterior abdominal wall between it and the descending colon. Carefully remove the fat and clean the exposed structures, including the sympathetic nerves and lymph nodes associated with the vessels [Fig. 146].

Inferior Mesenteric Artery

This artery supplies the intestine from the left part of the transverse colon to the inferior part of the rectum. It arises from the front of the aorta posterior to the horizontal part of the duodenum. It descends, surrounded by the inferior mesenteric plexus of nerves, on the left of the aorta and posterior to the peritoneum, and divides into sigmoid and superior rectal arteries anterior to the middle of the left common iliac artery.

Branches [Fig. 139]. Arteries that cross the posterior abdominal wall behind the peritoneum to supply the gut tube, do so because of fusion of their mesenteries with that wall. All of them, therefore, lie anterior to the posterior abdominal wall, and to the kidneys, ureters, and gonadal vessels which lie on it.

The **left colic artery** arises a short distance below the duodenum, and passing to the left, divides into ascending and descending branches which form part of the **marginal artery**. The ascending branch crosses the lower pole of the left kidney, and anastomosing with the middle colic artery, supplies the end of the transverse colon and the left flexure. The descending branch supplies the descending colon and anastomoses with the sigmoid arteries.

The **sigmoid arteries** are two or more vessels which pass inferiorly and to the left, and branching, anastomose with each other and with the descending branch of the left colic artery to continue the marginal artery. They supply the descending colon in the left iliac fossa and the sigmoid colon.

The lowest sigmoid artery also sends a branch to anastomose with the superior rectal artery, but this is smaller than the other anastomoses and is not adequate to maintain the blood supply to the rectum if the superior rectal artery is tied at operation.

The superior rectal artery will be seen in the pelvis.

Inferior Mesenteric Vein [Fig. 146]

This vein is the continuation of the superior rectal vein. It ascends lateral to the inferior mesenteric artery, and receives tributaries corresponding to the branches of the artery which pass either anterior or posterior to it.

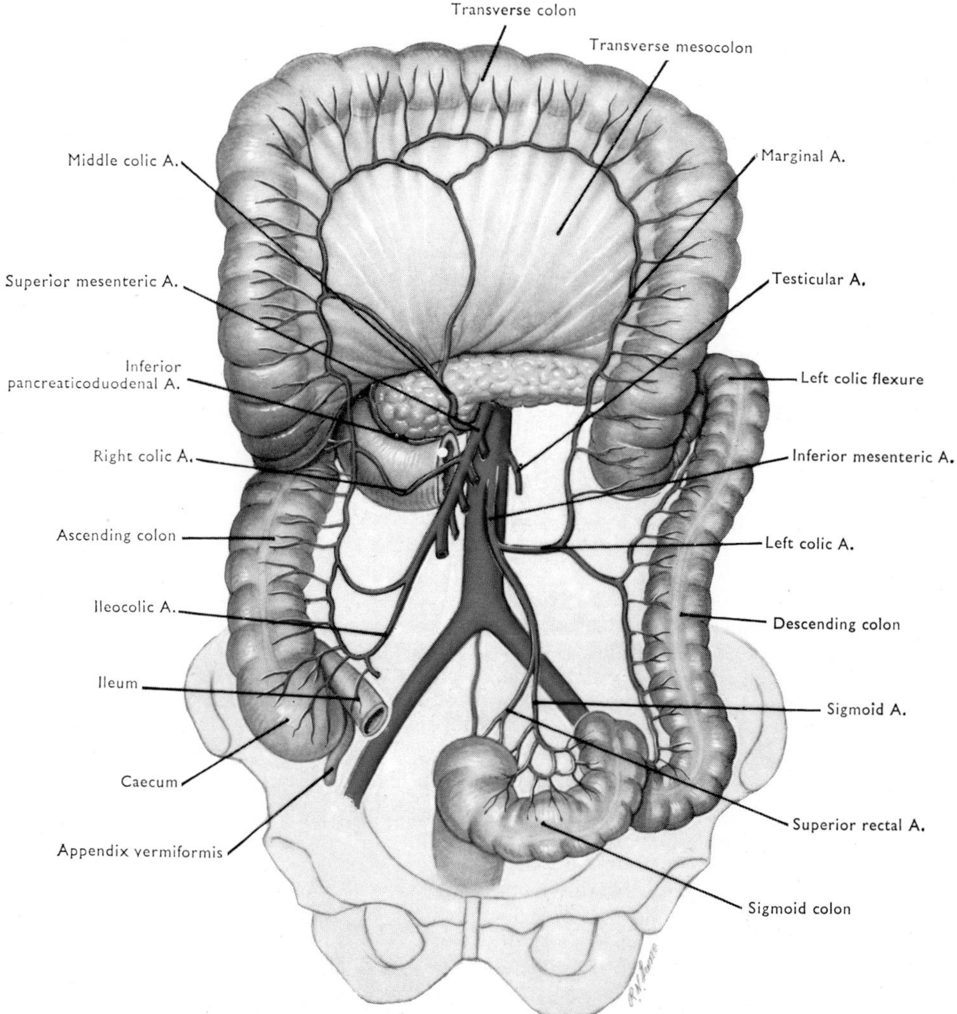

FIG. 139 The branches of the superior and inferior mesenteric arteries to the large intestine. Usually there is more than one sigmoid artery

The vein then passes lateral to the duodeno-jejunal flexure and anterior to the left renal vein, to enter the splenic vein posterior to the pancreas. It may deviate to the right and pass posterior to the horizontal part of the duodenum to enter either the superior mesenteric vein or its junction with the splenic vein.

Arterial Anastomoses on Gastro-intestinal Tract

Each of the three vessels that supply the gut tube in the abdomen (coeliac trunk, superior and inferior mesenteric arteries) give branches which anastomose with each other and with the artery or arteries supplying the adjoining territories. Thus there are anastomoses between the two pancreaticoduodenal arteries (coeliac trunk and superior mesenteric), and between the middle and left colic arteries (superior and inferior mesenteric). In addition the branches of the middle and left colic arteries anastomose with the gastro-epiploic arteries in the greater omentum. Thus blockage of a single vessel or even of a group of vessels is not followed by degeneration of any part of the intestine. If a loop of intestine is compressed at the neck of a hernial sac or twisted upon itself (volvulus) none of the anastomoses can be effective, and death of the intestinal loop with rupture of its wall will follow unless the condition is treated.

Abdominal Aortic Plexus

This consists of two or three intercommunicating strands of nerve fibres which descend over each side of the abdominal aorta. They arise in the coeliac and superior mesenteric plexuses (q.v.), and are reinforced by three or four branches from each lumbar sympathetic trunk **(lumbar splanchnic nerves)**. These descend obliquely at the sides of the aorta, and forming a single cord, unite with the lowest part of the plexus. The plexus gives extensions on to all the branches of the abdominal aorta below the superior mesenteric artery. Below the bifurcation of the aorta, it forms a single plexus on the front of the fifth lumbar vertebra and the left common iliac vein, the **superior hypogastric plexus** (presacral nerve). On the sacral promontory, this plexus divides into right and left **inferior hypogastric** (pelvic) **plexuses,** which pass to surround the corresponding internal iliac arteries, and are distributed with its branches to the pelvic viscera.

Structure of Small Intestine

The small intestine has the same four layers as the stomach.

The outer, peritoneal or **serous layer** is tightly bound to the muscular layer by a thin but tough layer of extraperitoneal tissue.

The **muscular layer** consists of a complete outer, longitudinal layer, and an inner, thicker, circular layer of smooth muscle. It is sometimes stated that both these layers are spirally arranged, but this cannot be determined with certainty in a sheet of small, spindle-shaped muscle fibres. The layers are separated by a little connective tissue in which lies a plexus of nerve cells and fibres, the **myenteric plexus.** This is responsible for the contraction of the muscle layers which together produce a peristaltic wave.

The **submucous layer** consists of areolar tissue containing blood vessels and the **submucous plexus** of nerve cells and fibres.

The **mucous layer** is very different from that in the stomach. The functions of the small intestine are to complete digestion and to absorb from the fluid, digested contents. The maximum area for absorption is achieved by three structural arrangements.

1. There are permanent, circular **folds** of the whole thickness of the mucous membrane, including the muscularis mucosae [Figs. 140, 142].

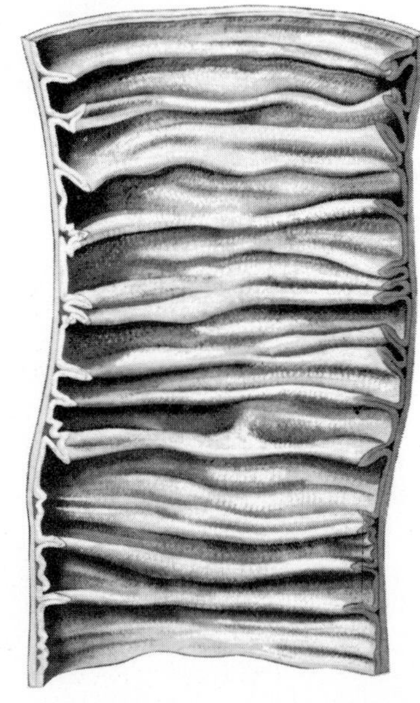

Fig. 140 A part of the interior of the jejunum to show the numerous circular folds of its lining.

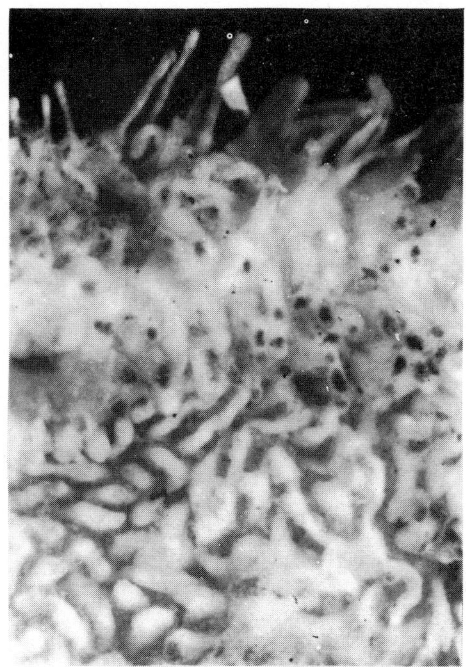

FIG. 141 A photograph of the surface of the mucous membrane of the human duodenum. Note the long villi which project from the entire surface, but which are only clearly seen at the edge.

2. The internal surface is covered with minute leaf-shaped or finger-shaped projections (**villi,** 0·5 mm. or less in length) which are visible with a hand lens and give the surface of the mucous membrane a velvety appearance. Each villus contains a fine mesh of reticular fibres and cells, a central lymph vessel (lacteal), a capillary loop, and some longitudinal muscle fibres which allow it to contract and relax; a function which may aid the discharge of lymph in the lacteal [FIG. 141].

3. The individual columnar cells which cover the villi as a single layer have a **brush border.** This consists of minute villous processes of the cell surface which are only clearly visible under the electron microscope, but greatly increase the surface which the cells present to the intestinal contents.

Between the villi are the **crypts.** These are simple tubular glands that dip into the mucous membrane and secrete digestive enzymes and mucus. In the upper part of the **duodenum** there are complex mucous glands which extend into the submucosa and open into the crypts. Their alkaline mucus plays an important part in the neutralization of the acid in the stomach contents delivered to the duodenum. Elsewhere the crypts are limited to the mucous membrane. The epithelial cells deep in the crypts show a high level of mitotic activity, and it has been shown by radioactive tracer techniques that the cells formed here are passed out of the crypts and over the surface of the villi, eventually to be shed from the tips of the villi. In this way the complete epithelial lining

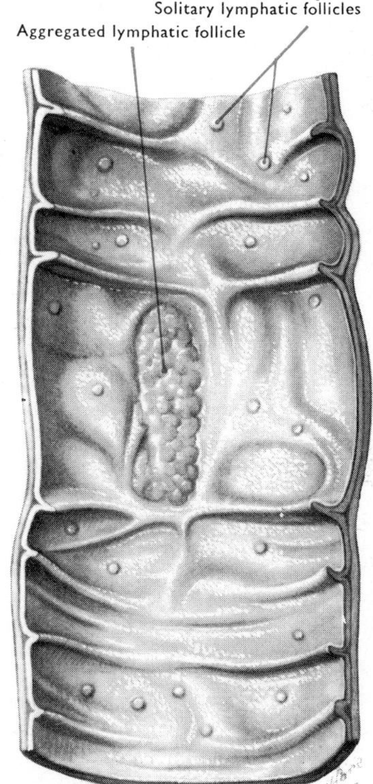

FIG. 142 The internal surface of part of the ileum for comparison with FIG. 140. Note the small, sparse, circular folds and the solitary and aggregated lymphatic follicles.

of the small intestine is replaced every two to four days.

In addition to the absorptive cells, many cells on the villi develop into **goblet cells.** These contain a central accumulation of mucus which is discharged into the lumen to protect the surface and reduce friction.

The mucous membrane also contains aggregations of **lymphoid tissue.** These may appear as solitary lymphatic follicles 1–2 mm. in diameter, but larger collections **(aggregated lymphatic follicles)** are occasionally found, especially on the antimesenteric wall of the ileum [FIG. 142].

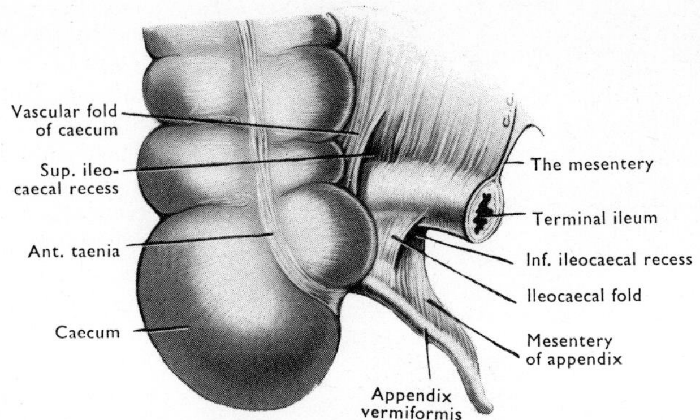

FIG. 143 The anterior surface of the ileocaecal region.

DISSECTION. Examine the jejunum and ileum. Note the greater diameter and thickness of the jejunum, the smaller amount of fat in its mesentery, and the fact that the lumen is usually empty.

Divide the jejunum close to the duodenojejunal flexure and the ileum close to the caecum, both between ligatures. Cut through the mesentery close to the intestine, remove the intestine and wash it out with water. Remove a few inches of the jejunum and open it longitudinally with scissors. Pin this out and remove the peritoneal coat to expose the longitudinal muscle layer. Next examine the mucosal surface. Note the folds of the mucous membrane and the fact that they are not removed by stretching the wall of the intestine. Identify the villi with a hand lens.

Strip the mucous membrane and submucosa from the wall of the intestine and identify the circular layer of muscle.

Open the whole length of the remaining part of the intestine and note the gradual change in structure of the mucous membrane along its length. The circular folds (which are largest and most numerous in the duodenum) become progressively smaller and less numerous, and are missing from the terminal ileum. There are more and larger villi in the jejunum than in the ileum, but the latter contains the aggregated lymphatic follicles. These are best seen in children, and when viewed by transmitted light. They are difficult to demonstrate in the aged where all the lymphoid tissues are atrophied.

THE LARGE INTESTINE

[FIGS. 118, 146, 147]

The large intestine extends from the right iliac fossa to the perineum, and surrounds the centrally placed small intestine. It is much shorter (1·5 m.) than the small intestine, and also decreases in diameter from the caecum to the descending colon, but all parts of it are capable of considerable distension.

The parts of the large intestine are: the caecum and vermiform appendix; the ascending, transverse and descending parts of the colon joined by the right and left flexures; the sigmoid colon; the rectum and anal canal.

CAECUM

This is the blind end of the large intestine in the right iliac fossa. It is approximately 5–7 cm. in length and width. Superiorly it joins the ascending colon and terminal ileum [FIG. 143].

It lies on the iliopsoas muscle and on the nerves (genitofemoral, femoral, and lateral cutaneous of thigh) and blood vessels (testicular or ovarian) on its surface, and frequently overlaps the external iliac artery.

It is a relatively mobile organ which may lie in the lesser pelvis. It is almost completely surrounded by peritoneum [FIG. 144], but is often attached to the peritoneum of the iliac fossa laterally and medially, thus isolating a wide, **retrocaecal, peritoneal recess** which may ascend posterior to the inferior part of the ascending colon, and which usually has the appendix vermiformis lying in it [FIG. 124]. Rarely the caecum may lie at the level of the

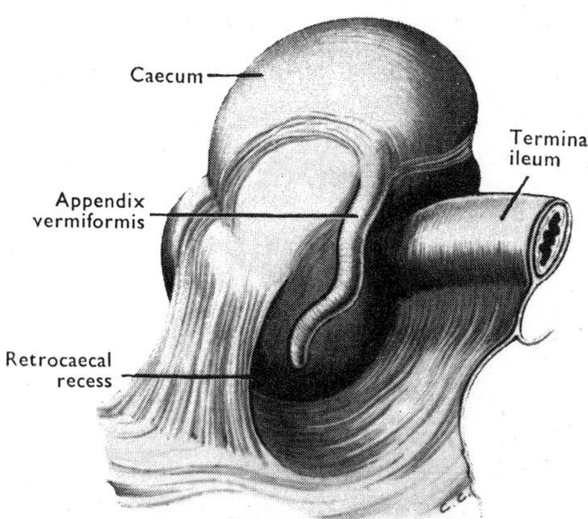

FIG. 144 The inferior surface of the ileocaecal region. The caecum has been pulled forwards to open the retrocaecal recess in which the appendix vermiformis commonly lies.

right colic flexure, in which case the ascending colon is absent.

Vermiform Appendix

The appendix is attached to the postero-medial surface of the caecum, 2–3 cm. infero-lateral to the ileocaecal junction. It is a blind tube of very variable length (5–15 cm., more or less) and about 5 mm. in diameter. It is attached by a small mesentery to the postero-inferior surface of *the* mesentery, and has no fixed position. Most commonly it lies in the retrocaecal recess, but it may extend into the lesser pelvis and lie close to the ovary and ureter [FIG. 146].

Structurally it has the same peritoneal and muscle coats as the small intestine, and the longitudinal coat is continuous at its base with the three taeniae of the caecum and colon, which diverge from it. The lumen is very narrow and is easily blocked by inflammation.

The mucous membrane consists mainly of **lymphatic follicles** lined by columnar epithelium which contains many goblet cells and forms crypts which pass between the follicles.

Vessels and Nerves. The caecum and appendix are supplied by branches of the ileocolic artery, that to the appendix passing into its mesentery posterior to the terminal ileum. Their **lymph vessels** pass to nodes in the mesentery of the appendix and scattered along the ileocolic artery up to the duodenum. The **nerves** pass along the branches of the ileocolic artery from the superior mesenteric plexus.

DISSECTION. Turn the caecum upwards and clean the structures posterior to it. Cut away the lateral wall of the caecum and examine the ileocaecal and appendicular orifices. Examine the relation of the terminal ileum to the caecum, and trace the three taeniae to the root of the appendix.

Ileocaecal Orifice. The ileocaecal orifice is very variable in appearance in the cadaver, mainly because of post-mortem changes and fixation. Normally the ileum enters obliquely through a horizontal slit guarded above and below by folds of the wall of the gut tube produced by the invagination of the ileum into the caecum (**ileocaecal valve**). The folds meet medially and laterally in single ridges, the **frenula of the valve** [FIG. 145]. The muscle in the human ileocaceal valve is poorly developed

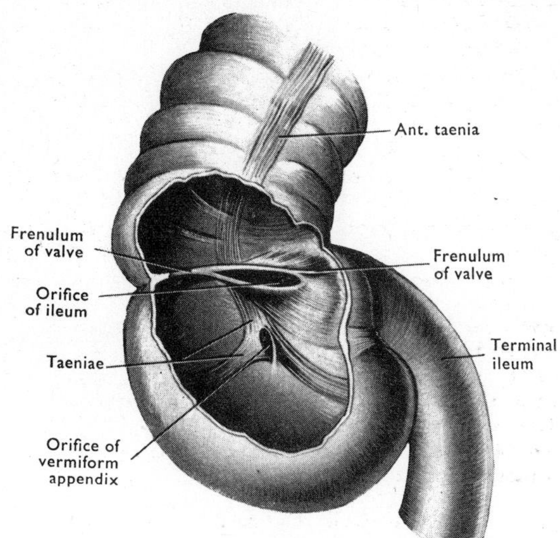

FIG. 145 A dried distended caecum opened to show the ileocaecal orifice and valve.

and probably plays little if any part in preventing the reflux of caecal contents into the ileum. Reflux is prevented mainly by the contraction of the circular muscle of the ileum, assisted by the fact that distension of the caecum tends to compress the obliquely entering ileum, and tightening the frenula, draws the lips of the valve together.

ASCENDING COLON

The ascending colon is 12–20 cm. long. It begins at the level of the entry of the ileum in the right iliac fossa, on the anterior surface of iliacus. It ascends over the iliac crest and quadratus lumborum in the paravertebral gutter, and crosses the **lateral cutaneous nerve of the thigh,** the **ilioinguinal,** and **iliohypogastric nerves.** It ends on the anterior surface of the inferior part of the right kidney, posterior to the liver. Here it turns sharply to the left, and forms the right flexure which is continuous with the transverse colon.

The peritoneum covers the front and sides of the ascending colon, and binds it to the posterior abdominal wall. Sometimes the peritoneum may surround it to form a short

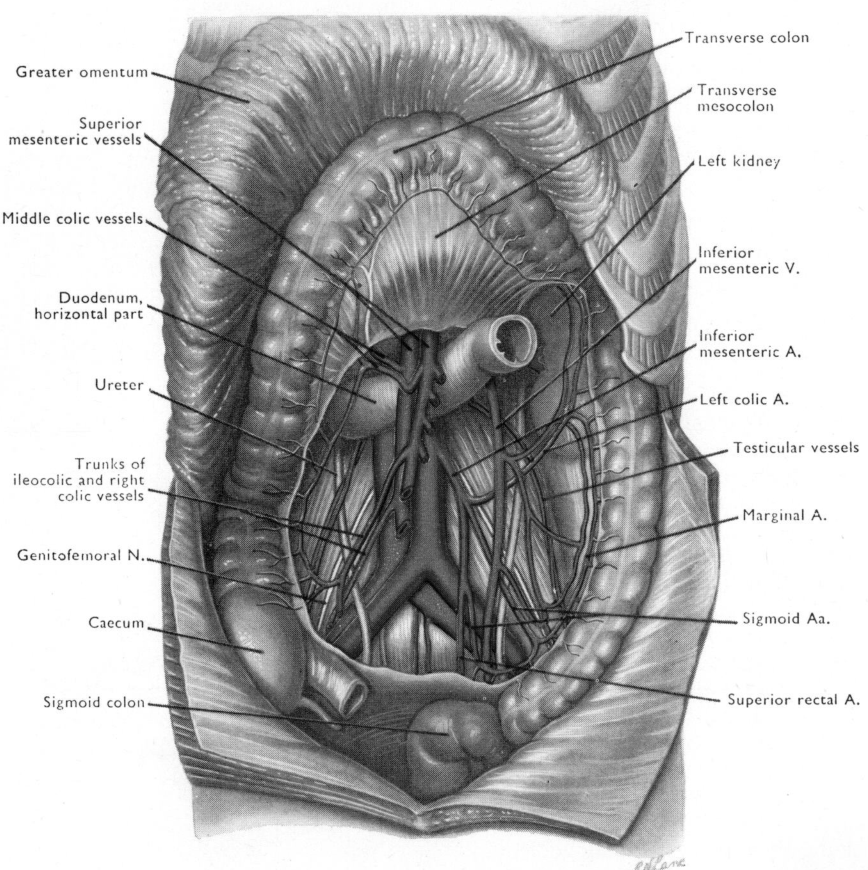

FIG. 146 Structures on the posterior wall of the infracolic compartment of the abdomen. The greater omentum and transverse colon are turned upwards, and the jejunum, ileum, *the* mesentery. and peritoneum covering the posterior wall are removed. See also FIGS. 118, 148, 175.

ascending mesocolon. The anterior abdominal wall is immediately in front of it, but the greater omentum and small intestine may intervene.

The **right flexure** is in direct contact with the right kidney posteriorly, but elsewhere is covered with peritoneum [FIG. 168]. The right lobe of the liver overlaps it anterosuperiorly and laterally.

Vessels and Nerves. The ascending colon and the right flexure are supplied by the **ileocolic** and **right colic arteries,** along which run the nerves from the superior mesenteric plexus. The **lymph vessels** end in nodes on the medial side of the colon and along its vessels.

TRANSVERSE COLON

This is usually the longest (40–50 cm.) and most mobile part of the colon. It begins at the right flexure, and suspended by the transverse mesocolon, arches across the abdomen with its convexity antero-inferiorly. It ends in the left flexure on the lateral margin of the left kidney, immediately inferior to the spleen. The lowest part of its convexity may reach well below the umbilicus in the erect position, but is usually immediately superior to it in the recumbent position. If the intestines are distended, it may be pushed superiorly either posterior or anterior to the stomach. In the latter case it may, if distended with gas, make the upper abdomen tympanitic to percussion and partly mask the dullness of the liver to percussion, thus mimicking the presence of gas in the peritoneal cavity.

The transverse colon is suspended by the transverse mesocolon behind the omental bursa [FIG. 123], and is fused to the posterior surface of the greater omentum except at its extremities where the mesocolon is short [FIG. 133]. The transverse colon begins anterior to, and sometimes directly in contact with, the

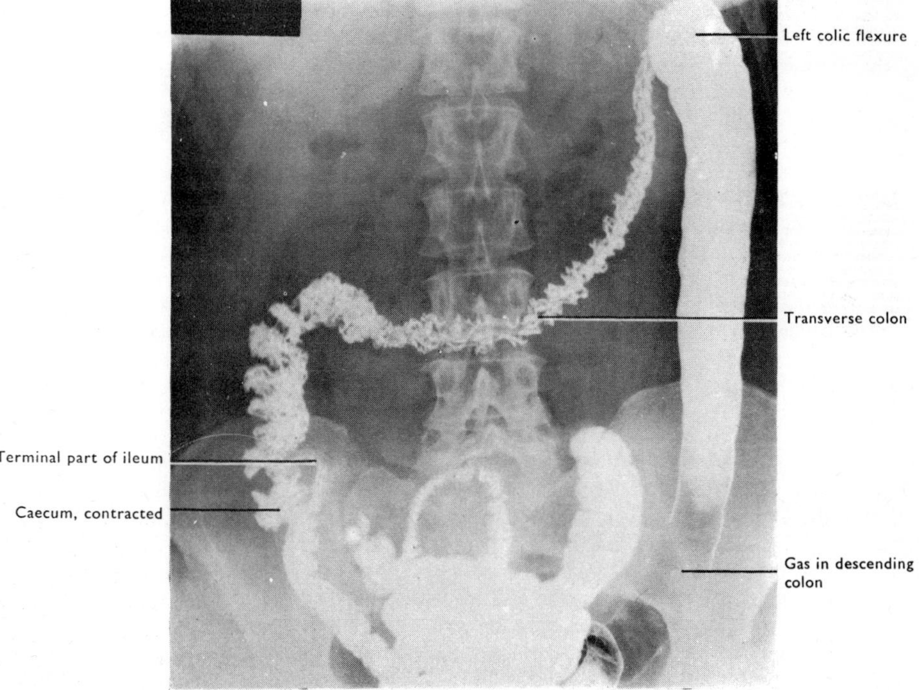

FIG. 147 A radiograph of the partially emptied colon outlined by barium introduced as an enema.

descending part of the duodenum and the head of the pancreas, and posterior to the liver and fundus of the gall-bladder. It then crosses anterior to the horizontal part of the duodenum and coils of the jejunum. On the left it extends up to the spleen, anterior to the left kidney and posterior to the greater curvature of the stomach or the left margin of the greater omentum.

The **transverse mesocolon** (mostly fused with the greater omentum) extends posterosuperiorly from the transverse colon to a linear attachment to the descending part of the duodenum, the head and lower margin of the body of the pancreas, and the anterior surface of the left kidney [Fig. 124]. It contains the middle colic vessels and branches of the left and right colic vessels with their accompanying nerves and lymph vessels. The latter enter nodes scattered along the vessels.

The **left flexure** lies at a slightly higher level, is more acute, and further lateral than the right flexure. It lies on the lateral margin of the left kidney [Fig. 168] and is attached to the diaphragm by peritoneum (**phrenicocolic ligament**) below the spleen. Occasionally it has a short mesentery.

Vessels and Nerves. The transverse colon is mainly supplied by the middle colic vessels, but its extremities and the corresponding flexures are supplied by the right and left colic vessels. The nerves accompany the arteries from the superior and inferior mesenteric plexuses. In addition to the sympathetic fibres which both plexuses contain, the former carries a number of vagal fibres, while the latter transmits pelvic parasympathetic fibres. The lymph nodes lie in the mesocolon along the blood vessels.

DESCENDING COLON

The descending colon (30 cm.) passes inferiorly from the left flexure to the margin of the superior aperture of the lesser pelvis. It is attached by peritoneum to the posterior abdominal wall in the left paravertebral gutter and iliac fossa. At first anterior to the diaphragm and lateral surface of the left kidney, it passes over transversus abdominis, quadratus lumborum, and the iliac crest, in front of the same nerves as the ascending colon [p. 154]. It then crosses the left iliac fossa to the anterior superior iliac spine, and turning medially, superior to the inguinal ligament, crosses iliacus, the testicular or ovarian vessels and the femoral nerve, psoas and the genitofemoral nerve, and joins the sigmoid colon anterior to the external iliac vessels [Fig. 146].

The pressure of the lowest part of the descending colon on the testicular and external iliac veins may partly account for the greater frequency of varicose veins in the spermatic cord and leg on the left side.

Vessels and Nerves. The blood supply is by the left colic and upper sigmoid branches of the inferior mesenteric vessels. These, together with the lymph vessels and nodes and the nerves which accompany them, lie anterior to the other structures of the posterior abdominal wall [Fig. 175].

DISSECTION. Divide the peritoneum along the lateral margin of the descending colon, and turn it medially. Clean the structures that lie posterior to it.

SIGMOID COLON

This part of the colon varies greatly in length (15–80 cm., usually approximately 30 cm.) and extends from the end of the descending colon to the pelvic surface of the third piece of the sacrum where it joins the rectum. When of normal length, it lies free in the lesser pelvis inferior to the small intestine, but when long it may lie in any part of the abdomen that the length of its mesentery (sigmoid mesocolon) allows.

The **sigmoid mesocolon** has a Λ-shaped attachment. It begins at the end of the descending colon and ascends on the external iliac vessels to the middle of the common iliac artery, then turns sharply downwards and to the right across the lesser pelvis to the third piece of the sacrum [Fig. 124]. Just lateral to the apex of the Λ, a pocket-like extension (the intersigmoid peritoneal recess) extends upwards, posterior to the root of the mesocolon, in front of the **ureter.** The **inferior mesenteric artery** divides near the apex of the Λ, and the **superior rectal artery** enters the right limb of the mesocolon, while the sigmoid arteries enter the left limb. Rarely the mesocolon begins at the iliac crest and runs directly to the third piece of the sacrum. In this case the sigmoid colon could be said to start at the iliac crest, where the blood supply by the sigmoid arteries begins.

Taeniae Coli

These are three ribbon-like thickenings of the otherwise thin layer of longitudinal muscle in the caecum and colon. They diverge from the longitudinal muscle of the appendix vermiformis, and end by spreading out on the terminal part of the sigmoid colon to become continuous with the longitudinal muscle of the rectum. They are uniformly spaced around the circumference of the colon, and the wall of the colon and caecum between them forms three rows of puckered pouches. In the ascending and descending colon the positions of the taeniae are anterior, posteromedial, and posterolateral, but in the transverse colon, which is turned down, the corresponding positions are posterior, superior and anterior.

Lymph Nodes of Large Intestine

Small nodes lie along the mesocolic border of the large intestine and on the blood vessels passing to it. The lymph from the territory supplied by branches of the superior mesenteric artery passes through these nodes to the intestinal trunk in the root of *the* mesentery, while that from the territory of the inferior mesenteric artery drains to the lumbar lymph nodes beside the aorta. Both reach the cisterna chyli [Fig. 176].

DISSECTION. Divide the colon between ligatures at the junction of the descending and sigmoid parts. Remove the caecum and colon in one piece, dividing the blood vessels close to them.

Wash out the colon, examine its external surface, and open it longitudinally. Cut a transverse section through the appendix, and examine the cut surface with a hand lens.

Structure of Large Intestine

The same four layers are present as in the stomach and small intestine.

The **serous layer** of peritoneum is firmly bound to the muscle, and is complete except in the ascending and descending colon and the upper part of the rectum, which are applied to the abdominal and pelvic walls. The inferior third of the rectum has no contact with the peritoneum.

The **appendices epiploicae** are small pouches of peritoneum filled with fat. These project from all parts except the caecum, appendix, and rectum, and are most numerous on the sides of the sigmoid colon and the posterior surface of the transverse colon.

The **muscular layers** consists of a thin, outer, longitudinal layer in which lie the taeniae coli. This layer is uniform and thick in the appendix, rectum, and anal canal. The internal, circular layer is nearly uniform, but is thickened between the sacculations, and especially where it forms the **internal sphincter of the anus.**

The **submucous layer** does not differ significantly from that of the ileum.

The **mucous layer** is arranged in a number of crescentic folds which increase the surface area for absorption. It consists of numerous simple tubular glands (crypts) united by a very delicate connective tissue which is permeated by large numbers of cells of the lymphocyte series. These are so placed as to come into immediate contact with bacteria which may enter through abrasions of the epithelium. (The contents of the large intestine, unlike those of the upper part of the small intestine, contain large numbers of bacteria.) Many small, solitary lymphatic follicles bulge the mucous membrane, but neither villi nor aggregated lymphatic follicles are present.

The vermiform appendix has complete muscle layers, a minute lumen, and numerous lymphatic follicles which make up the greater part of the mucous membrane. The muscularis mucosae is poorly developed.

DISSECTION. Clean the anterior surface of the pancreas, and trace the duodenum from the pylorus to the duodenojejunal flexure.

DUODENUM

This is the widest and most fixed part of the small intestine It is approximately 25 cm. long, and forms a C-shaped curve, the concavity of which faces upwards and to the left and is filled by the pancreas. The duodenum passes posterior to the transverse mesocolon, and therefore connects the supracolic and infracolic parts of the gut tube. It lies astride the vertebral column, and extends posteriorly on to the medial aspect of the right kidney in the paravertebral gutter [FIGS. 124, 168].

The **superior part** of the duodenum passes upwards and backwards from the pylorus. It lies superior to the pancreas, passes anterior to the portal vein (with the gastroduodenal artery and bile-duct between them), and then crosses the right sides of the portal vein and inferior vena cava. It lies posterior to the quadrate lobe of the liver, and ascends to the level of the neck of the gall-bladder where it turns sharply downwards to form the descending part. The superior part is approximately 5 cm. long but appears much shorter (duodenal cap) in an anteroposterior radiograph

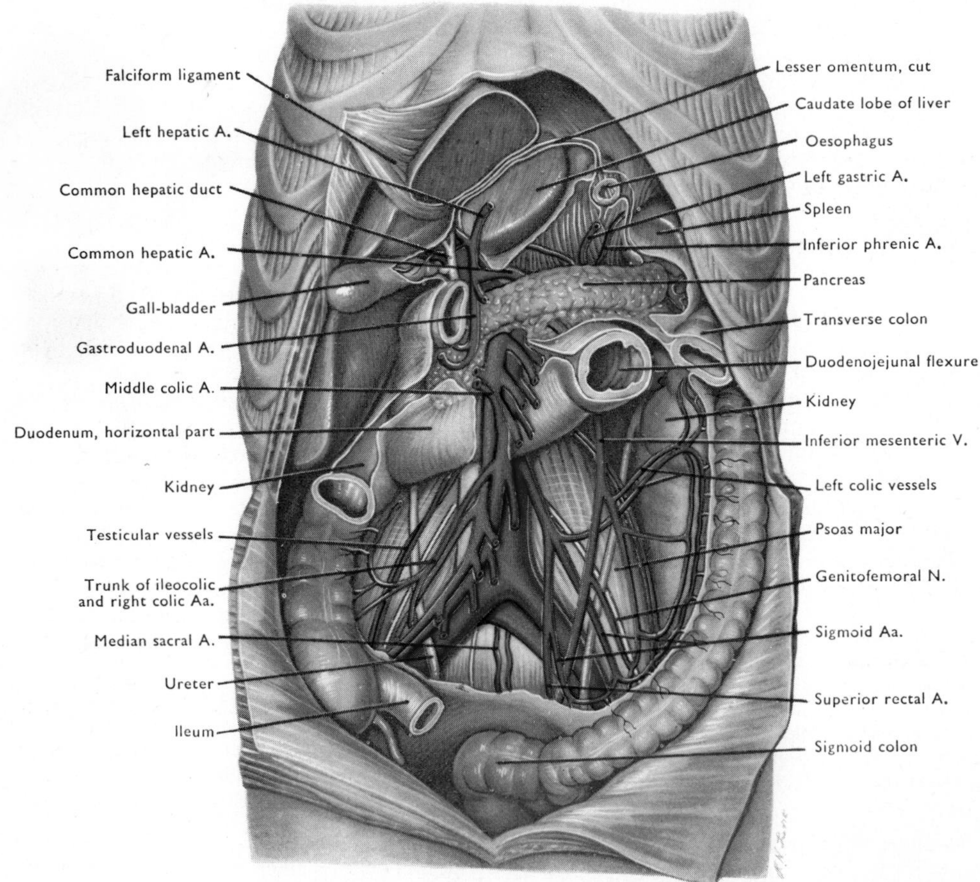

FIG. 148 Structures on the posterior abdominal wall.

[FIG. 132] because of its oblique direction. The first half is enclosed in the peritoneum of the lesser and greater omenta, and lying anterior to the right extremity of the omental bursa, is free to move with the stomach. The second half is adherent to the structures on its medial side.

The **descending part** is 8 cm. long, has no mesentery, but lies directly on the medial part of the right kidney and psoas major (anterior to the renal vessels and ureter) down to the level of the third lumbar vertebra.

At first posterior to the liver and gall-bladder, it passes behind the beginning of the transverse colon, and is covered by part of the jejunum in the infracolic compartment [FIG. 133].

Medially it is applied to the head of the pancreas, and the bile- and pancreatic ducts enter its posteromedial aspect slightly inferior to the middle [FIG. 153].

The **horizontal part,** also adherent to the posterior abdominal wall, is nearly 10 cm. long. It lies almost at right angles to the descending part, and passes to the left, inferior to the pancreas and anterior to the vertebral column, the psoas major muscle, and the structures lying on them (*i.e.*, the right ureter, testicular or ovarian artery, inferior vena cava, and the aorta with the inferior mesenteric artery arising from it). The anterior and inferior surfaces are covered with peritoneum except where the root of *the* mesentery and the contained superior mesenteric vessels cross it anteriorly [FIG. 146].

The **ascending part** passes upwards to the left of the aorta and the head of the pancreas on to the left psoas major, and bends anteriorly to form the duodenojejunal flexure 2–3 cm. to the left of the median plane at the level of the second lumbar vertebra. It, therefore, crosses the sympathetic trunk and testicular or ovarian artery on the left [FIG. 146].

The position of the duodenum is variable. The first half of the superior part is highly mobile. The horizontal part may ascend to the duodenojejunal flexure without a recognizable ascending part, and the entire duodenum may lie at a higher or lower level.

Vessels and Nerves. The superior part receives small branches from the hepatic (supraduodenal), right gastric, right gastro-epiploic, and gastroduodenal (retroduodenal) arteries. In most cases these are small, anastomose poorly with each other, and are said not to anastomose across the pylorus with the gastric vessels. The remainder of the duodenum is supplied by the superior and inferior **pancreaticoduodenal arteries.** These anastomose with each other and form arcades anterior and posterior to the head of the pancreas on the duodenum.

The **lymph vessels** drain to nodes that lie between the duodenum and pancreas. These send efferent vessels to nodes around the origin of the coeliac trunk and the superior mesenteric artery. The **nerves** reach the duodenum on the arteries, and originate in the coeliac and superior mesenteric plexuses.

DISSECTION. Divide the peritoneum along the convex surface of the duodenum, and turn the duodenum on to the anterior surface of the pancreas. Clean the structures thus exposed.

Replace the duodenum, and separating the ascending part from the pancreas, remove the fat between them. This exposes the inferior mesenteric vein and part of the left renal vein. Posterior to these is a slender fibromuscular band which passes from the right crus of the diaphragm to the duodenojejunal flexure (the suspensory muscle of the duodenum).

The **suspensory muscle of the duodenum** arises from the diaphragm on both sides of the oesophageal orifice [FIG. 174], and descending on the anterior surface of the left crus of the diaphragm, is attached to the duodenojejunal flexure. It is easily demonstrated in the child, but becomes a loose ligamentous structure which is difficult to identify in the adult.

DISSECTION. Open the entire length of the duodenum by cutting along its convex surface. Clean the interior with a sponge.

Structure of Duodenum

The duodenum has the same four layers as the other parts of the intestine.

The **serous,** peritoneal layer is incomplete except in the first 2–3 cm.

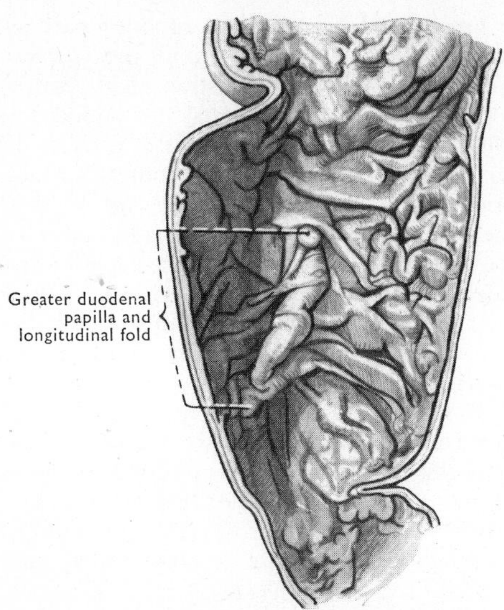

FIG. 149 The internal surface of the posterior wall of the descending part of the duodenum. The greater duodenal papilla lies at the upper end of a longitudinal fold, and is hooded by a circular fold.

The **muscular layer** is arranged in the same way as that in the rest of the small intestine.

The **submucous layer** is thick and contains compound, mucous, **duodenal glands.** These are present in the proximal third of the duodenum, but disappear progressively in the distal two thirds, though a few may be found in the proximal jejunum. Their ducts pierce the muscularis mucosae and enter the duodenal crypts. If the serous and muscle layers are carefully removed from a small area of the duodenum, the duodenal glands will be seen as small, reddish-grey bodies approximately 1 mm. in diameter. These glands are known to secrete an alkaline mucus, but there may be other constituents.

The **mucous layer** is similar to that of the jejunum, but the villi are short and broad. The **circular folds** begin approximately 2 cm. from the pylorus. At first small and irregular, they become large and numerous further distally. On the posteromedial wall of the descending part, note a longitudinal fold which ends superiorly in the **greater duodenal papilla** frequently hidden by a circular fold [FIG. 149]. On the summit of the papilla is the common opening of the bile and pancreatic ducts. The papilla and longitudinal fold are variable, and the former may be difficult to find if the latter is poorly marked; their position can be confirmed when the bile-duct is traced to the duodenum.

Superior and anterior to the greater papilla, the **lesser duodenal papilla** may be found where the accessory pancreatic duct enters the descending part of the duodenum.

DISSECTION. Lift the tail of the pancreas from the spleen, and ease the body from the posterior abdominal wall. Identify the splenic vein on the posterior surface of the pancreas, and trace it to the superior mesenteric vein. Follow the inferior mesenteric vein to its termination posterior to the pancreas, and the superior mesenteric vessels as they pass upwards anterior to the uncinate process of the pancreas and posterior to the junction of its body and head. Free the horizontal part of the duodenum and the uncinate process from the posterior abdominal wall.

Trace the portal vein downwards to its junction with the superior mesenteric vein, posterior to the pancreas.

PORTAL VEIN
[FIG. 150]

This vein drains the abdominal part of the alimentary canal (except the lowest part of the rectum and anal canal), the spleen, pancreas, and gall-bladder. It enters the porta hepatis, and is peculiar in that it breaks up into branches which discharge their blood into the sinusoids of the liver where it is only separated from the liver cells by a single layer of phagocytic endothelial cells. The portal vein carries the products of digestion of carbohydrates and proteins (fats are mostly transported through the lacteals to the thoracic duct) to the liver, and contains in its various tributaries and branches up to one third of the total volume of blood in the body.

The portal vein begins posterior to the junction of the body and head of the pancreas by the union of the splenic and superior mesenteric veins. It ascends posterior to the superior part of the duodenum, where it is joined by a **pancreaticoduodenal vein,**

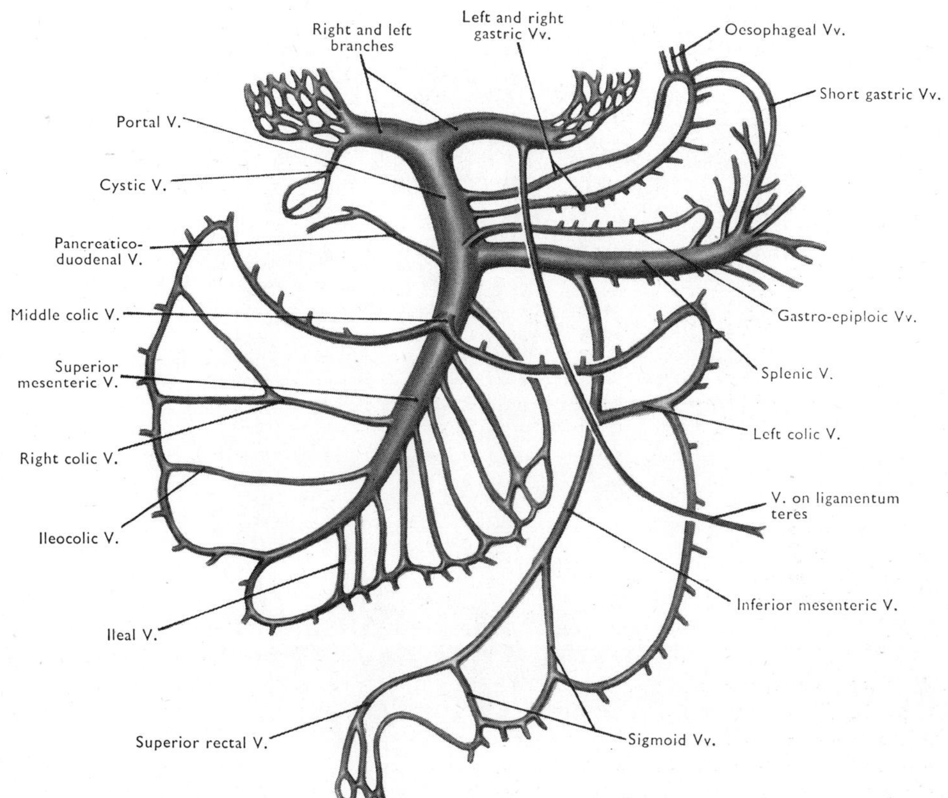

FIG. 150 A diagram of the portal venous system.

and passing anteriorly, receives the right and left **gastric veins** as it enters the free edge of the lesser omentum, through which it passes to the porta hepatis. Here it divides into right and left branches. The **right branch** receives the cystic vein from the gall-bladder and enters the right lobe of the liver. The **left branch** passes to the left end of the porta hepatis, unites with the **ligamentum teres** and the **ligamentum venosum,** and enters the left lobe of the liver. The left branch is united to the umbilicus both by the ligamentum teres and by some small **para-umbilical veins** which pass along the ligament.

Throughout its length the portal vein lies anterior to the **inferior vena cava,** though separated from it in the free edge of the lesser omentum by the epiploic foramen. From the superior part of the duodenum upwards, the bile-duct and first the gastroduodenal artery and later the hepatic artery lie anterior to it.

Communications. The portal vein [FIG. 152] communicates with the **systemic venous system:** (1) at the gastro-oesophageal junction through the oesophageal veins; (2) at the umbilicus through the para-umbilical veins; and (3) in the rectum through the superior rectal vein. In obstruction of the portal vein these communications may be greatly enlarged, and bleeding may occur from the distended submucous venous plexuses in the lower oesophagus.

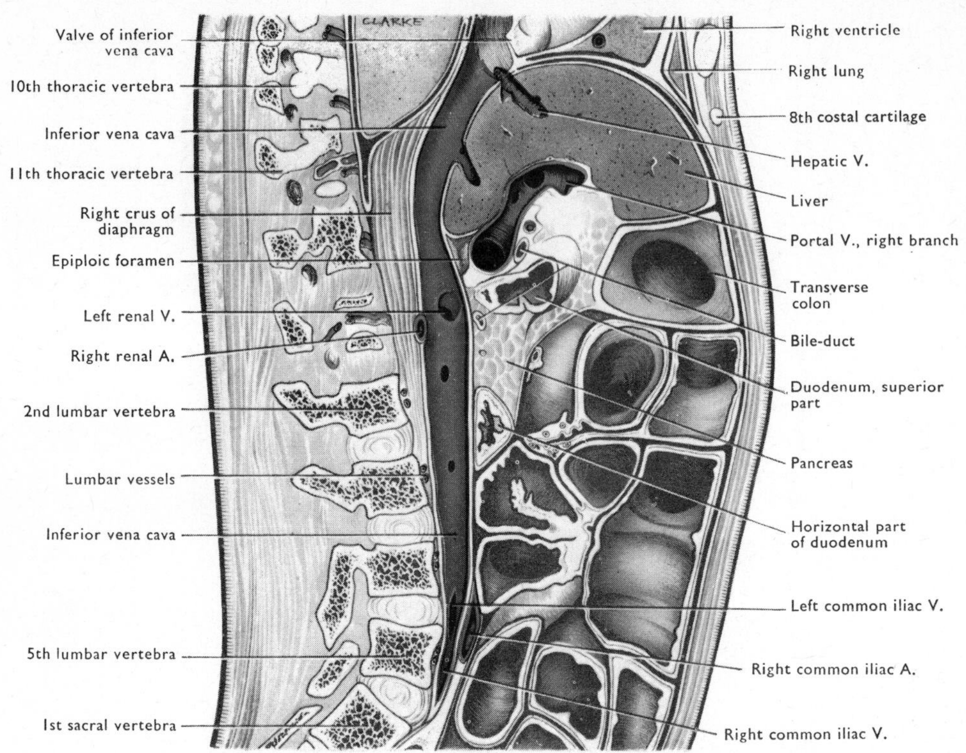

FIG. 151 A sagittal section through the abdomen along the inferior vena cava.

The back pressure on the splenic vein usually causes considerable enlargement of the spleen.

Splenic Vein

This vein is formed by five or six tributaries which emerge from the hilus of the spleen. It passes to the right on the posterior surface of the pancreas, at first in the lienorenal ligament and then anterior to the left kidney, left psoas, left crus of the diaphragm, and aorta, the latter between the origins of the superior mesenteric artery and the coeliac trunk. It ends by joining the superior mesenteric vein anterior to the inferior vena cava.

Tributaries. In addition to those from the spleen, it receives veins corresponding to the branches of the splenic artery (short gastric, left gastro-epiploic, and small pancreatic veins) and the inferior mesenteric vein which usually joins it in its last 5 cm.

DISSECTION. Turn the descending part of the duodenum and the head of the pancreas to the left, and look for a pancreaticoduodenal vein and the bile-duct on the posterior surface of the pancreas. The vein runs to the portal vein on the medial side of the bile-duct which lies in a groove on the posterior surface of the head of the pancreas. Trace the bile-duct inferiorly from the lesser omentum, and find its union with the pancreatic duct close to the duodenum. Clean the structures posterior to the head of the pancreas.

DUCTS OF LIVER

The liver is formed as a branching, hollow outgrowth of the epithelial lining of the duodenum, and its cavity forms the system of bile-

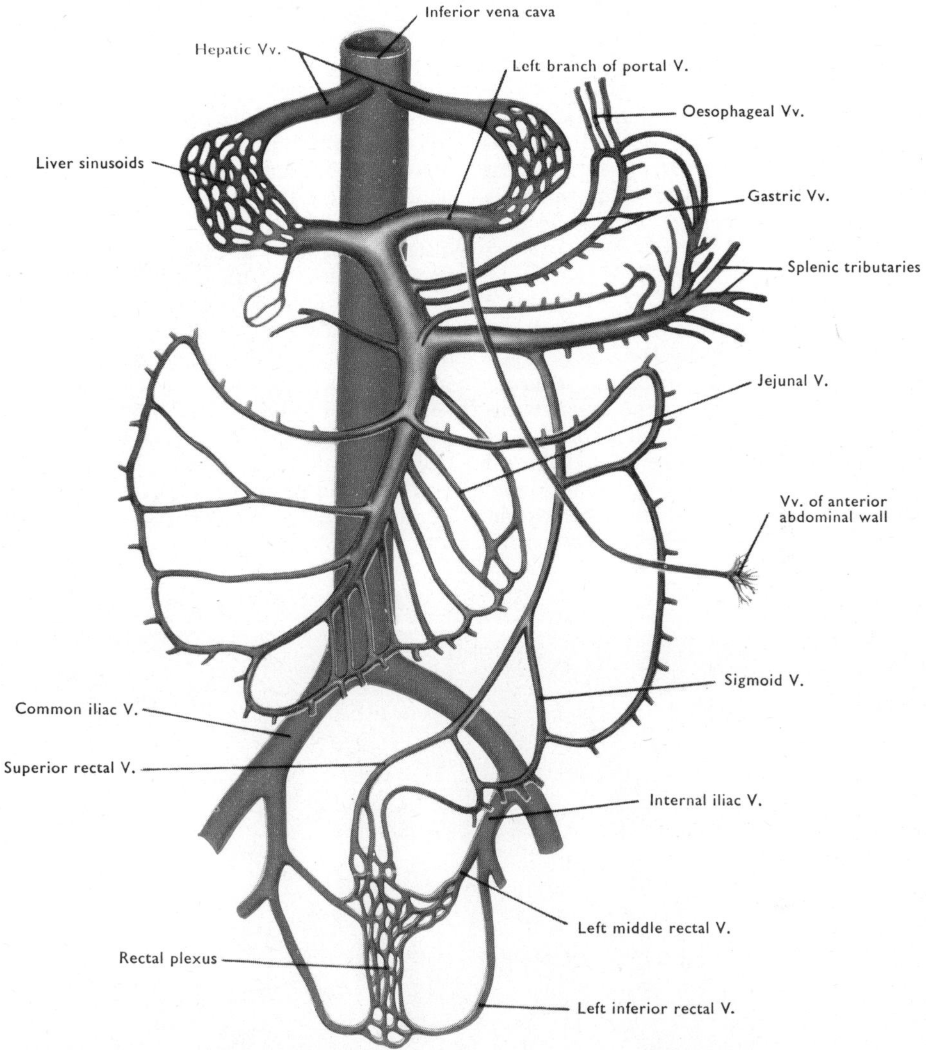

FIG. 152 A diagram of the portal venous system (grey) to show its anastomoses with the systemic venous system (blue).

ducts which drains into the duodenum. The terminal branches (consisting of a double row of cells with a minute extension of the cavity, the **bile canaliculus,** between them) form the substance of the liver, and each is surrounded by the blood sinusoids into which the portal vein and hepatic arteries discharge. The canaliculi join to form interlobular ductules. These unite and emerge from the porta hepatis as the right and left **hepatic ducts,** which join to form the **common hepatic duct** almost immediately. The common hepatic duct is directly continuous with the bile-duct where the **cystic duct** from the gall-bladder (a blind diverticulum of the biliary system) unites with it.

Bile produced in the liver thus flows either directly to the duodenum, or into the gall-bladder when the sphincter of the bile-duct (which lies at the entry into the duodenum) is closed. Bile is concentrated within the gall-bladder.

Bile-duct [FIG. 160]

This duct is approximately 10 cm. long and 0·5 cm. wide. It begins by the union of the cystic and common hepatic ducts, and descending through the free edge of the lesser omentum, passes posterior to the superior part of the duodenum, anterior to the portal vein and lateral to the hepatic and gastro-duodenal arteries. It then deviates slightly to the right in a groove on the posterior surface of the head of the pancreas, and enters the postero-medial surface of the descending part of the duodenum a little inferior to its middle.

The duct passes obliquely through the duodenal wall, expanding to form the **ampulla** [FIG. 154] which bulges the mucous membrane of the duodenum inwards (the duodenal papilla) where the duct pierces it. The **pancreatic duct** runs with the bile-duct for a short distance and joins it either before or during its passage through the duodenal wall. Here a **sphincter** of circular muscle controls the release of bile and pancreatic secretions into the duodenum. The strongest part of the sphincter surrounds the bile-duct alone, and lies proximal to the ampulla and the junction with the pancreatic duct. When this contracts, bile passes along the cystic duct to the gall-bladder, but does not enter the pancreatic duct. The remainder of the bile-duct contains very little muscle.

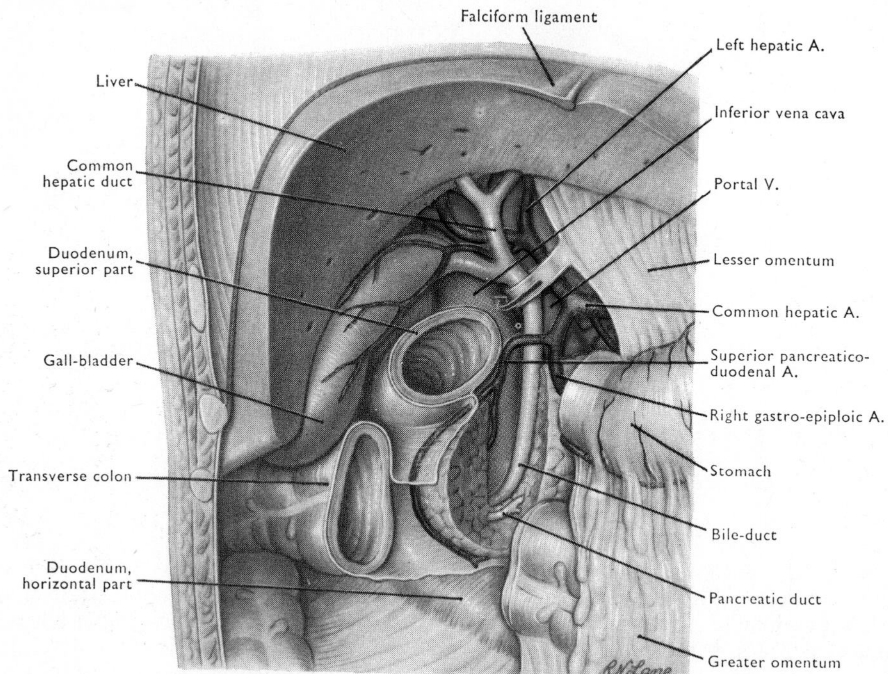

FIG. 153 A dissection to show the extrahepatic biliary system. The arrow indicates the epiploic foramen.

The point of junction of the cystic and common hepatic ducts is very variable, but is usually close to the porta hepatis. The arrangement of the bile- and pancreatic ducts is also variable, and they commonly do not join but open together on the duodenal papilla [FIG. 155].

DISSECTION. Remove the spleen, pancreas, and duodenum from the abdomen in one piece. Lift the spleen forwards, dividing the left wall of the lienorenal ligament, and strip the pancreas from the posterior abdominal wall, dividing: (1) the inferior mesenteric vein at its junction with the splenic vein; (2) the splenic and superior mesenteric arteries 1–2 cm. from their origins, and the superior mesenteric vessels at the lower border of the duodenum; and (3) the gastroduodenal artery, bile-duct, and portal vein at the upper border of the duodenum. Clean the structures posterior to the pancreas, and study the pancreas in the block of tissue removed.

PANCREAS

This elongated gland lies across the upper part of the posterior abdominal wall from an expanded head, lying in the concavity of the duodenum, to a blunt tail which often reaches the spleen. The transverse mesocolon is attached to the pancreas which is, therefore, at the junction of the supracolic and infracolic compartments of the peritoneal cavity. It is a compound gland that secretes into the duodenum a considerable number of different enzymes that break down proteins, starches, and fats in alkaline conditions. The gland also contains minute islands (**islets**) of cells which are not connected with the duct system, but secrete insulin and glucagon directly into the blood stream for the control of the blood sugar level, etc.

The gland consists of lobules of secretory tissue held loosely together by delicate areolar tissue, and is very pliable in life.

The **head** lies in the concavity of the duodenum (overlapping the descending and horizontal parts), and is anterior to the inferior vena cava [FIG. 151], to the bile-duct (in a groove on the superolateral part), and to the aorta where the inferomedial part (**uncinate process**) extends posterior to the superior

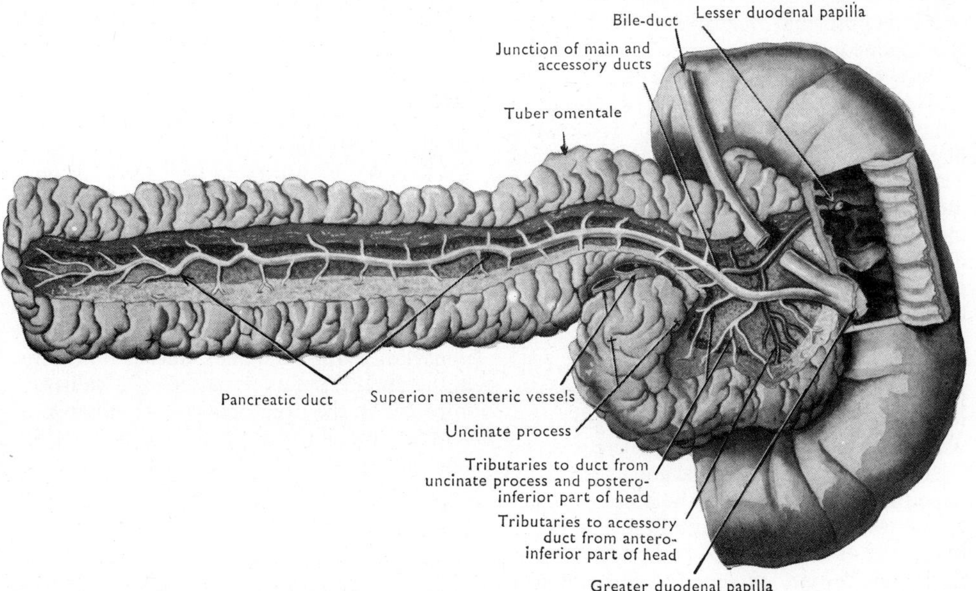

FIG. 154 A dissection of the posterior surface of the pancreas to show its ducts.

mesenteric vessels. The head is covered anteriorly by the transverse colon or its mesentery, and superiorly by the first 2–3 cm. of the duodenum where the head of the pancreas joins the body, anterior to the portal vine.

The **body** passes to the left across the aorta (anterior to the origin of the superior mesenteric artery), left crus of the diaphragm, psoas major, the left renal vessels and kidney [Fig. 115]. It lies posterior to the omental bursa and stomach, but anterior to the aorta it is in contact with the lesser omentum (**tuber omentale**) immediately inferior to the coeliac trunk. The splenic artery runs a sinuous course along its upper margin, while the splenic vein lies on its posterior surface and is joined by the inferior and superior mesenteric veins.

The **tail** of the pancreas is the blunt, terminal part of the body. It lies in the lienorenal ligament and may touch the hilus of the spleen [Fig. 128].

Vessels and Nerves. The pancreaticoduodenal arteries and veins supply the head, while the splenic vessels supply the remainder. Lymph nodes lie along its superior border (pancreaticosplenic nodes) and on the pancreaticoduodenal vessels.

Ducts [Fig. 154]. Developmentally the pancreas arises as two separate, hollow, branching outgrowths from the duodenum. The smaller of these (ventral pancreas) arises in common with or close to the hepatic outgrowth (bile-duct), while the other (dorsal pancreas) arises more proximally. These two rudiments subsequently fuse, the ventral pancreas (posterior part of the head and uncinate process) and the bile-duct passing into a position dorsal to the dorsal pancreas (the remainder of the pancreas). Their ducts (the stems of the outgrowths) join, and the duct of the ventral pancreas forms the duodenal end of the main duct, while the duct of the dorsal pancreas forms the remainder. The duodenal end of the dorsal pancreatic duct remains as the accessory duct. It therefore usually communicates with the main duct of the pancreas, and opens into the duodenum 2–3 cm. proximal to the main duct.

The main **duct** begins in the tail, runs through

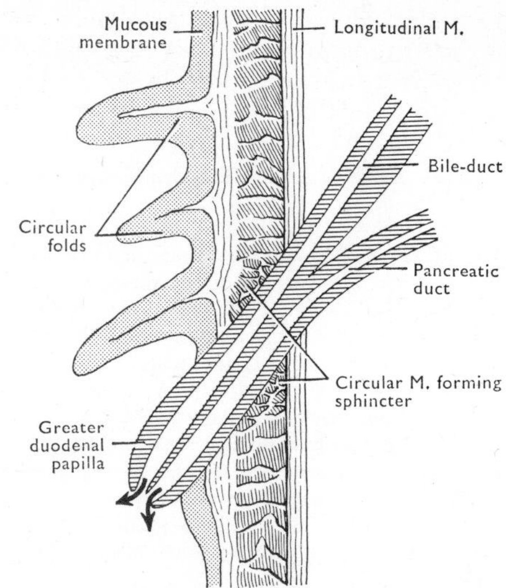

Fig. 155 A diagrammatic section through the duodenal wall to show one arrangement of the ducts in the greater duodenal papilla.

the body slightly anterosuperior to the centre, and receives small tributaries throughout. At the head it bends inferiorly, communicates with the accessory duct, then drains the uncinate process and posterior part of the head of the pancreas, and runs along the medial side of the bile-duct, joining it as it pierces the duodenal wall [Fig. 154].

The **accessory pancreatic duct** passes through the upper part of the head, and receives tributaries from it and from the anterior part of the head. Normally it connects the main duct to the duodenum, but it may be a tributary of the main duct without separate entry to the duodenum. This is a matter of some importance when the main duct is obstructed at the duodenum, as it may be by a gall-stone impacted in the hepatopancreatic ampulla.

Where the pancreatic duct joins the bile-duct, weak **sphincters** are found on the pancreatic duct and on the combined channel.

DISSECTION. Make a parallel cut along the posterior surface of the body of the pancreas close to each border. Pick away the lobules of the gland between the cuts, and expose the greyish-white duct. Trace the

duct in both directions, taking particular care in the head of the pancreas to expose the accessory duct and the tributaries. Follow the accessory duct to the duodenum, and find its point of entry on the internal surface.

THE LIVER

[FIGS. 156–158]

The liver is the largest gland in the body. It is responsible for: (1) the metabolism of the products of digestion which reach it through the portal vein (principally degradation products of proteins and carbohydrates); (2) the storage and release of substances (principally glucose) so as to maintain a constant level in the blood: and (3) the synthesis, conjugation, and transformation of substances (*e.g.*, formation of proteins, detoxication of poisonous substances, production of carbohydrates from proteins). All these are endocrine functions which alter the composition of the blood passing the liver cells, but it also has an exocrine or secretory function, the formation of bile. **Bile** is an important agent in digestion, especially of fats, and it is secreted into the bile canaliculi on the sides of the liver cells opposite to those exposed to the blood stream. Bile contains a large number of substances, the most obvious of which are the bile pigments. These accumulate in the blood stream (jaundice) in cases of liver damage in which the cells are unable to excrete the waste products of red cell destruction that reach them via the portal vein from the spleen. Jaundice can also arise from the excessive destruction of red blood cells or from the blockage of the biliary tract.

The greater part of the liver lies under cover of the ribs and costal cartilages, and is in contact with the **diaphragm** which separates it from the pleural cavity and lung. With one hand in the pleural cavity and the other in the peritoneal cavity, examine the position of the liver. Note that the liver ascends to the level of the fifth rib in the mid-clavicular line, filling the right dome of the diaphragm and part of the left dome. The right lobe of the liver is separated from the **costodiaphragmatic recess** of the pleura by the diaphragm, but posteriorly the upper part of the **right kidney** and suprarenal gland intervene between the liver and the diaphragm.

DISSECTION. Pull the liver downwards, and divide the anterior layers of the coronary and left triangular ligaments [p. 132], avoiding injury to the inferior vena cava. Clean the inferior vena cava between the liver and the diaphragm, and identify and divide the hepatic veins entering the vena cava. Strip the liver downwards from the inferior vena cava, identifying and dividing the remaining peritoneal connexions of the liver to the diaphragm. If the inferior vena cava is deeply buried in the posterior surface of the liver, divide it and remove a segment with the liver.

The liver is a dark brown, highly vascular, soft organ which is readily ruptured or torn in abdominal injuries, giving rise to severe intra-abdominal bleeding. It is approximately one-fiftieth of the body weight in the adult, but is proportionately larger (one-twentieth of the body weight) in the new-born, and partly accounts for the protuberant abdomen in young children.

The **shape** of the liver is determined by the surrounding organs, but once fixed *in situ*, it retains the shape of a blunt wedge (with its rounded base to the right) which is indented by the organs in contact with it. It has two surfaces: (1) the **diaphragmatic surface** which is divisible into superior, anterior, right, and posterior parts, all of which are continuous parts of the curved surface applied to the diaphragm; (2) the postero-inferior or **visceral surface** meets the right and anterior parts of the diaphragmatic surface at a sharp inferior margin, but is less distinctly separated from it posteriorly.

Fissures of Liver. On the visceral and posterior parts of the diaphragmatic surface, a deep fissure extends almost vertically from the attachment of the falciform ligament at the inferior margin, to the groove for the oesophagus at the junction of the posterior and superior parts of the diaphragmatic surface [FIG. 156]. The fissure lodges the ligamentum teres of the liver to the left of the **quadrate lobe;** the superior part contains the **ligamentum venosum,** has the upper part of the lesser omentum attached in its depths,

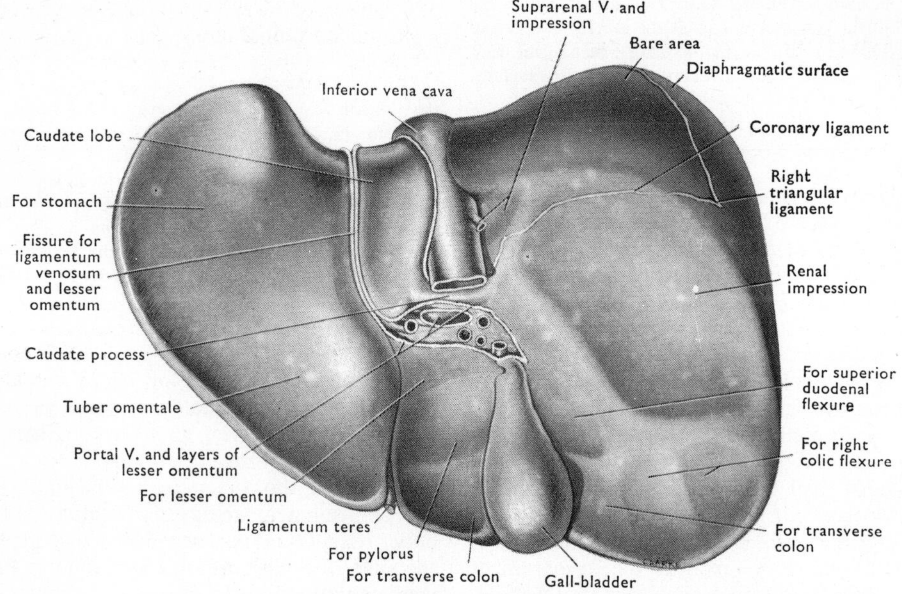

FIG. 156 The postero-inferior (visceral) surface of the liver.

and lies to the left of the **caudate lobe.** This fissure marks the separation of the liver into **right** and **left lobes.** It passes through the left extremity of a short transverse fissure, the **porta hepatis.**

At the porta hepatis the two layers of peritoneum of the lesser omentum leave the fissure and pass to the right around the structures in the porta hepatis (branches of the hepatic artery and portal vein, the hepatic ducts, nerves, and lymph nodes and vessels), to meet in the free edge at the neck of the gall-bladder. The porta separates the **quadrate lobe** [FIG. 158] antero-inferiorly from the **caudate lobe** superiorly [FIG. 156], and the right borders of these two lobes are formed, respectively, by the gall-bladder in its fossa, and the inferior vena cava in its sulcus. The latter does not form a complete right margin to the caudate lobe, a small strip of which extends to the right between the inferior vena cava and the porta hepatis, the **caudate process.** The peritoneum which covers the caudate process is the superior wall of the epiploic foramen [FIG. 156].

The ligamentum teres and the ligamentum venosum are fibrous remnants of the (left) umbilical vein and the ductus venosus of the foetus respectively, and both join the left branch of the portal vein at the porta hepatis. In the foetus the ductus venosus forms a by-pass through which the oxygenated umbilical venous blood passes directly to the inferior vena cava and the right atrium without traversing the liver. It curves to the right at the upper border of the caudate lobe to join the inferior vena cava. It is relatively large in the early foetus, but becomes progressively smaller in the later stages.

Surfaces of Liver. The **right part** of the **diaphragmatic surface** lies between the seventh and eleventh ribs in the mid-axillary line, and is separated by the diaphragm from the pleura down to the tenth rib, and from the lung down to the eighth rib.

The **anterior part** of the diaphragmatic surface is triangular. A considerable part of it is in contact with the anterior abdominal wall between the right and left costal margins [FIG. 111], but a small part to the left and a large

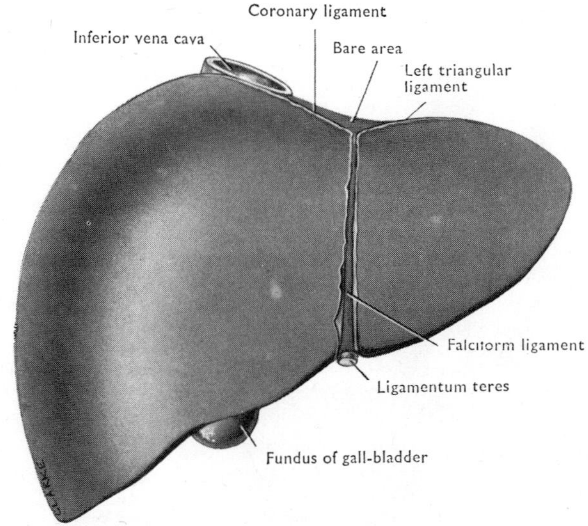

FIG. 157 The liver viewed from the front.

the anterior wall of the superior recess of the omental bursa, and is separated by the bursa and diaphragm from the lowest part of the thoracic aorta. Inferiorly the caudate lobe abuts on the porta hepatis and unites with the remainder of the right lobe through the **caudate process.**

The **inferior vena cava** lies in a deep groove (occasionally buried in the liver) immediately to the right of the caudate lobe. Here the peritoneum on the caudate lobe turns posteriorly on to the diaphragm to form the right and posterior walls of the superior recess of the omental bursa. The two main hepatic veins enter the inferior vena cava at the upper end of the groove, while smaller veins enter it at a lower level. To the right of the inferior vena cava the posterior part of the diaphragmatic surface is broad, and much of it is not covered by peritoneum (**bare area**) where it lies between the superior and inferior layers of the coronary ligament [FIG. 158]. A slight depression in the bare area immediately to the right of the inferior vena cava marks the position of the right suprarenal gland [FIG. 158]. The

part to the right are in contact with the diaphragm. The **falciform ligament** is attached vertically to this surface from a notch on the inferior margin to the superior part of the diaphragmatic surface. It marks the division of the liver into right and left lobes anteriorly.

The **superior part** of the diaphragmatic surface is ovoid and convex. It rises almost to the level of the right nipple and to the level of the fifth rib in the left mid-clavicular line. It is slightly flattened inferior to the pericardium to form the **cardiac impression,** and in the left lobe it meets the visceral surface posteriorly at a sharp edge [FIG. 158].

The **posterior part** of the diaphragmatic surface is narrow in the left lobe, but widens at the fissure for the ligamentum venosum, and is grooved by the oesophagus at the upper end of the fissure. To the right of the fissure is the **caudate lobe** which forms

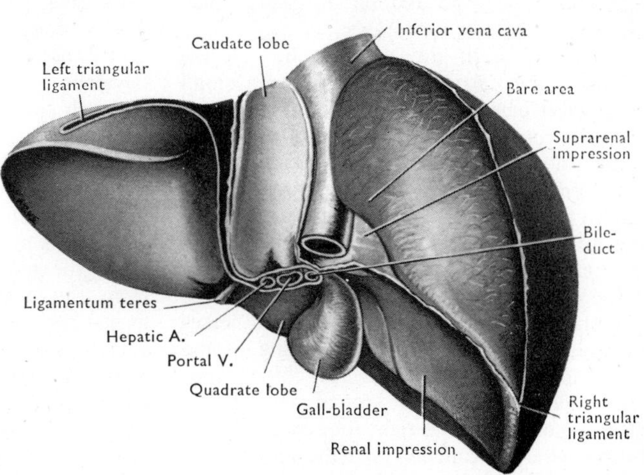

FIG. 158 The liver viewed from behind.

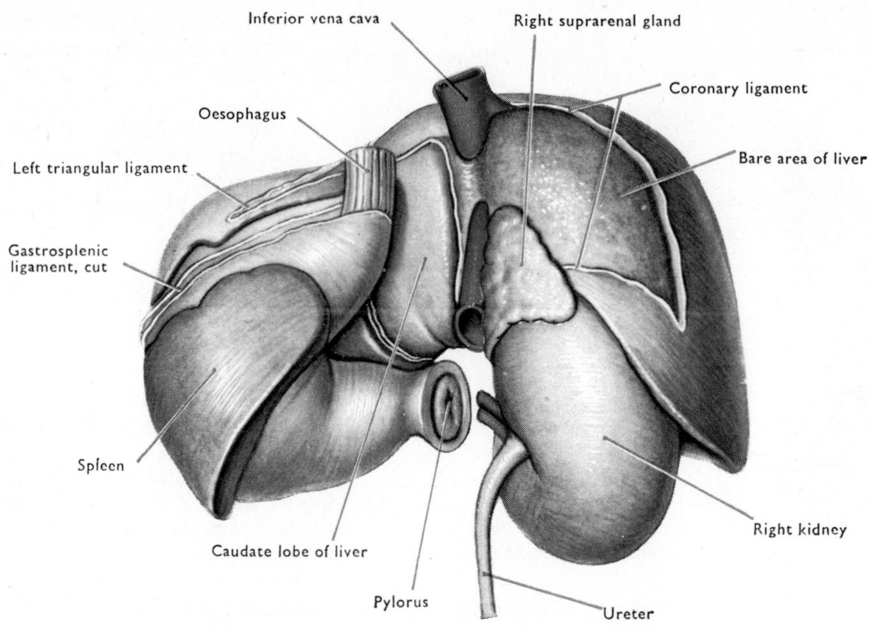

FIG. 159 The liver, right kidney, spleen, and stomach, as seen from behind

remainder of the bare area is directly in contact with the inferior vena cava and diaphragm, through which some lymph vessels and small veins may pass.

The **visceral surface** [FIG. 156] is irregular in shape to fit the upper abdominal viscera which lie postero-inferior to it.

This surface of the left lobe lies on the stomach and oesophagus except for a small part (**tuber omentale**) which is in contact with the lesser omentum close to the porta hepatis.

The most obvious feature on the right lobe is the **gall-bladder.** This extends from the right end of the porta hepatis to a shallow notch on the inferior margin. It overlies the descending part of the duodenum and the transverse colon. The quadrate lobe, to the left of the gall-bladder, therefore overlies the lesser omentum, the pylorus, the beginning of the duodenum, and the transverse colon from above downwards. The remainder of the visceral surface of the right lobe is in contact through the peritoneum with the junction of the superior and descending parts of the duodenum, the upper part of the right kidney, and the right flexure of the colon [FIG. 156].

Peritoneum of Liver. The liver is completely covered by peritoneum except in the bare area, which includes the groove for the inferior vena cava, and the fossa for the gall-bladder. The peritoneal reflexions of the liver are readily understood if it is appreciated that the liver develops in the ventral mesentery of the stomach and upper duodenum, and that it splits this into a part connecting these organs to the liver and a part connecting the liver to the anterior abdominal wall (falciform ligament). Initially the part linking the liver to the stomach is a thick sheet, in the right part of which the inferior vena cava extends forwards from the posterior abdominal wall to the liver. The formation of the epiploic foramen and the superior recess of the omental bursa in the substance of this mesentery, posterior to the caudate process and lobe, splits this part of the mesentery into: (1) the **lesser omentum** below and to the left; and (2) the **mesentery of the inferior vena cava** to the right. Superiorly the liver abuts directly on the diaphragm producing the bare area. This interrupts the direct continuation of the lesser omentum and mesentery of the inferior vena cava with the falciform ligament, which would have existed had the liver been entirely enclosed between the layers of the ventral mesentery.

Vessels and Nerves. The liver is supplied both by the hepatic artery and by the portal vein, and it transmits a large volume of blood when the mesenteric arteries are dilated. The venous blood drains into the inferior vena cava principally through the right and left hepatic veins, but also by some smaller veins.

The branches of the portal vein and hepatic artery, and the tributaries of the right and left hepatic veins and ducts enter or leave the corresponding lobes of the liver; though all of the quadrate lobe, and part of the caudate lobe are supplied and drained by the vessels of the left lobe.

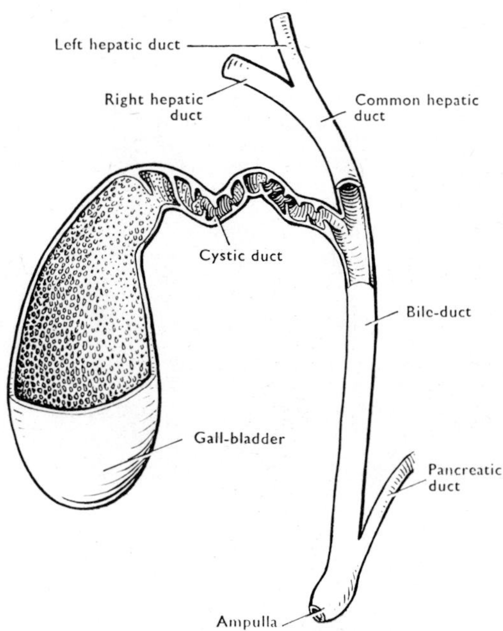

FIG. 160 A diagram of the extrahepatic parts of the biliary system.

The left hepatic vein usually emerges from the upper end of the fissure for the ligamentum venosum, and runs with the ligament along the upper margin of the caudate lobe to the inferior vena cava.

The **nerves** are derived from the coeliac plexus and the gastric branches of the vagi. Some sensory fibres in the phrenic nerve appear to reach the biliary tract.

The **lymph vessels** either emerge through the porta hepatis to nodes in the porta and lesser omentum, or through the bare area to the pancreaticosplenic nodes and through the diaphragm to nodes in the thorax.

GALL-BLADDER

This is a piriform storage chamber of 30–60 ml. capacity, in which bile is concentrated, and from which it is discharged into the duodenum by muscular contraction. X-ray-opaque substances which are excreted in the bile are also concentrated, and this is used to demonstrate the cavity of the gall-bladder and its ability to contract [FIG. 161].

The gall-bladder lies in a shallow fossa on the visceral surface of the liver, along the right edge of the quadrate lobe. Usually it is held directly in contact with the liver substance by peritoneum and a few small veins, but it may be partly buried in the liver, or suspended from it by a short mesentery.

Antero-inferiorly, the rounded fundus protrudes below the inferior margin of the liver, touching the anterior abdominal wall approximately where the right linea semilunaris meets the ninth costal cartilage. The fundus lies on the transverse colon, and through the body (anterosuperior to the descending part of the duodenum) is continuous with the narrow neck which lies close to the right extremity of the porta hepatis on the junction of the superior and descending parts of the duodenum [FIGS. 153, 156].

Vessels and Nerves. The gall-bladder is supplied by the cystic artery (from the right hepatic artery) and vein, and its lymph vessels pass to nodes on the cystic duct and in the porta hepatis. Nerves reach it along the

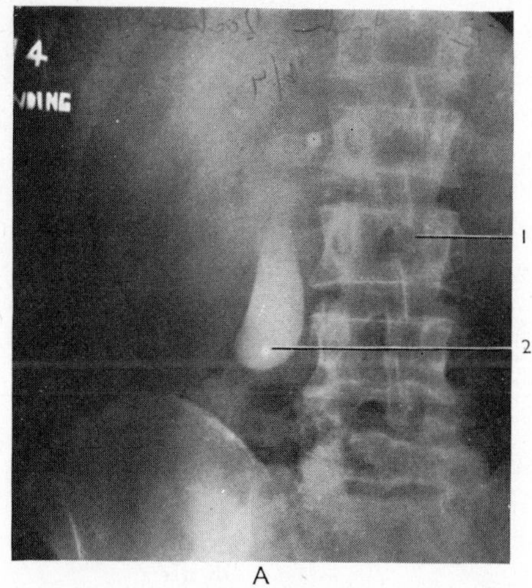

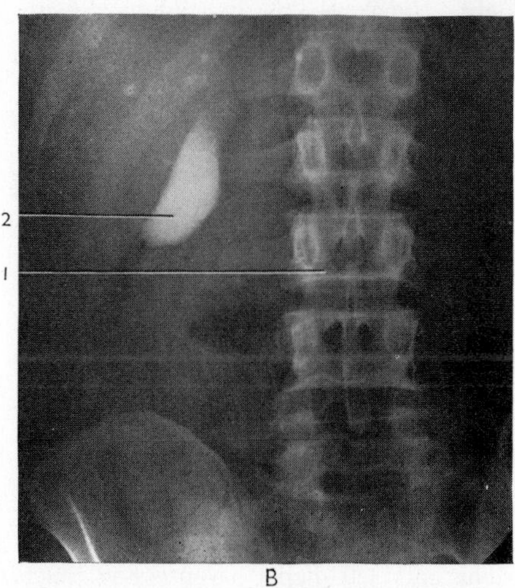

FIG. 161 Two radiographs to show the changing position of the gall-bladder in different positions of the body. The gall-bladder is filled with an X-ray-opaque material which is excreted by the liver in the bile. A is taken in the standing position, B in the lying position.

1 3rd lumbar vertebra 2 Gall-bladder

artery from the coeliac plexus (sympathetic), the vagus (parasympathetic), and the right phrenic nerve (sensory).

Cystic Duct [FIG. 160]

This duct is 2 cm. or more in length. It descends from the neck of the gall-bladder to run in the lesser omentum with the **common hepatic duct** joining it to form the **bile-duct.**

DISSECTION. Clean the structures in the porta hepatis, and follow them to their entry into the liver. The arrangement of these structures is very variable, and may not correspond to the following description.

Structures in Porta Hepatis

As these structures enter the liver they are enclosed in a fibrous sheath which is reflected over them from the surface of the liver. This **perivascular fibrous capsule** extends around their branches and tributaries into the substance of the liver, and forms the fibrous capsule which separates the surface of the liver from the peritoneum.

Near the porta hepatis the common hepatic duct, hepatic artery, and the portal vein divide into right and left branches, and these pass together into the corresponding lobes of the liver with the hepatic ducts anterior to the arteries, and both in front of the veins. The **right branch of the portal vein** receives the cystic vein and enters the right lobe of the liver almost immediately. The **left branch** passes medially between the caudate and quadrate lobes, supplying both, and sinks into the left lobe. The left branch of the portal vein unites with the ligamenta venosum and teres before it disappears into the liver.

DISSECTION. Trace a branch of the portal vein for some distance into the liver with the artery and hepatic duct. Note the branches which they give simultaneously to the liver substance. In a similar manner trace one hepatic vein from the inferior vena cava into the liver, and inspect the cut surface of a slice of liver with a hand lens.

Structure of Liver

Within the liver the complicated branches of the structures in the porta hepatis (surrounded by extensions of the perivascular fibrous capsule) interdigitate with similar tributaries of the hepatic veins, but are separated from them by a narrow space filled with strands of liver cells (the terminal branches of the biliary system) which pass radially from the lobular branches of the hepatic ducts (interlobular ductules) towards the surrounding tributaries of the hepatic veins (central venules). Between the strands of liver cells are the **sinusoids** which connect the terminal branches of the hepatic artery and portal vein to the central venules, while the bile canaliculi lie in the strands of liver cells. Various **lobules** have been described in the liver, and these may be centred either on a central venule or on a portal tract (the terminal branch of the perivascular fibrous capsule and its contained structures). In most animals no clear cut lobular pattern exists, though in the pig, sheets of the perivascular fibrous capsule join the various portal tracts and outline lobules, each of which has a centrally placed venule. From the point of view of the biliary system, the lobule is the volume of liver that drains into a single interlobular ductule. The central venules arranged around it each drain several parts of adjacent hepatic lobules. Since the terminal branches of each hepatic artery lie with the interlobular ductules in the portal tracts, the oxygen tension is highest close to these and lowest in the liver tissue adjacent to the central venules. Thus anything that slows the rate of the hepatic circulation will affect the cells round the central venules, while poisons entering the liver through the portal vein tend to damage the cells immediately round the portal tracts.

DISSECTION. Make a longitudinal incision through the wall of the gall-bladder and cystic duct, clean the interior with a jet of water and examine the lining.

Structure of Gall-bladder and Cystic Duct

The gall-bladder is lined with columnar epithelial cells which are of the absorptive type with numerous microvilli on their internal surfaces. The mucous membrane is complexly folded to increase the surface area, and has a honeycomb appearance to the unaided eye. There is no muscularis mucosae, and the mucous membrane lies directly on a thin smooth muscle layer which consists of interlacing bundles running in many directions; a feature which is found in all hollow organs of this type, and allows them to contract uniformly and force the contents through a single aperture.

From the neck of the gall-bladder a prominent fold of mucous membrane runs spirally along the cystic duct, the **spiral fold.** It may help to control the flow of bile from the gall-bladder [FIG. 160].

ABDOMINAL STRUCTURES IN CONTACT WITH DIAPHRAGM

The **right dome of the diaphragm** is filled by the right lobe of the liver, the right kidney and suprarenal gland, the **left dome** by the left lobe of the liver, the stomach, the spleen, and the left kidney and suprarenal gland. Parts of all these organs are separated from the pleura by the diaphragm, *i.e.*, the upper parts of both kidneys and stomach, the greater part of the diaphragmatic surface of the liver, the suprarenal glands, and the spleen. The parts of the diaphragmatic surface of the liver not adjacent to the pleura are: (1) the parts of the superior surfaces of the right and left lobes which lie inferior to the pericardium; (2) the part in contact with the anterior abdominal wall; and (3) the part of the posterior surface which is anterior to the right kidney. To a lesser extent the liver, stomach, and spleen are also associated with parts of the pleural cavities which normally contain the lungs.

Replace the upper abdominal organs that were removed, and confirm their position relative to the pleural cavities.

DISSECTION. Find a coeliac ganglion on each side of the coeliac trunk. They lie in the coeliac plexus of nerves on the aorta and the corresponding crus of the diaphragm. Trace branches of the ganglia to the suprarenal glands, to the coeliac trunk, and inferiorly along the aorta to the superior and inferior mesenteric arteries, to form the corresponding plexuses on these vessels. The aortic plexus receives the lumbar splanchnic nerves, and its inferior part has been seen already [p. 150].

THE AUTONOMIC NERVOUS SYSTEM

The general arrangement of this system has been described already [p. 29]. Motor cells in peripherally situated ganglia innervate various organs of the body, especially smooth muscle and glands, through their axons (**postganglionic fibres).** These motor cells are stimulated by the axons (**preganglionic fibres)** of nerve cells within the central nervous system. The latter leave the central nervous system though the thoracic and upper two lumbar nerves (**sympathetic** preganglionic fibres), and also through certain cranial nerves (including the vagus) and the third and fourth sacral nerves (**parasympathetic** preganglionic fibres). Both pass to separate groups of ganglion cells, the former some distance from the organs they supply and usually associated with the arteries, the latter in or near all parts of the gut tube and the structures developed from it.

SYMPATHETIC NERVOUS SYSTEM

The main parts are: (1) the sympathetic **trunks;** and (2) the sympathetic **plexuses.**

The **sympathetic trunks** extend from the upper cervical region to the coccyx on the anterolateral surfaces of the vertebral column. The cells of the ganglia on each trunk send their axons principally to the spinal nerves (**grey rami communicantes**) for the supply of the body wall, but bundles of preganglionic fibres (**splanchnic nerves)** from the white rami communicantes continue through the trunks to the visceral plexuses and ganglia around the aorta and its branches, which they reach at levels much inferior to their origins. Thus the **thoracic splanchnic nerves** pierce the crura of the diaphragm and reach the coeliac (greater and lesser splanchnic nerves) and renal plexuses (lowest splanchnic nerve); the **lumbar splanchnic nerves** join the inferior part of the abdominal aortic plexus, and the **sacral splanchnic nerves** join the inferior hypogastric plexuses. The latter are also joined by the pelvic splanchnic nerves (visceral branches of the third and fourth sacral nerves) which transmit preganglionic parasympathetic fibres to the pelvic organs and the descending colon through the hypogastric plexuses.

The abdominal and pelvic sympathetic plexuses are the coeliac, renal, superior and inferior mesenteric, and the superior and inferior hypogastric.

Coeliac Plexus

This plexus lies on the aorta and the crura of the diaphragm around the coeliac trunk. It is therefore posterior to the omental bursa and partly overlapped by the pancreas and, on the right, by the inferior vena cava.

The large, nodular **coeliac ganglia** lie on each side of the coeliac trunk, and give rise to most of the nerves in the plexus which are therefore postganglionic. Some preganglionic fibres pass through the ganglia directly to the suprarenal glands and to the ganglia on the branches of the coeliac trunk and the superior mesenteric artery. The plexus is also joined by vagal (preganglionic parasympathetic) fibres from the **posterior vagal trunk,** and by **phrenic fibres** (sensory) which reach it along the inferior phrenic arteries, and pass to the suprarenal gland and to the biliary apparatus, the latter by way of the hepatic plexus on the common hepatic and hepatic arteries.

The coeliac plexus is continuous with the **abdominal aortic plexus** (of which it is really a part), and through it with the **superior** and **inferior mesenteric plexuses** on the corresponding arteries. The abdominal aortic plexus is continued inferiorly as the **superior hypogastric plexus** between the two common iliac arteries, and this splits as it enters the pelvis to pass with the internal iliac arteries and their branches as the **inferior hypogastric plexuses.**

The **renal plexuses** form subsidiary plexuses along the gonadal arteries and the ureter. Ganglia of various sizes are found scattered through all the plexuses, and even in the walls of the viscera.

DISSECTION. Remove the fat and fascia from the anterior surface of the left kidney and suprarenal gland. Find the left suprarenal vein and the left testicular or ovarian vein, and trace both to the left renal vein. Clean the latter vein from the inferior vena cava to the left kidney, and note its tributaries. Displace the vein

and clean the left renal artery, following its branches to the left suprarenal gland and ureter. Clean the remainder of the ureter in the abdomen.

Turn the left kidney medially, clean the posterior surfaces of the kidney, its vessels and the ureter, and the muscles, vessels, and nerves that lie posterior to the kidney.

On the right side carry out the same dissection, but note that the testicular (or ovarian) and suprarenal veins join the inferior vena cava directly.

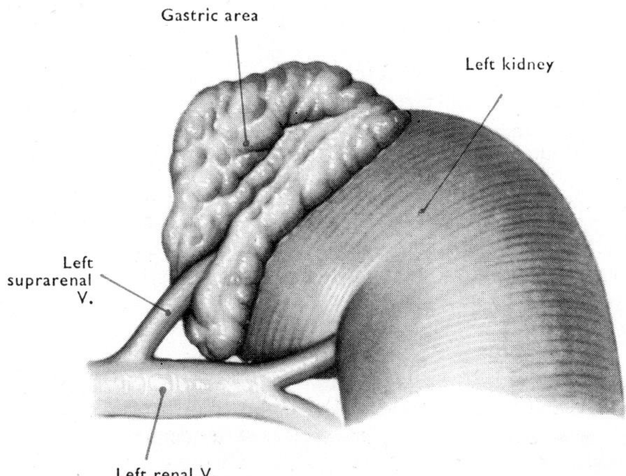

FIG. 163 The anterior surface of the left suprarenal gland.

SUPRARENAL GLANDS

These important endocrine glands each consist of two parts, the **cortex** (developed from the mesodermal lining of the peritoneal cavity) and the **medulla** (developed from the neural crest and equivalent to a group of sympathetic ganglion cells).

The cortex secretes a considerable number of steroid hormones which are responsible for: (1) the control of electrolyte and water balance; (2) the maintenance of blood sugar concentration and of liver and muscle glycogen stores; and (3) the control of inflammatory reactions and of connective tissues in general.

The medulla secretes adrenaline and noradrenaline into the blood stream. These sympathomimetic catecholamines are similar to those released by postganglionic sympathetic nerve fibres, and they are stored in quantity in the medulla. They are readily oxidized to a dark brown colour by potassium bichromate, and thus the medulla forms part of the chromaffin tissue of the body.

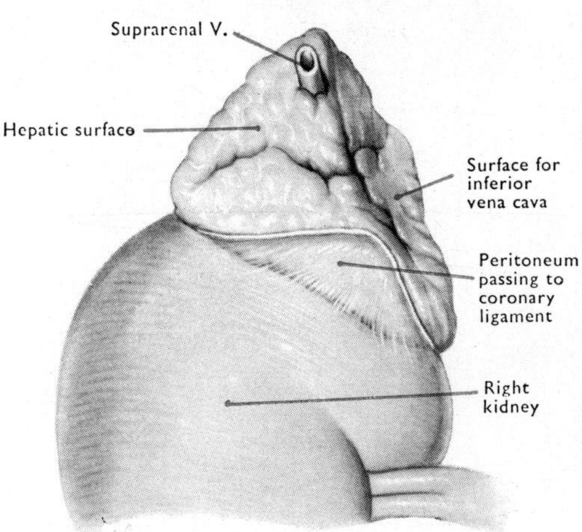

FIG. 162 The anterior surface of the right suprarenal gland.

Position [FIGS. 133, 168, 175]

Each gland lies against the superomedial surface of the corresponding kidney, and is separated from it by a little fatty connective tissue, but is enclosed in the same fascial sheath (**renal fascia,** p. 106).

The **right gland** is pyramidal in shape and is wedged between the diaphragm posteromedially, the inferior vena cava anteromedially, the liver anteriorly, and the kidney inferolaterally. The superior part of the gland lies directly against the bare area of the liver, but the inferior part is separated from it by peritoneum [FIG. 162].

The **left gland** is crescentic in shape, and lies between the diaphragm posteromedially, the stomach anteriorly (separated by the omental bursa and inferiorly by the pancreas and the splenic artery), and the kidney inferolaterally.

Vessels. The very large blood supply is achieved by a considerable number of small **arteries** that enter the surface of the glands at different points. These arise from the **renal arteries,** the **aorta,** and the **inferior phrenic arteries.** The suprarenal arteries pierce the cortex, supply it, and pass into the medulla. The **veins** run inwards from the cortex to the medulla and a single vein leaves each gland; the right at the superomedial part of the gland immediately enters the inferior vena cava, while the left leaves the inferomedial part of the gland and enters the left renal vein.

DISSECTION. Make a series of sections through the right gland. Follow the left suprarenal vein into the gland, and cut away the anterior surface of the gland to display the extent of the medulla. Examine the cut surfaces with a hand lens.

Structure. The cortex consists of three layers: (1) the outer, **zona glomerulosa** composed of nests or clumps of cells; (2) the **zona fasciculata,** formed of parallel columns of cells; (3) the **zona recticularis,** a mesh of interlacing cords of cells. It may be that the different layers each has a different function, but it seems clear that new cells can be formed at the junction of the outer two layers, and that the cortex may be regenerated from it. In the foetus the cortex is very large but of unknown function. After birth, this foetal cortex degenerates and is replaced by the remaining outermost layer. The medulla consists of cells arranged in strands or clumps (chromaffin cells) with several sympathetic ganglion cells scattered through it.

THE KIDNEYS

These organs are responsible for the removal of excess water, salts, and waste products from the blood, and for maintaining its pH. To achieve this the blood flow through the wide renal vessels is approximately one quarter of the resting cardiac output, *i.e.,* 1·2–1·4 litres per minute.

The kidneys are reddish brown in colour and approximately 10 cm. long, 5 cm. wide, and 2·5 cm. thick. They are ovoid in outline, and the lateral and medial borders are convex, but the medial is deeply indented and concave at its middle. Here a wide, vertical cleft (the **hilus**) transmits the structures entering and leaving the kidney, and leads into a space within it, the **sinus** of the kidney. The hilus lies approxi-

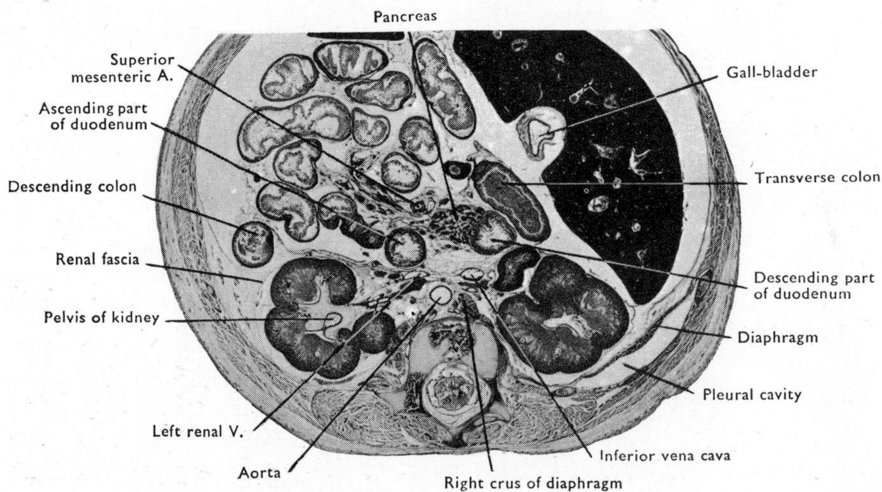

FIG. 164 A horizontal section through the abdomen of a seven-month human foetus. The levels of the various structures are not identical with those in the adult, but the absence of dense connective tissue makes the structures more obvious.

mately at the level of the first lumbar vertebra.

The upper end of the ureter expands into the **pelvis** of the kidney, and this passes through the hilus to become continuous with some short, funnel-like tubes (**calyces**) which unite it to the kidney tissue in the sinus. The amount of the pelvis enclosed in the sinus is variable. The renal vessels lie anterior to the pelvis of the kidney, but some of their branches and tributaries pass posterior to it. Lymph vessels and nerves also pass through the hilus into the sinus which is packed with fat.

The kidneys lie obliquely in the upper parts of the paravertebral gutters (posterior to the peritoneum) against the structures covering the sides of the vertebrae from the last thoracic to the third lumbar. The superior extremities are medial to the inferior extremities, and the medial and lateral borders face anteromedially and posterolaterally [FIG. 125]. Thus the **anterior** and **posterior surfaces** face anterolaterally and posteromedially respectively.

The superior extremity of the right kidney lies at a lower level (eleventh intercostal space) than the left (eleventh rib) because of the presence of the liver [FIGS. 167, 171].

The kidney is enclosed in a dense **fibrous capsule** which is readily stripped from its surface. At the hilus, the capsule passes into and lines the sinus of the kidney, becoming continuous with the walls of the calyces where they are attached to the kidney. The fibrous capsule is surrounded by a **fatty capsule** (perirenal fat), and this fills the space inside the

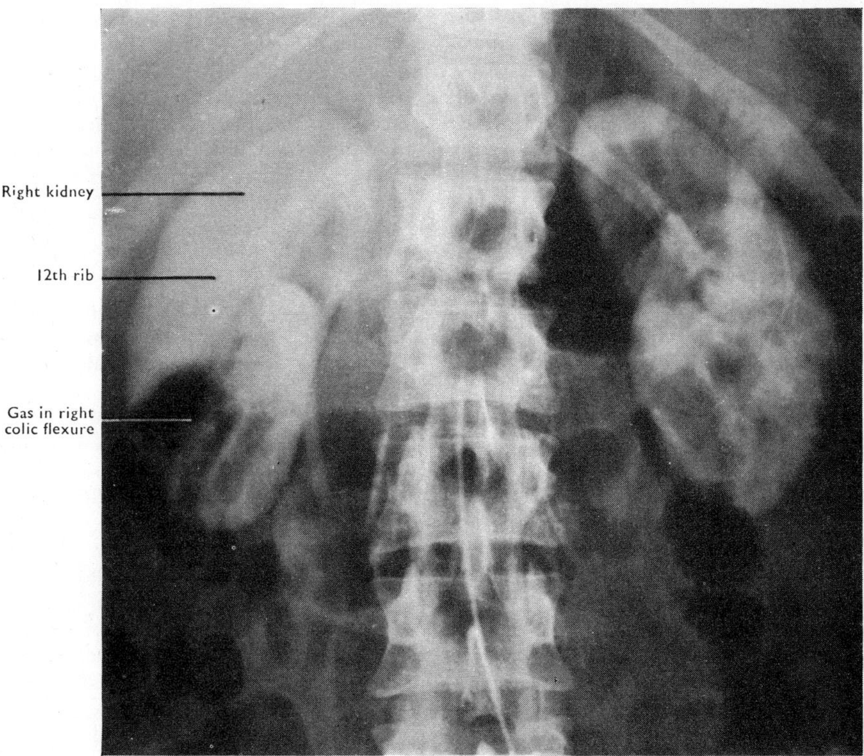

FIG. 165 An anteroposterior radiograph of the upper abdomen shortly after the injection of contrast material into the aorta, at the level of the renal arteries. The kidneys are outlined by the contrast material in their capillaries.

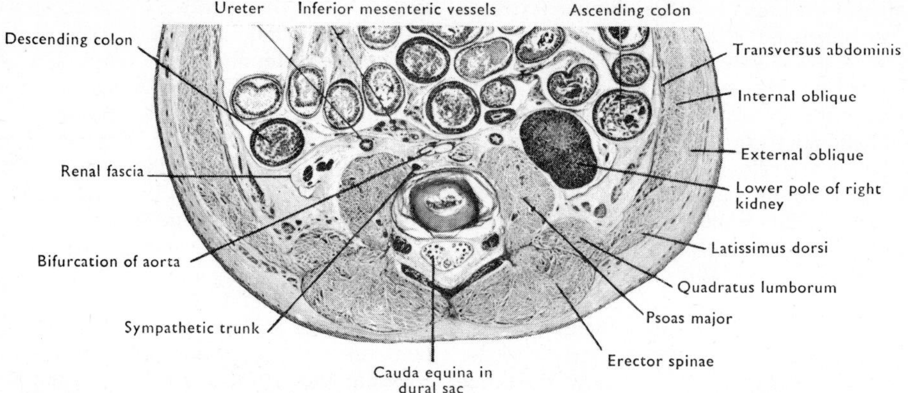

FIG. 166 A horizontal section through the abdomen of a seven-month human foetus at the level of the bifurcation of the aorta.

loosely fitting sheath of renal fascia which encloses it with the kidney and suprarenal. The layers of the **renal fascia** fuse with each other, and become continuous laterally with the transversalis fascia, superiorly with the diaphragmatic fascia, and medially fuse around the renal vessels. Inferiorly the layers of the renal fascia are only loosely united, and may be separated for some distance below the kidney [FIGS. 164, 166]. Abscesses may form in the fatty capsule and cause a swelling of the loin. The kidney may descend to an unusually low level if the supporting fatty capsule is absorbed; the renal vessels are then its only support. Such a descent may lead to kinking of the ureter and failure of the urine to drain freely down it.

Developmentally the kidney is first formed in the pelvis and ascends to its final position. Its ascent may be arrested at any point, and thus the kidney may be found near the superior aperture of the lesser pelvis. As it ascends, the kidney receives a different blood supply at each level, thus **accessory renal arteries** from the aorta may be found entering the lower pole of a normally placed kidney. When first formed, the rudiments of the two kidneys are close together and may fuse anterior to the aorta, forming a **horseshoe kidney.** Such a kidney cannot ascend beyond the level of origin of the inferior mesenteric artery which bars its ascent.

There may be a considerable collection of fat (**pararenal fat**) between the peritoneum and the renal fascia, and air injected into the loose retroperitoneal tissues anterior to the sacrum ascends to the level of the kidneys, and surrounding them, makes their outlines readily visible on X-ray examination.

Structures in Contact with Kidney [FIGS. 124, 166–168]

Posteriorly these are similar on the two sides, and consist of the diaphragm (superiorly), psoas major (medially), quadratus lumborum and transversus abdominis (laterally). The subcostal vessels and nerve and the iliohypogastric and ilioinguinal nerves lie posterior to the kidney and anterior to quadratus lumborum and the anterior layer of the thoracolumbar fascia [FIG. 177].

The diaphragm separates the upper part of the kidney from the pleura and twelfth rib, though occasionally there is a defect in the diaphragm between its costal origin and that from the lateral arcuate ligament [FIG. 174] when the kidney may be in direct contact with the pleura and the last rib.

The **right kidney** is wedged between the posterior abdominal wall and the visceral surface of the liver [FIG. 164]. It is separated from the liver by the suprarenal gland supero-

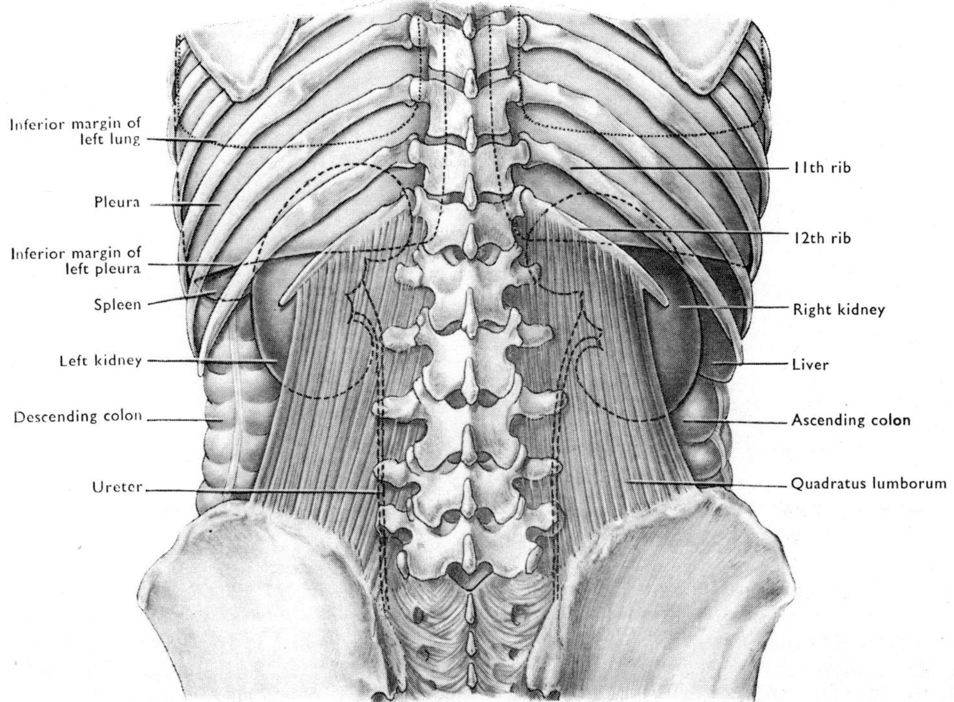

FIG. 167 A dissection from behind to show the relation of the two pleural sacs to the kidneys.

medially, the descending part of the duodenum medially, and the right flexure of the colon inferiorly. Inferior to the latter it may be in contact with a loop of jejunum.

The upper part of the **left kidney** lies posterior to the stomach and the omental bursa, but is separated from them by the suprarenal gland superomedially, by the spleen and lienorenal ligament superolaterally, and by the body of the pancreas at the level of the hilus [FIG. 133]. With the pancreas are the associated blood vessels and the attachment of the transverse mesocolon. Thus, inferior to the pancreas, the kidney lies in the infracolic compartment with the descending colon along its lateral border, the jejunum anterior, and the duodenojejunal flexure medial to the kidney. Only the descending colon, pancreas, and suprarenal gland are not separated from it by peritoneum.

DISSECTION. Remove the anterior wall of the renal sinus piecemeal from the hilus laterally. Divide the vessels that enter the wall, and separate the calyces that are attached to it. Clean the contents of the sinus, and then remove the anterior part of the kidney by making a clean coronal slice from the borders into the sinus.

The **sinus of the kidney** is a considerable space which takes up a large part of the interior of the kidney, and is more extensive than the hilus. It contains the greater part of the pelvis of the kidney, the calyces, vessels, and nerves.

Structure of Kidney [FIG. 169]. On the cut surface note the outer, paler, **cortex** adjacent to the capsule. This has a uniform granular appearance, while the medulla contains darker, triangular masses (the **renal pyramids**) which show radial striations and are separated from each other by extensions of the cortical tissue,

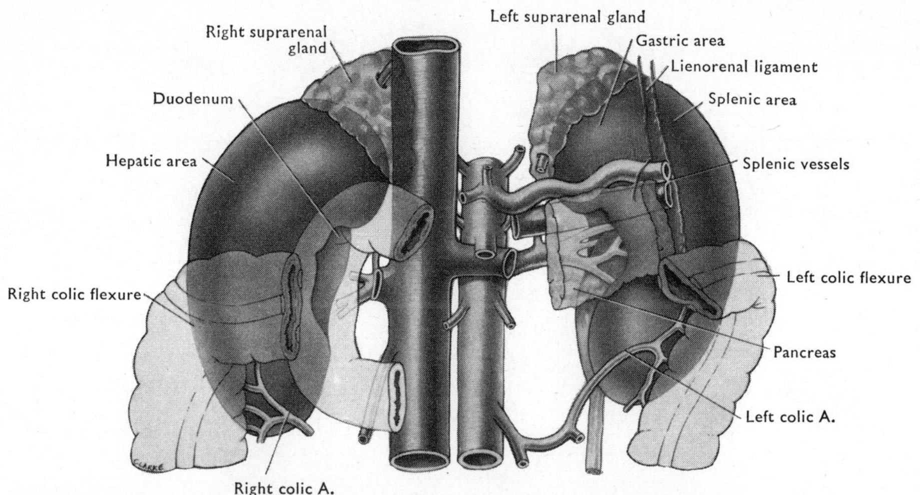

FIG. 168 A diagram to show the structures in contact with the anterior surfaces of the kidneys. The pancreas, colon, suprarenal glands, and duodenum are shown as though transparent.

the **renal columns.** The apex of each pyramid extends into the sinus as a small, conical projection (**renal papilla**) covered by the end of a lesser calyx attached around the base of the papilla. Here the fibromuscular wall of the calyx becomes continuous with the fibrous capsule lining the sinus, while the epithelial lining is continued over the surface of the papilla. On the papilla the epithelium is pierced (**foramina papillaria**) by the collecting tubules that discharge urine into the calyx from a **lobe of the kidney** (one pyramid with its covering of cortical tissue). The collecting tubules pass radially through the pyramid into the cortex where they take part in the formation of radial striations (the **medullary rays**) with other renal tubules, and receive the urine from the excretory units of the kidney, the **nephrons.** Each nephron consists of a filter or **renal corpuscle.** This is a tuft of capillaries with perforated endothelial walls (**glomerulus**) invaginated into the blind, expanded end (**glomerular capsule**) of a long tubule which leaves the renal corpuscle to form a **proximal convoluted tubule** in the cortex. In this tubule certain substances are reabsorbed (glucose, salt, etc.) and some are excreted by the epithelial lining. The proximal convoluted tubule leads into the **straight tubule** which loops down into the pyramid and back to the cortex, to become continuous with the **distal convoluted tubule,** which opens into a **collecting tubule.** This is common to a number of nephrons, and passes through the pyramid towards the papilla, through which it enters a calyx. In the latter parts, the urine is concentrated and other substances are added and removed by the tubular epithelium. In addition the distal convoluted tubule comes into close association with the afferent glomerular arteriole, and the cells of both are modified to form the juxtaglomerular apparatus. This is thought to be responsible for the release of substances which raise the blood pressure and thereby maintain the renal blood flow.

Vessels of Kidney. The renal artery divides into four or five branches close to the hilus. The majority pass anterior to the pelvis of the kidney (but one or two pass posterior to it), and giving off twigs to the structures in the sinus, branch into **lobar arteries,** one to each papilla. These divide into **interlobar arteries** which enter the kidney substance near the papilla, and ascending at the sides of the

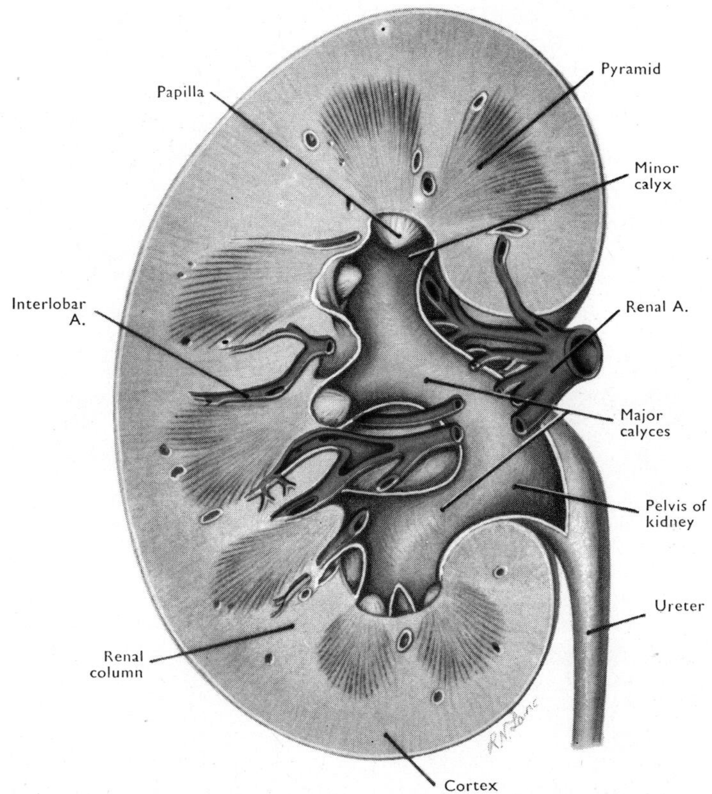

FIG. 169 A coronal section of the kidney. Note the papillae projecting into the minor calyces.

pyramid, divide into arcuate arteries at the corticomedullary junction. The **arcuate arteries** run parallel to the surface of the kidney between the pyramid and its cortical cap. They do not anastomose with adjacent arcuate arteries, but send branches vertically towards the surface of the kidney, the **interlobular arteries.** Afferent arterioles pass from these to the glomeruli. The efferent arterioles from the glomeruli either pass to another group of capillaries around the convoluted tubules, or run as **straight arterioles** into the medulla from the glomeruli close to the medulla. The capillaries drain into interlobular veins, and thence to the **interlobar veins,** which begin deep to the renal capsule as **stellate veins,** and pass through the kidney tissue to the sinus.

Pelvis of Kidney and Calyces [FIGS. 169–171]

The calyces are short, funnel-like tubes. They are the remnants of the main branches of the ureteric bud of the embryo, which forms the ureter, pelvis of the kidney, calyces, and collecting tubules. There are two orders of calyces, greater and lesser. Each **lesser calyx** (approximately ten in number) embraces a renal papilla and receives the urine from the collecting tubules. Their renal extremities are therefore cup-shaped, though they are more complicated when they surround more than one papilla. The lesser calyces are branches of two or three **greater calyces** which arise from the renal pelvis. The volume of pelvis and calyces together does not exceed 8 ml.,

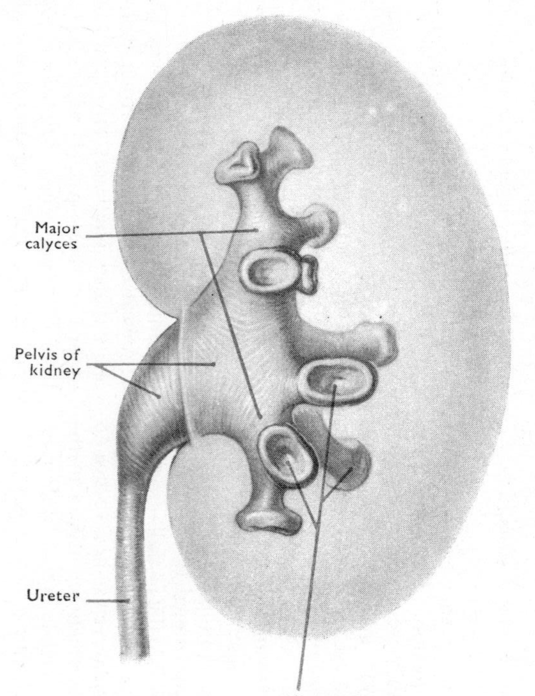

Fɪɢ. 170 The pelvis and calyces of the kidney, from a cast. The cupped appearance of the lesser calyces is due to each having a renal papilla inserted into it.

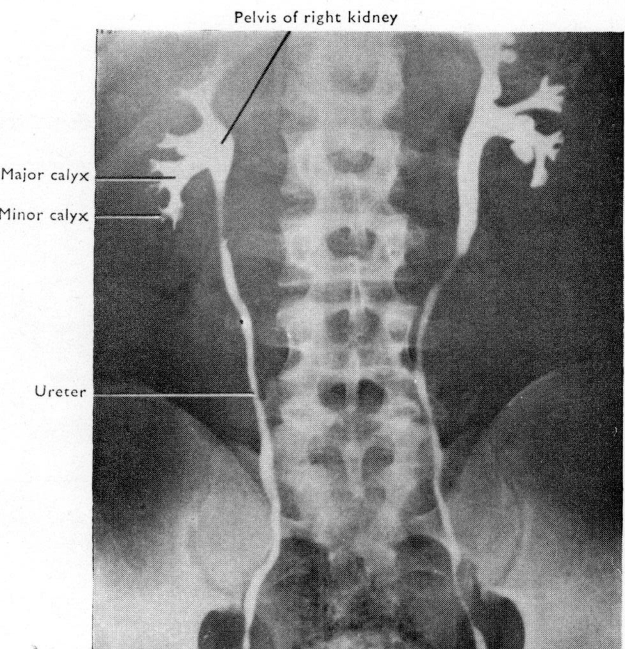

Fɪɢ. 171 A pyelogram. This radiograph shows the ureters, pelvis, and calyces of the kidneys outlined by a contrast medium filling their lumina.

and if more than this volume of X-ray-opaque material is injected through the ureter to outline these cavities, the pressure may tear the epithelial junction of the minor calyces with the papillae, and the material enters the adjacent renal veins.

The renal pelvis and calyces are surrounded by fat, vessels and nerves in the renal sinus. The pelvis emerges through the lower part of the hilus, and tapering downwards on psoas major, joins the ureter near the inferior extremity of the kidney. The extrarenal part of the right pelvis is covered by the descending part of the duodenum and the renal vessels, while on the left the renal vessels and pancreas partially cover it [FIG. 168].

URETER

This expansile, muscular tube is 25 cm. long by 5 mm. wide. From a slight constriction at its junction with the pelvis of the kidney, it descends almost vertically along the line of the tips of the lumbar transverse processes to its mid-point which lies on the origin of the external iliac artery. Here the ureter enters the lesser pelvis [FIG. 148].

The ureter is adherent to the posterior surface of the peritoneum anterior to psoas major and the genitofemoral nerve, but it is separated from the peritoneum by the testicular (or ovarian) vessels and those passing to the colon. On the right these are the right colic, ileocolic, and superior mesenteric vessels, and on the left, the left colic and sigmoid vessels. The left ureter runs parallel and lateral to the inferior mesenteric vein [FIG. 146].

DISSECTION. Remove a small part of the ureter, slit it open, and pinning it out under water, dissect its walls layer by layer.

Structure. There is an outer layer of connective tissue. The muscle layer is complex and consists of bundles of smooth muscle separated by connective tissue. Throughout most of the ureter the muscle layers are inner longitudinal and outer circular, but a further longitudinal layer appears externally in the inferior part, and the circular layer disappears as the ureter reaches the bladder. In the pelvis of the kidney and the calyces, the muscle is mainly circular. The mucous membrane contains much elastic tissue and is lined by transitional epithelium (also elastic in character) which is also found in the calyces, pelvis of the kidney, and the bladder.

Blood Supply. The ureter receives branches from all the arteries with which it is related (renal, testicular or ovarian, aorta, common and internal iliac, vesical, and uterine) and these form longitudinal anastomoses on it. Lymph vessels drain to lumbar, common and internal iliac nodes.

DISSECTION. Strip the peritoneum from the diaphragm, and clean the crura on the anterior surfaces of the lumbar vertebrae. Identify the arcuate ligaments from which the diaphragm arises anterior to the aorta, psoas, and quadratus lumborum [Fig. 173]. Clean the slips of the diaphragm arising from the remaining costal cartilages, and identify the nerves and vessels entering the abdominal wall between them. Review the anterior attachments of the diaphragm.

THE DIAPHRAGM

[FIGS. 173, 174]

This thin, fibromuscular partition between the thoracic and abdominal cavities is an important muscle of respiration. It increases the vertical extent of the thoracic cavity by partially flattening its dome and compressing the abdominal contents when it contracts. The median part of the diaphragm is slightly depressed by the heart, and thus it has right and left domes. The **right dome,** supported by the liver, lies at a slightly higher level (a little inferior to the nipple) than the left, and may rise to the level of the fourth rib, superior to the nipple, on full expiration.

Attachments

The muscle fibres arise from the margins of

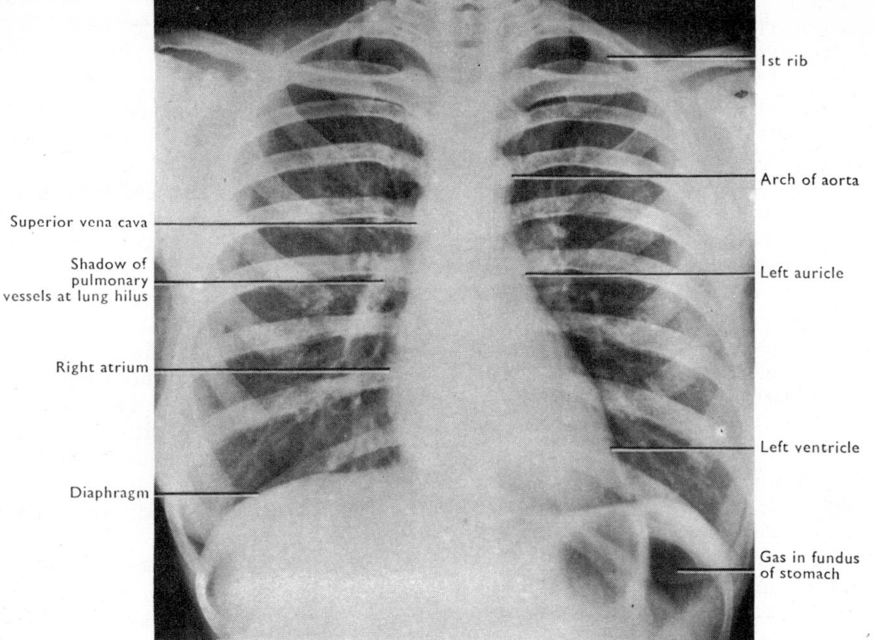

FIG. 172 An anteroposterior radiograph of the thorax in inspiration.

the inferior aperture of the thorax, and pass superomedially to the edges of the flat, C-shaped **central tendon.** The anterior fibres are nearly horizontal, but the posterior fibres pass almost vertically upwards and leave a deep recess between the thoracic wall and the diaphragm (costodiaphragmatic recesses and lower part of posterior mediastinum).

The **sternal origin** consists of two small slips from the back of the xiphoid process.

The **costal origin** is by wide, obliquely placed slips from the lower six costal cartilages, with the slips of transversus abdominis fitted between them.

The **vertebral origin** is by the crura and the arcuate ligaments.

Crura. These are thick, fleshy bundles that taper inferiorly to be attached to the anterior surfaces of the upper two (left) or three (right) lumbar vertebral bodies and the intervening discs by tendinous slips which arch over the lumbar vessels on the vertebral bodies. The muscle fibres of the right crus deviate to the left as they pass towards the central tendon, and thus surround the oesophageal hiatus.

Arcuate Ligaments. Superiorly the medial sides of the two crura are united by a tendinous band (the **median arcuate ligament**) over the anterior surface of the aorta, at the level of the twelfth thoracic vertebra. Laterally the tendinous part of each crus is connected to the transverse process of the first (or second) lumbar vertebra by a tendinous thickening of the fascia over psoas major, the **medial arcuate ligament.**

The **lateral arcuate ligament,** a linear thickening of the anterior layer of the thoracolumbar fascia over quadratus lumborum [FIG. 177], passes from the medial arcuate ligament over the anterior surface of quadratus lumborum to the twelfth rib.

All three ligaments give rise to muscle fibres of the diaphragm, though there are relatively few from the lateral ligament, and

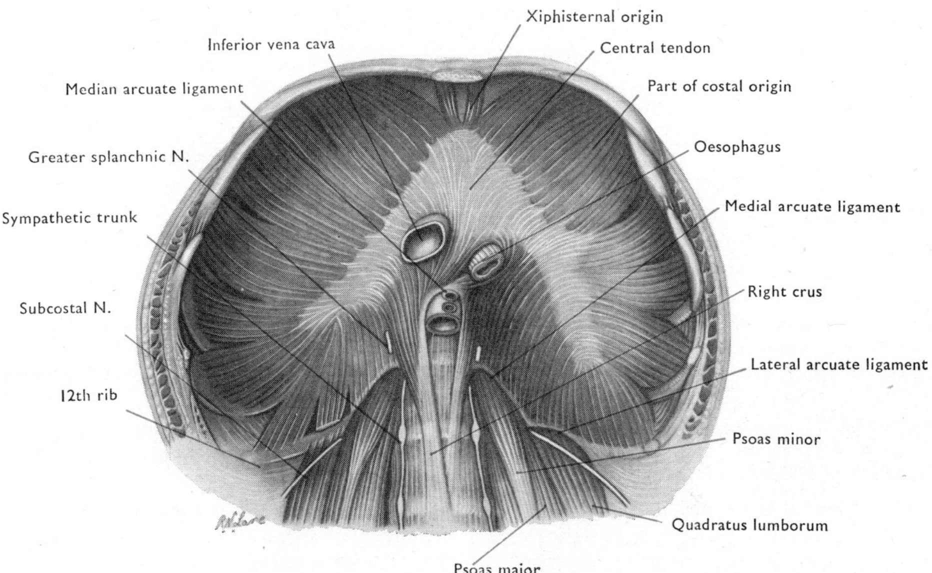

FIG. 173 The abdominal surface of the diaphragm.

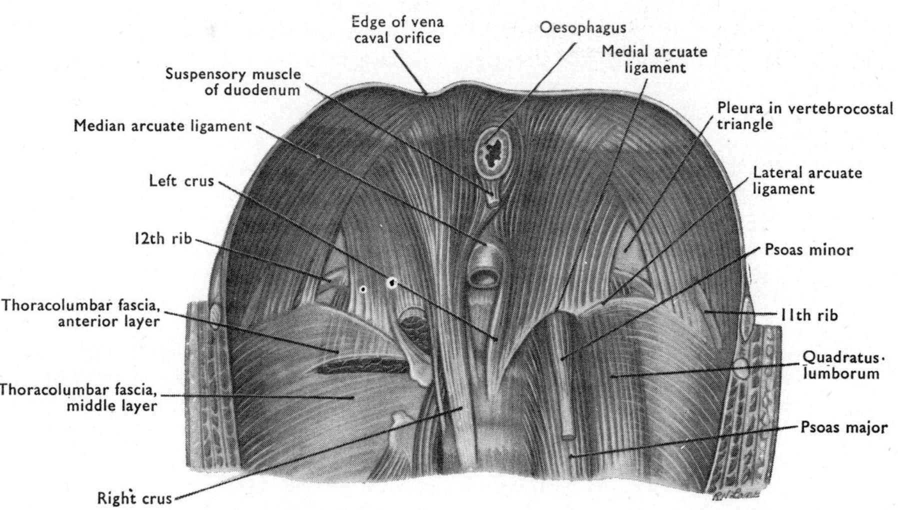

FIG. 174 The posterior origin of the diaphragm, seen from in front. The vertebrocostal triangles are particularly well marked.

they may be absent laterally (**vertebrocostal triangle,** FIG. 174), thus leaving the pleura almost directly in contact with the kidney, and making a potential site for the herniation of the abdominal contents into the thorax. This triangle is thought to represent the position of the embryonic pleuroperitoneal canal which is closed by the union of the parts of the diaphragm derived from the dorsal mesentery and the pleuroperitoneal membrane.

All the muscle fibres of the diaphragm converge on the strong C-shaped **central tendon** which is composed of interlacing tendinous bundles. It has right and left horns which curve posteriorly into the corresponding halves of the diaphragm, while the median part expands anteriorly towards the xiphoid process, and is the largest part.

Foramina in Diaphragm

A number of structures pass between the thorax and abdomen, but only the inferior vena cava and oesophagus form large foramina in the diaphragm, while the aorta passes behind its free posterior edge (median arcuate ligament).

The **inferior vena cava** pierces and fuses with the central tendon of the diaphragm 2–3 cm. to the right of the median plane, approximately at the level of the eighth thoracic vertebra. When the diaphragm contracts, it compresses the abdominal viscera, lowers the intrathoracic pressure, and pulls the inferior vena cava open, thus facilitating the flow of blood from the abdomen into the thorax. Slender branches of the right phrenic nerve and some lymph vessels from the liver also pass through the foramen for the vena cava [FIG. 48].

The **oesophagus** passes obliquely through an oval hiatus in the muscular part of the diaphragm, 2–3 cm. to the left of the median plane, and posterior to the central tendon. This hiatus lies approximately at the level of the tenth thoracic vertebra, and also transmits the anterior and posterior vagal trunks, oesophageal branches of the left gastric artery, and communications between the gastric and oesophageal veins.

The **aortic hiatus** lies between the upper ends of the two crura, posterior to the median arcuate ligament, and anterior to the twelfth thoracic vertebra. In addition to the aorta, the hiatus transmits the **thoracic duct,** the **azygos vein,** and **lymph vessels** which descend to the cisterna chyli (the saccular origin of the thoracic duct) from the thorax.

In addition to the three main apertures, a number of other structures pass from the thorax to the abdomen mainly at the margins of the diaphragm:

1. The **phrenic nerves,** the right lateral to the inferior vena cava, the left lateral to the pericardium.
2. The **superior epigastric vessels,** between the sternal and costal origins.
3. The **musculophrenic vessels,** between the slips from the seventh and eighth costal cartilages.
4. The lower five **intercostal nerves,** between the slips from the last six costal cartilages.
5. The **subcostal vessels** and **nerves,** posterior to the lateral arcuate ligaments.
6. The **sympathetic trunks,** posterior to the medial arcuate ligaments.
7. The **splanchnic nerves** pierce the crura, and the hemiazygos vein pierces the left crus.

Vessels and Nerves. The motor supply to the diaphragm is from the **phrenic nerves,** which ramify on its inferior surface, and arise from the third to fifth cervical ventral rami (mainly the fourth). The sensory supply comes via the phrenic and lower intercostal nerves.

The **arteries** are numerous, but the principal vessels are the inferior phrenic from the aorta, the musculophrenic from the internal thoracic, and the pericardiacophrenic which accompany the phrenic nerves through the thorax.

The high level of origin of the phrenic nerves is due to the caudal movement of the diaphragm and viscera relative to the vertebral column during development. The oblique course of the splanchnic nerves and the cervical cardiac branches of the sympathetic and vagus is similarly produced.

THE POSTERIOR ABDOMINAL WALL

VESSELS

DISSECTION. Clean the abdominal aorta and the inferior vena cava. Identify the lymph nodes that lie adjacent to them, and clean the sympathetic trunks which lie on each side of the aorta on the anterior margins of the psoas muscles; the right posterior to the inferior vena cava. Trace the branches of the sympathetic trunks, and clean the proximal parts of the lumbar arteries. Expose the cisterna chyli and vena azygos between the right crus of the diaphragm and the aorta. Trace the cisterna chyli to the thoracic duct and the azygos vein to the posterior surface of the inferior vena cava at the level of the renal veins. Clean the testicular or ovarian vessels.

THE ABDOMINAL AORTA

This median vessel extends from the aortic hiatus in the diaphragm to its bifurcation into the common iliac vessels, slightly to the left of the median plane on the fourth lumbar vertebra, at the level of the highest points on the iliac crests.

It lies on the anterior longitudinal ligament, the vertebral bodies, intervertebral discs, and the left lumbar veins crossing the median plane to enter the inferior vena cava. Superiorly it is between the crura of the diaphragm; inferiorly between the sympathetic trunks. The inferior vena cava lies on its right side, but is separated from it superiorly by the right crus of the diaphragm, while the ascending part of the duodenum and the coils of the jejunum lie on its left side inferiorly.

Several structures lie immediately anterior to the aorta in addition to those which partially surround it (the sympathetic plexuses, lymph vessels and nodes), and the visceral branches that arise from its anterior surface. From above downwards these are: (1) the pancreas and splenic vein, partly separated from the aorta by the superior mesenteric artery; (2) the left renal vein between the aorta and the superior mesenteric artery; (3) the horizontal part of the duodenum; (4) the root of the mesentery; and (5) the peritoneum separating it from coils of small intestine. In a slim person the inferior part of the abdominal aorta is very close to the anterior abdominal wall, and it may readily be compressed against the convexity of the lumbar vertebral column by firm pressure on the anterior abdominal wall in the region of the umbilicus.

BRANCHES

There are three sets of branches, **unpaired visceral branches** which have been seen already, **paired lateral branches** to the structures derived from the intermediate mesoderm of the embryo (the suprarenal glands, the kidneys, and the ovaries or testes), and **paired posterolateral branches** to the abdominal wall [p. 196].

The unpaired branches are the coeliac trunk, the superior and inferior mesenteric arteries, and the median sacral artery. The latter arises from the posterior surface of the extremity of the aorta and enters the lesser pelvis.

Paired Branches [Fig. 175]

Inferior Phrenic Arteries. These pass superolaterally over the crura of the diaphragm around the superior margins of the suprarenal glands (to which they send many small **superior suprarenal arteries),** and ramify on the inferior surface of the diaphragm. The corresponding veins enter the inferior vena cava, though the left may enter the left suprarenal vein.

Middle Suprarenal Arteries. These small vessels arise near the origin of the superior mesenteric artery, and pass laterally to the suprarenal glands. The right passes posterior to the inferior vena cava.

The **suprarenal veins,** one on each side, drain into the left renal vein and inferior vena cava respectively. Occasionally the left vein drains across the anterior surface of the aorta into the inferior vena cava.

Renal Arteries. These large arteries arise opposite the upper part of the second lumbar vertebra, and crossing the corresponding crus of the diaphragm and psoas muscle, reach the kidneys. Here each branches to supply the kidney [p. 180] and sends small arteries to the ureter and suprarenal gland (**inferior suprarenal artery**). The right renal artery passes posterior to the inferior vena cava and the corresponding vein, the left is posterior to its vein [FIG. 168].

An **accessory renal artery** is not uncommon. It usually arises from the lower part of the aorta, and passing anterior to the ureter (and the inferior vena cava if right-sided), enters the antero-inferior part of the kidney.

Renal Veins. These enter the inferior vena cava on the right of the median plane, and thus the right renal vein is much shorter than the left. Both veins lie anterior to the corresponding artery. The **right vein** passes posterior to the descending part of the duodenum, and may be overlapped by the right margin of the head of the pancreas. The long **left vein** is joined by the suprarenal, testicular or ovarian veins, and usually by the hemiazygos vein close to the kidney. The inferior mesenteric vein lies anterior to the left renal vein. The latter passes medially, posterior to the inferior border of the pancreas, and crosses the median plane in the angle between the aorta and the superior mesenteric artery [FIG. 175].

The difference in arrangement of the suprarenal and testicular or ovarian veins on the right and left sides (they join the inferior vena cava on the right) is due to the fact that the part of the left renal vein immediately to the left of the aorta is all that remains of the left inferior vena cava. This usually disappears early in development, but may persist from the level of the left renal vein downwards.

Testicular and Ovarian Vessels. The **testicular arteries** are long slender vessels that arise from the front of the aorta a short distance inferior to the renal arteries, and run inferolaterally to enter the inguinal canals, each through the corresponding deep inguinal ring. They lie anterior to the posterior abdominal wall and the urinary structures lying on it, but posterior to the gut tube and the mesenteric vessels. Thus the right testicular artery crosses the inferior vena cava, psoas, and ureter, and lies on the external iliac artery, but it is crossed by the duodenum, and by the right colic, ileocolic, and superior mesenteric vessels. The left testicular artery has the same structures posterior to it, except that it crosses the sympathetic trunk and not the inferior vena cava. It is crossed by the duodenum, the inferior mesenteric vein, the left colic and sigmoid arteries, and the inferior part of the descending colon [FIG. 146].

The **ovarian arteries** are exactly similar to the testicular arteries except that they enter the lesser pelvis by crossing the external iliac arteries 2–3 cm. inferior to their origins [FIG. 175].

Each **testicular** or **ovarian vein** arises from a pampiniform plexus, the one at the deep inguinal ring, the other at the margin of the superior aperture of the pelvis. These veins accompany the corresponding arteries, and the left enters the left renal vein, while the right enters the inferior vena cava just inferior to the renal vein.

Lumbar Arteries. Four pairs of these arteries arise from the posterior surface of the abdominal aorta in series with the intercostal arteries, and pass laterally on the surfaces of the vertebral bodies [p. 196].

THE INFERIOR VENA CAVA

This is the widest vein of the body. It drains venous blood directly from the lower limbs, most of the abdominal wall, and the urogenital apparatus. The venous blood from the remaining abdominal viscera enters the inferior vena cava after circulating through the liver.

It begins by the union of the two common iliac veins on the front of the fifth lumbar vertebra, posterior to the right common iliac artery [FIG. 175]. It ascends, 2 cm. to the right of the median plane, at first between the aorta and the right ureter, anterior to the vertebral column, psoas, the sympathetic trunk, and the lumbar arteries. It then lies between the right crus of the diaphragm and the kidney and suprarenal gland, and arches anteriorly in front of the right crus, the right renal artery, the right coeliac ganglion and middle suprarenal

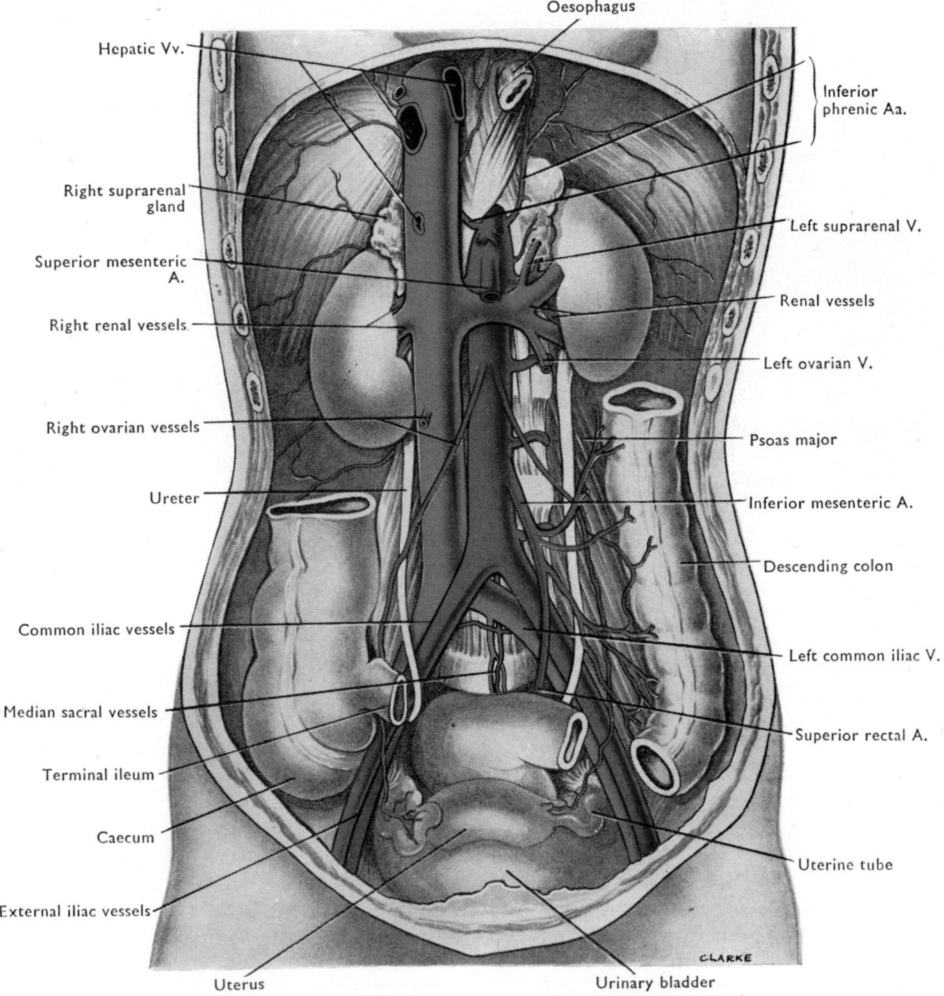

FIG. 175 The inferior vena cava and the abdominal aorta.

artery, the medial part of the right suprarenal gland, and the posterior part of the diaphragm [FIG. 116]. The latter part of the vein is embedded in the liver between the right and caudate lobes [FIG. 158].

Anterior to the inferior vena cava as it ascends are: (1) the superior mesenteric vessels in the root of the mesentery; (2) the leocolic and right colic vessels; (3) the horizontal part of the duodenum and the right testicular or ovarian artery; (4) the head of the pancreas and the bile-duct; (5) the portal vein, at first posterior to the duodenum, and then anterior to the epiploic foramen in the lesser omentum; and (6) a deep groove in the liver tissue between the caudate and right lobes. Here it receives the hepatic veins, then piercing the central tendon of the diaphragm and the pericardium, enters the postero-inferior part of the right atrium [FIG. 48].

TRIBUTARIES

(1) Common iliac veins. (2) Third and fourth lumbar veins. (3) Right testicular or ovarian vein. (4) Renal veins. (5) Right supra-renal vein. (6) Inferior phrenic veins. (7) Hepatic veins. (8) The azygos vein.

Common Iliac Arteries [FIGS. 146, 175]

These terminal branches of the abdominal aorta arise on the anterior surface of the fourth lumbar vertebra, and each passes inferolaterally to the superior surface of the sacro-iliac joint, where it divides into internal and external iliac arteries. *Both* common iliac arteries are crossed by branches of the corresponding sympathetic trunk passing to the hypogastric plexuses, the *left* by the superior rectal vessels and some sigmoid arteries. The *right* common iliac artery lies on the end of the inferior vena cava and the corresponding vein, while the *left* crosses the sympathetic trunk and the medial margin of psoas on the fourth and fifth lumbar vertebrae.

Common Iliac Veins [FIG. 175]

These veins begin on the medial surface of psoas by the union of the internal and external iliac veins, and they end by uniting in the inferior vena cava 2 cm. to the right of the median plane on the fifth lumbar vertebra. Each receives an **iliolumbar vein,** and the **median sacral vein** joins the left common iliac vein.

The right vein is posterior to the corresponding artery, while the left is infero-medial to the artery and runs a longer course to reach the inferior vena cava.

External Iliac Arteries. These arteries begin immediately anterior to the sacro-iliac joints as the direct continuation of the common iliac arteries. Each passes inferolaterally along the margin of the superior aperture of the lesser pelvis, at first medial and then anterior to psoas, and enters the thigh, as the **femoral artery,** posterior to the inguinal ligament at the mid-inguinal point. The deep circumflex iliac and the inferior epigastric arteries arise immediately superior to the inguinal ligament, and are the only branches.

The artery is at first anterior and then lateral to its vein, and is crossed proximally by the ureter and distally by the ductus deferens (or the round ligament of the uterus) and the deep circumflex iliac vein. The genital branch of the genitofemoral nerve runs on the distal part of the artery, and the ovarian vessels cross it 2–3 cm. inferior to its origin [FIG. 209]. On the right the caecum and appendix may overlie it; on the left, the end of the descending colon is directly in contact with its inferior part.

External Iliac Veins. Each of these veins begins posterior to the inguinal ligament on the medial side of the artery. Medial to psoas it ascends to the posterior surface of the artery, and passing lateral to the internal iliac artery, unites with the internal iliac vein. It receives the **inferior epigastric** and **deep circumflex iliac veins,** and is crossed by the same structures as the artery.

THE LYMPH NODES OF THE POSTERIOR ABDOMINAL WALL [FIGS. 176, 228]

These are scattered along the iliac vessels and the aorta and inferior vena cava.

The **external iliac nodes** lie along the free surfaces of the external iliac vessels. Inferiorly the medial nodes receive lymph from the free lower limb and pelvic viscera, while the lateral nodes drain the territories of the inferior epigastric and deep circumflex iliac arteries. This lymph passes upwards through other external iliac nodes to the **common iliac nodes.** These consist of: (1) lateral groups along the common iliac arteries, which drain the lower limbs and pelvis through the external and internal iliac nodes; and (2) a median group between the arteries. These drain the pelvic viscera directly and through the internal iliac and sacral nodes. The common iliac nodes send their efferent vessels to the lumbar nodes.

The **lumbar nodes** are scattered around the aorta (particularly on its left side) and the inferior vena cava. They receive lymph directly from adjacent structures, and along the testicular or ovarian vessels from the testes or from the ovaries, uterine tubes, and uterus. Lymph drains into these nodes through other nodes from: (1) the remainder of the abdominal contents (except the small intestine, p. 148); and (2) from the pelvis and lower limbs. Their efferent vessels form the **lumbar lymph trunks,** one on each side, and these drain to the cisterna chyli.

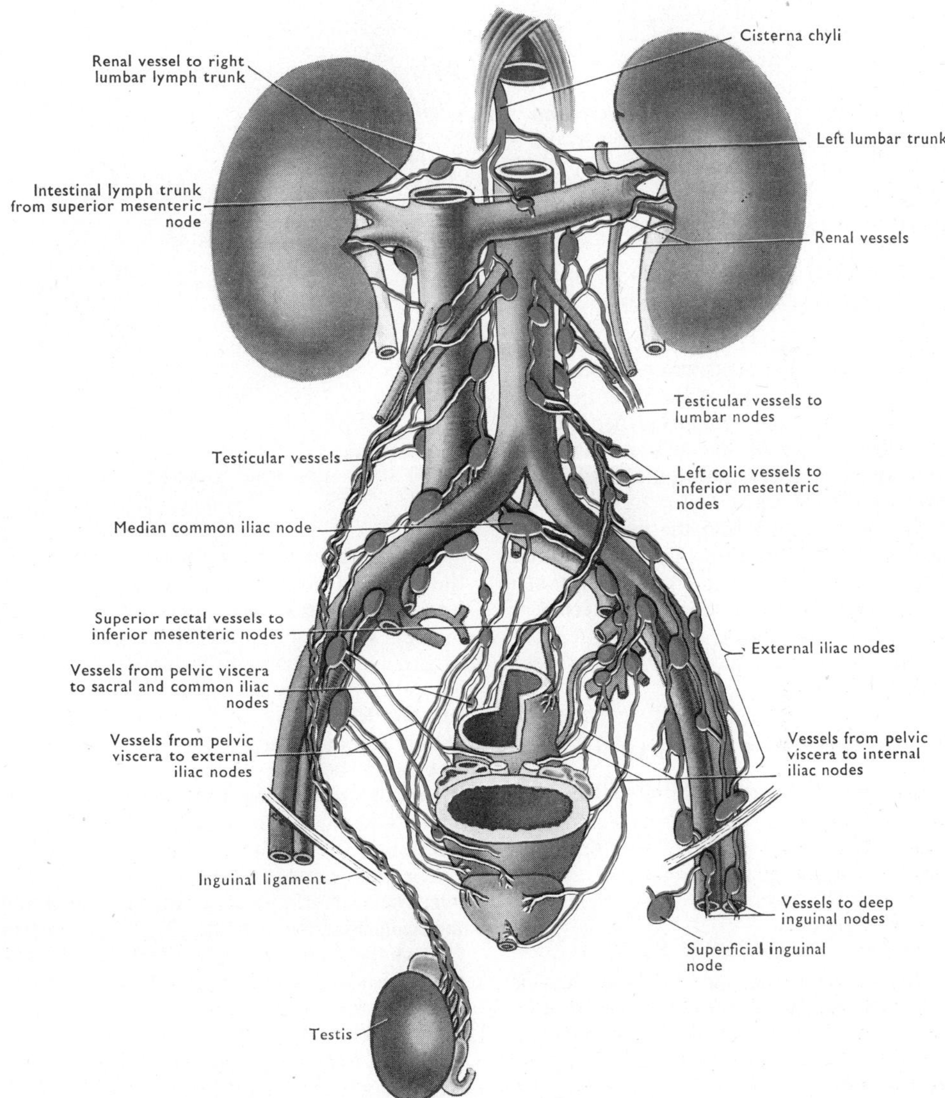

FIG. 176 A diagram to show the lymph vessels and nodes of the male pelvis and abdomen.

THE CISTERNA CHYLI

This long (5 cm.), white lymph sac, approximately 4 mm. wide in the cadaver, is often tortuous and branched. It lies on the upper two lumbar vertebrae between the aorta and azygos vein, hidden by the right crus of the diaphragm. It receives the **lumbar lymph trunks** inferiorly, the **intestinal lymph trunk** (which drains the small intestine) about the middle, and two lymph trunks from the lower **intercostal nodes** superiorly. Above it narrows to the thoracic duct, which passes through the aortic hiatus in the diaphragm between the aorta and the azygos vein [Fig. 75].

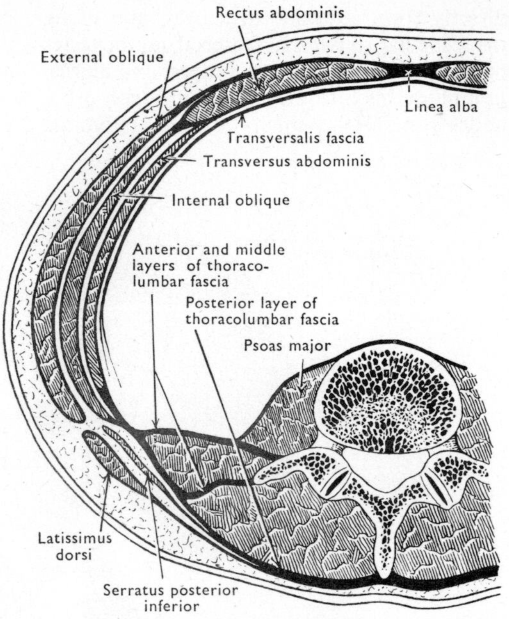

Fig. 177 A horizontal section through the abdominal walls at the level of the second lumbar vertebra, to show the thoracolumbar fascia.

THE AZYGOS AND HEMIAZYGOS VEINS

These veins usually begin in the abdomen, the azygos from the posterior surface of the inferior vena cava at the level of the renal veins, and the hemiazygos from the posterior surface of the left renal vein. They ascend into the thorax, the azygos vein through the aortic hiatus to the right of the thoracic duct, and the hemiazygos through the left crus of the diaphragm. Either or both veins may arise from the union of the **subcostal** and **ascending lumbar veins**; the latter ascending in the substance of psoas, anterior to the lumbar transverse processes [Fig. 180].

THE MUSCLES AND FASCIA OF THE POSTERIOR ABDOMINAL WALL

Three muscles on each side form the greater part of the posterior abdominal wall, and each is covered with fascia.

Quadratus Lumborum [Figs. 91, 167, 174]

This muscle arises from the iliolumbar ligament, the adjacent part of the iliac crest, and the last two to four lumbar transverse processes. It ascends, narrowing slightly, and passing posterior to the lateral arcuate ligament, is inserted into the medial part of the anterior surface of the twelfth rib, posterior to the lowest part of the pleura. It is also inserted into the transverse processes of the upper four lumbar vertebrae, posterior to the slips of origin. Nerve supply: direct branches from the ventral rami of the upper four lumbar nerves. Action: It is a lateral flexor of the lumbar vertebral column, and a muscle of inspiration. The latter because it helps to elongate the thorax by preventing the twelfth rib rising either with the other ribs, or with the contraction of the diaphragm.

The quadratus lumborum is enclosed between the anterior and middle layers of the **thoracolumbar fascia** [Fig. 177]. These layers fuse at the lateral margin of quadratus lumborum, and elsewhere are attached to the same structures as quadratus lumborum, but anterior and posterior to it. The **anterior layer** is thickened to form the **lateral arcuate ligament** and is thin superior to this where it is behind the pleura.

Psoas Major [FIGS. 173, 177]

This long muscle arises between the lower border of the twelfth thoracic vertebra (superior to the diaphragm) and the upper border of the fifth lumbar vertebra. Between these points it arises from: (1) the anterior surfaces of the lumbar transverse processes, medial to quadratus lumborum; and (2) the sides of the intervertebral discs and the adjacent margins of the vertebral bodies, and between these, from **tendinous arches** that bridge over the lumbar arteries.

The muscle passes inferolaterally along the margin of the superior aperture of the lesser pelvis, enters the thigh posterior to the inguinal ligament, and is inserted by a tendon into the lesser trochanter of the femur [FIG. 179]. Nerve supply: direct branches from the second to fourth lumbar ventral rami and from the femoral nerve. Action: see under iliacus.

Psoas Minor [FIG. 174]

This small muscle is present in only 60 per cent. of cases. It arises with the uppermost fibres of psoas major, passes on to the anterior surface of that muscle, and rapidly narrowing to a slender tendon, is inserted through the fascia on psoas major into the arcuate line of the ilium medial to psoas major [FIGS. 183, 231]. Nerve supply: the first lumbar nerve. Action: see under iliacus.

Iliacus [FIGS. 179, 231]

This muscle arises from the upper part of the floor of the iliac fossa. It converges on and fuses with the lower part of psoas major, and passing with it posterior to the inguinal ligament, is inserted partly with the tendon of psoas and partly into the femur immediately inferior to the lesser trochanter. Nerve supply: a branch of the femoral nerve.

Actions of Psoas and Iliacus. They are flexors and medial rotators of the hip joint, since they pass anterior to that joint and are inserted lateral to the axis of rotation of the femur. Acting from a fixed femur, they flex the trunk on the hip joint. Psoas major and minor flex the lumbar vertebral column laterally.

Fascia of Psoas and Iliacus. Superior to the iliac crest psoas is enclosed in a sheath of, fascia which is attached medially to the vertebral column with that muscle, and laterally blends with the anterior layer of the thoracolumbar fascia. It is thickened to form the **medial arcuate ligament,** and superior to this is continuous with the fascia over the anterior surface of the thoracic vertebral column. Below the iliac crest, the fascia is attached medially to the arcuate line of the ilium, but laterally it extends as a continuous layer over iliacus and is firmly attached to the internal lip of the iliac crest (iliac fascia). Inferiorly, the medial part of this common fascial sheet passes into the thigh posterior to the large vessels (**posterior wall of the femoral sheath,** FIG. 99), while the lateral part fuses with the transversalis fascia posterior to the inguinal ligament [FIG. 96].

The presence of a sheath of fascia stretching over psoas from the vertebral column to the groin makes a route for the spread of infected material from the vertebral column, so that this may first appear as an abscess in the groin

DISSECTION. Clean the muscles of the posterior abdominal wall by removing their fascial coverings. Avoid injury to the vessels and nerves related to the muscles (the main vessels lie anterior to the fascial layer while the nerves are posterior to it). The vessels on iliacus are branches of the iliolumbar artery.

THE NERVES OF THE POSTERIOR ABDOMINAL WALL

DISSECTION. Push the inferior vena cava laterally and expose the right sympathetic trunk. Trace both trunks superiorly to the medial arcuate ligament, and inferiorly, posterior to the common iliac vessels, into the pelvis. Find and trace the branches of both trunks to the superior hypogastric plexus [p. 150]. Detach psoas from the intervertebral discs and vertebral bodies, and trace the lumbar vessels and the rami communicantes from the sympathetic trunks posteriorly into the lumbar nerves.

Sympathetic Trunk [FIG. 173]

The thoracic part of each sympathetic trunk becomes the lumbar part posterior to the medial arcuate ligament. The trunk extends inferiorly in the groove between the anterior border of psoas major and the vertebral column (anterior to the lumbar vessels) to enter the pelvis by passing posterior to the common iliac vessels.

Branches. The **rami communicantes** [p. 29] are long and pass with the lumbar vessels to connect the ganglia to the ventral rami of the lumbar nerves. Both **white** and **grey** rami join the sympathetic trunk to the first two lumbar ventral rami, but there is only a grey ramus uniting it to the other lumbar and to the sacral nerves.

Visceral branches (lumbar splanchnic nerves) arise irregularly from the trunk, and pass to the aortic and hypogastric plexuses.

Subcostal Nerve

This is the ventral ramus of the last thoracic nerve. It sends a branch downwards in the upper part of psoas to join the first lumbar nerve, and then passing inferolaterally over the anterior surface of quadratus lumborum, it enters the abdomen posterior to the lateral arcuate ligament. At the lateral border of quadratus lumborum it pierces transversus abdominis, and passes into the abdominal wall between that muscle and the internal oblique [p. 102].

DISSECTION. Find the genitofemoral nerve [Fig. 179] on psoas, and trace it through that muscle to the lumbar nerves. Carefully complete the removal of psoas from the transverse processes of the lumbar vertebrae, disentangling the lumbar nerves from its substance. Clean these nerves and trace their branches.

LUMBAR NERVES

The five lumbar nerves emerge through the intervertebral foramina below the corresponding vertebrae, and their ventral rami pass into the posterior part of psoas major. They are connected to the sympathetic trunk by rami communicantes, and they give branches to supply the intertransverse muscles, quadratus lumborum and psoas. The ventral rami then divide, the upper branch of the **fourth lumbar nerve** joining with the branches of the first to third to form the **lumbar plexus,** while its inferior branch passes downwards to join the fifth lumbar ventral ramus and form the **lumbosacral trunk,** which passes to the **sacral plexus.** Because it divides in this manner to send nerve fibres into both plexuses, the fourth lumbar nerve is sometimes called the nervus furcalis.

Lumbar Plexus

This plexus is formed by the ventral rami of the first three lumbar nerves and part of the fourth, together with a contribution from the subcostal nerve. It lies in the substance of psoas major, and the ventral rami of the second, third, and fourth split into ventral and dorsal divisions which unite separately to form a series of nerves [Fig. 178].

The iliohypogastric nerve (L.1, T.12) emerges at the lateral border of psoas, and passing inferolaterally between quadratus lumborum and the kidney, pierces transversus abdominis a short distance superior to the iliac crest, and runs in the abdominal wall [p. 103].

The ilioinguinal nerve (L. 1) takes the same course as the iliohypogastric but on a slightly lower level. It has no lateral cutaneous branch.

The genitofemoral nerve (L. 1, 2; ventral divisions) passes anteriorly through psoas, and running inferiorly on that muscle, divides into femoral and genital branches.

The **femoral branch** runs along the lateral side of the external iliac artery, and enters the thigh posterior to the inguinal ligament. The **genital branch** pierces the fascia on psoas, and runs to enter the inguinal canal through the deep inguinal ring. In the male it supplies the cremaster muscle: in the female, sensory fibres to the round ligament of the uterus and skin of the labium majus.

The lateral cutaneous nerve of the thigh (L. 2, 3; dorsal divisions) emerges from psoas above the iliac crest, and passing obliquely across iliacus to the anterior superior iliac spine, enters the thigh posterior to the lateral end of the inguinal ligament.

The femoral nerve (L. 2, 3, 4; dorsal divisions) emerges from psoas below the iliac crest,

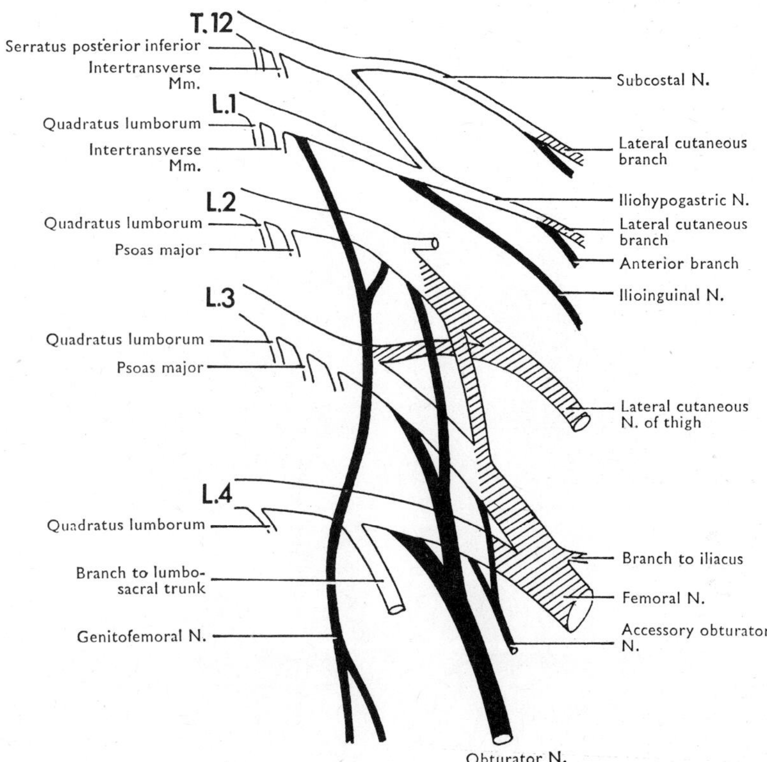

FIG. 178 A diagram of the lumbar plexus. Ventral divisions of the ventral rami, black; dorsal divisions, cross hatched. See also FIG. 229.

and descending in the groove between psoas and iliacus (posterior to the iliac fascia and the caecum or descending colon), enters the thigh lateral to the femoral sheath. It supplies psoas major and iliacus in the abdomen.

The obturator nerve (L. 2, 3, 4; ventral divisions) leaves the medial border of psoas major at the superior aperture of the lesser pelvis, and enters the pelvis by piercing the psoas fascia.

Occasionally an **accessory obturator nerve** arises either from the obturator nerve or from the third and fourth lumbar nerves. It enters the thigh along the medial side of psoas, gives branches to the hip joint and occasionally to pectineus, and joins the obturator nerve.

Lumbosacral Trunk. This is formed by the union of the ventral ramus of the fifth lumbar nerve with the inferior branch of the fourth. The latter descends through psoas over the medial part of the fifth lumbar transverse process, and uniting with the fifth, enters the lesser pelvis by passing over and grooving the ala of the sacrum, posterior to the common iliac vessels and psoas.

The roots of the obturator and femoral nerves cross the front of the **fifth lumbar transverse process.** Thus they, and the contribution from the fourth lumbar to the lumbosacral trunk, may be damaged in injuries of this process.

SUBCOSTAL AND LUMBAR VESSELS

The **subcostal artery** is the last parietal branch of the thoracic aorta. It passes with the

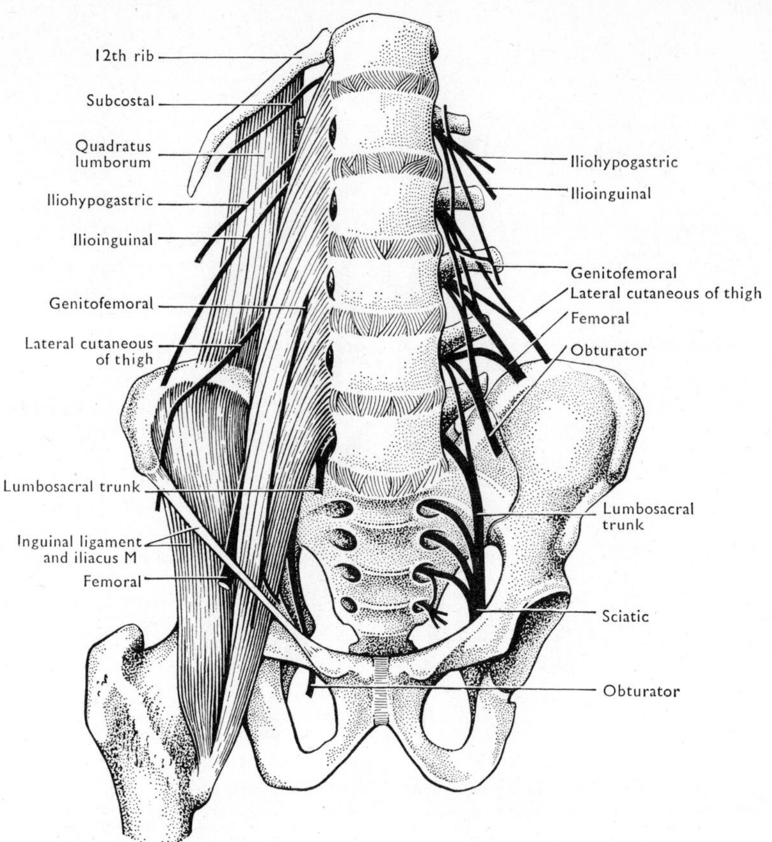

FIG. 179 A semidiagrammatic drawing of the lumbosacral plexus and the quadratus lumborum and iliopsoas muscles.

subcostal nerve, posterior to the lateral arcuate ligament and kidney, into the abdominal wall. The subcostal vein lies superior to the artery and enters either the azygos (right) or hemiazygos vein (left).

The **lumbar arteries.** The upper four pairs arise from the posterior surface of the aorta on the lumbar vertebral bodies. They curve over the vertebral bodies deep to the sympathetic trunk (and to cisterna chyli and the inferior vena cava on the right), and the fibrous arches that give origin to the crura of the diaphragm (upper two) and the psoas. The lumbar veins and the rami communicantes run with them. At the root of the transverse process, each artery gives off a posterior branch, and running posterior to quadratus lumborum, ends in a number of small branches between transversus abdominis and internal oblique muscles.

The **posterior branch** accompanies the dorsal ramus of the spinal nerve between the transverse processes, and sends branches into the erector spinae and the overlying skin. A **spinal branch** passes through the intervertebral foramen to supply the contents of the vertebral canal.

The small **fifth pair** of lumbar arteries arise from the median sacral artery or the iliolumbar arteries.

Lumbar Veins. These veins accompany the

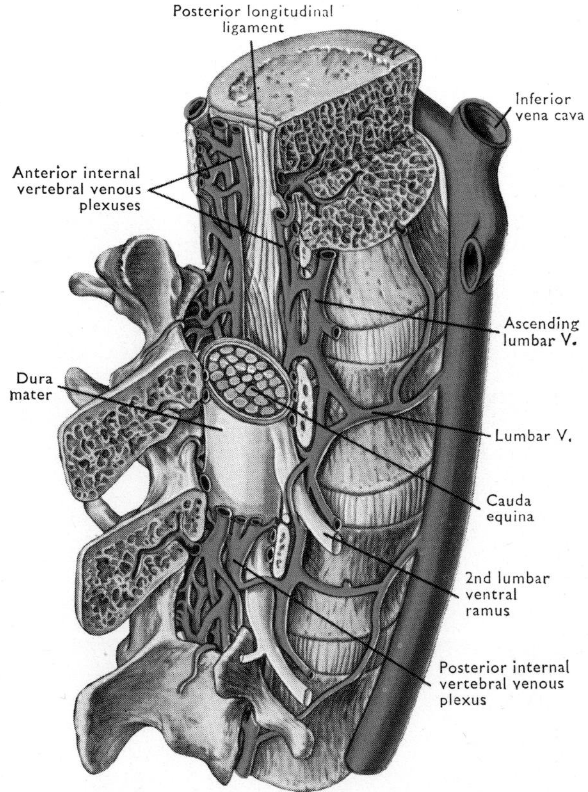

FIG. 180 Dissection of the upper four lumbar vertebrae to show the internal vertebral venous plexuses and their communications with the inferior vena cava.

lumbar arteries. The third and fourth enter the inferior vena cava (the left vessels passing posterior to the aorta), the first and second join the ascending lumbar vein on the lumbar transverse processes, while the fifth drains through the iliolumbar vein to the common iliac vein.

The **ascending lumbar vein** unites the lateral sacral, iliolumbar, and upper four lumbar veins to the subcostal vein. It lies in psoas major anterior to the lumbar transverse processes, and it drains into the azygos or hemiazygos vein through the subcostal vein. The major tributaries of this vein are the communications through the intervertebral foramina with the internal vertebral venous plexuses [FIG. 180].

DISSECTION. It is an advantage to remove the pelvis from the trunk at this stage, but this can only be done without damage if the erector spinae and the lumbar vertebral canal have been dissected. If this has not been done by dissectors of the head and neck, then pages 24 and 28–35 of Volume 3 of this 'Manual' should be read and the dissections carried out only on the lumbar and sacral regions.

Cut through the intervertebral disc between the third and fourth lumbar vertebrae and all the other soft structures on each side of the vertebral column at this level. Identify the joints between the articular processes, and dividing the ligaments uniting them, separate the pelvis and lower limbs from the remainder of the trunk.

THE INTERVERTEBRAL JOINTS

Examine the joints between the lumbar vertebrae, and with the help of dried vertebrae [FIGS. 85, 86], compare the arrangement in the lumbar region with those in the thoracic and cervical regions [p. 91]. Review the structure of the intervertebral discs [p. 87] and the arrangement of the ligaments uniting the vertebrae.

If the dissectors of the abdomen and pelvis are to proceed later to dissect the lower limb, *there is considerable advantage in dissecting the thigh and gluteal region before continuing with the pelvis.* If this is possible, then pages 129–169 of Volume 1 of this *Manual* should now be followed.

THE PELVIS AND PERINEUM

The bony structure of the pelvis consists of the two hip bones, the sacrum, and the coccyx, united by four joints: the two synovial sacro-iliac joints posterosuperiorly, the two fibro-cartilaginous joints—the pubic symphysis antero-inferiorly and the sacrococcygeal joint posteriorly.

In the erect position the pelvis lies with the upper margin of the pubic symphysis and the anterior superior iliac spines in the same coronal plane. This is the position taken up by an articulated pelvis placed with these three points touching a vertical surface.

The pelvis consists of two parts which are separated by the plane of the superior aperture of the lesser pelvis. This is an oblique plane passing from the sacral promontory to the upper surface of the pubic symphysis. The part anterosuperior to the plane, the greater pelvis, is formed by the iliac fossae and is part of the wall of the abdomen. The part postero-inferior to the plane is the lesser pelvis, to which the term pelvis is frequently applied.

THE LESSER PELVIS

The superior and posterior bony walls of the lesser pelvis together are formed by the curved sacrum and by the coccyx, while the antero-inferior wall lies below the level of the tip of the coccyx, and is short, consisting of the bodies of the pubic bones united in the midline by the pubic symphysis [FIG. 209].

The curved lateral wall is formed anteri-

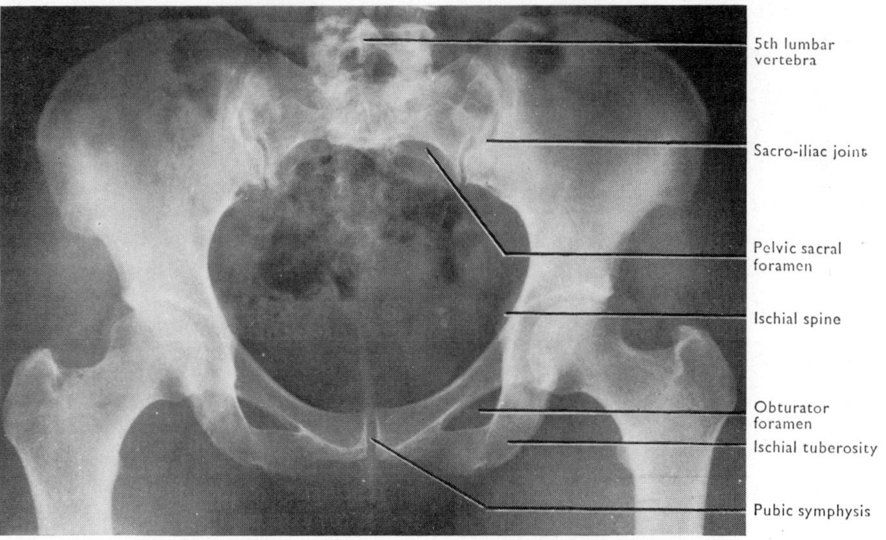

FIG. 181 An anteroposterior radiograph of the female pelvis.

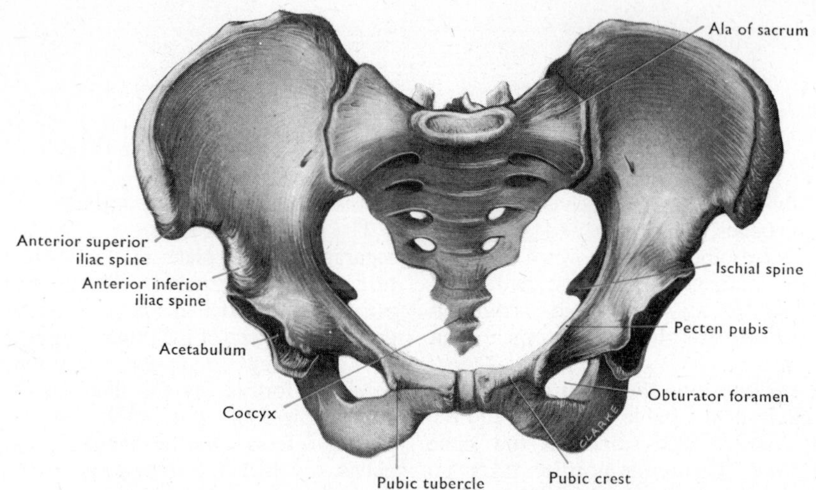

FIG. 182 The female pelvis seen from in front.

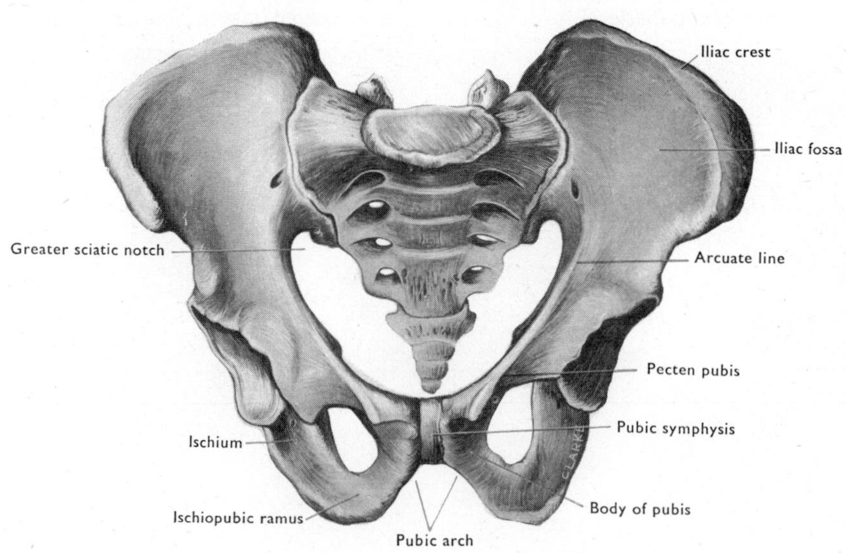

FIG. 183 The male pelvis seen from in front.

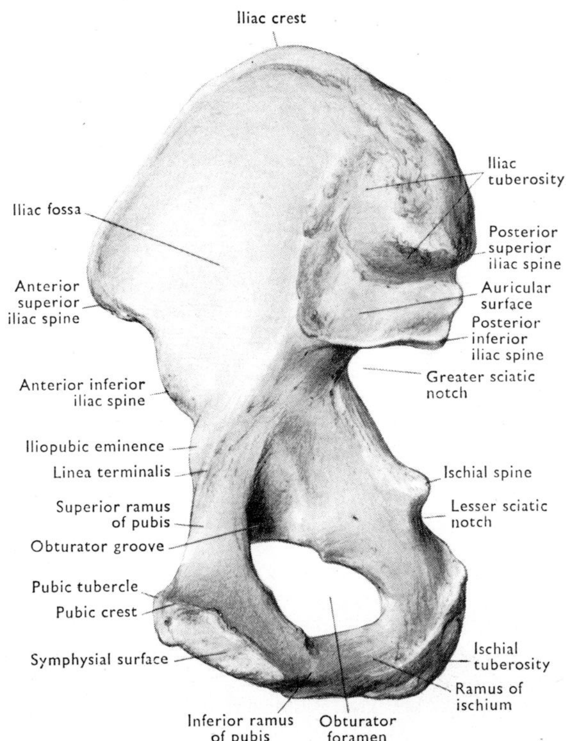

FIG. 184 Right hip bone seen from the medial side [FIG. 231].

orly by the rami of the pubis separated by the obturator foramen, laterally and below by the ischium which completes the obturator foramen, **and above by the union of the ilium, ischium, and pubis** (the medial wall of the acetabulum) [FIG. 207]. Posterosuperiorly the ilium forms a small part of the lateral wall, and curves medially to meet the sacrum in the **sacro-iliac joint.** Inferior to this the ilium and ischium are separated from the sacrum by a deep notch, which is partly divided by the projection of the spine of the ischium, into a larger, superior, **greater sciatic notch,** and a smaller, inferior, **lesser sciatic notch.** Inferior to the spine of the ischium, and separated from it by the lesser sciatic notch, is the **tuberosity of the ischium.** The **sacrospinous** and **sacrotuberous ligaments** [FIGS. 232, 233] pass from the sacrum and coccyx to the spine and tuberosity of the ischium. These convert the notches into the **greater** and lesser **sciatic foramina** respectively, forming part of the posterolateral wall of the lesser pelvis. The inferior part of the lateral wall is completed by the **obturator membrane,** which fills all but the anterior part of the obturator foramen where the obturator vessels and nerve leave the pelvis.

The walls of the lesser pelvis end above in the margins of the **superior aperture:** the sacral promontory and ala, the arcuate line of the ilium, the pecten pubis, the pubic crest, and the pubic symphysis. Inferiorly the walls end in the boundaries of the **inferior aperture** of the pelvis: *i.e.*, the coccyx, the sacrotuberous ligaments, the ischial tuberosities, the sides of the pubic arch (composed on each side by the ramus of the ischium and the inferior ramus of the pubic bone) and the pubic symphysis. These are also the boundaries of the perineum [FIGS. 192, 193].

The **inferior aperture** transmits the urethra, the vagina in the female, and the anal canal, but elsewhere is closed, anteriorly by the perineal membrane and certain muscles (in the pubic arch), and posteriorly by the levator ani muscles. The other walls of the pelvis are lined by muscles: piriformis on the sacrum, coccygeus on the sacrospinous ligament, obturator internus on the lateral wall. All of these are covered internally with a layer of **pelvic fascia.**

The **levator ani muscles** run postero-inferiorly from the fascia covering the obturator internus to meet one another along a line from the posterior surface of the urethra to the coccyx. Thus they form a V-shaped gutter which divides the cavity of the lesser pelvis into an upper part containing the pelvic viscera (the **pelvic cavity**) of which they form the sloping floor, and a lower part consisting of an **ischiorectal fossa** on each

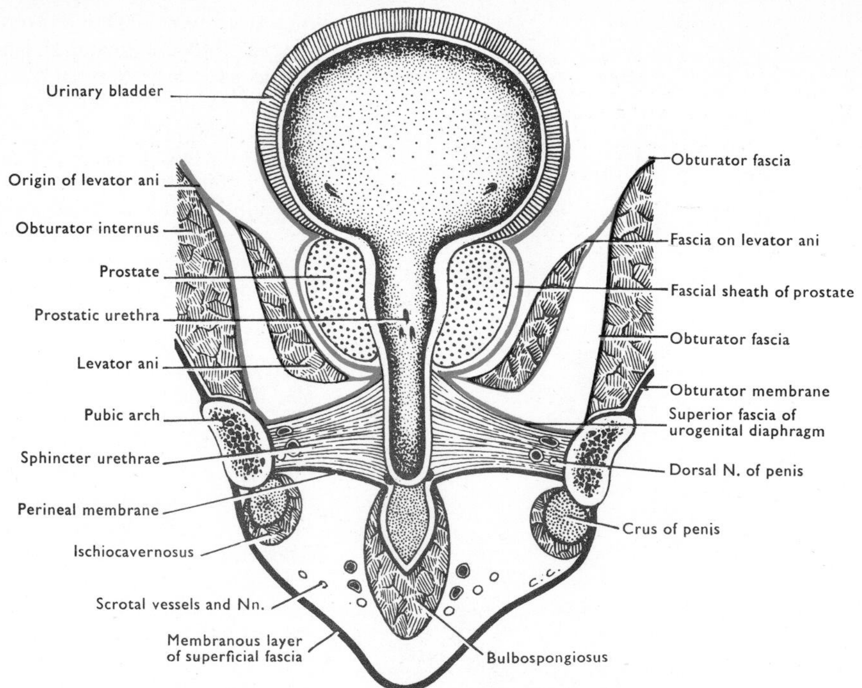

FIG. 185 A schematic coronal section through the male pelvis and perineum to show the arrangement of the parietal and visceral pelvic fascia (red).

side, roofed by the levator ani muscles [FIG. 198].

The **parietal pelvic fascia** lines the walls of the pelvic cavity. It is part of the fascial envelope of the abdomen, and is continuous at the superior aperture of the pelvis with the fascia iliaca laterally, and the fascia transversalis anteriorly. Inferiorly it covers the superior surfaces of the levator ani muscles, and becomes continuous with the loose fascial layer (**visceral pelvic fascia;** FIGS. 185, 195) that surrounds the pelvic viscera where these structures lie on, or pierce, levator ani. The **peritoneum** passes over the superior surfaces of the pelvic viscera and forms pouches between them. Elsewhere they are separated from the parietal pelvic fascia by fatty extraperitoneal tissue which contains the blood vessels. The nerves lie external to the parietal pelvic fascia.

DISSECTION. Clean the nerves and dura mater in the sacral canal, and follow each sacral nerve to its division into ventral and dorsal rami. Identify the sacral and coccygeal cornua, and trace the filum terminale, the coccygeal, and fifth sacral nerves through the lower end of the sacral canal [Fig. 187].

THE SACRAL CANAL

Contents. 1. The tubes of **dura mater** and **arachnoid** that surround the spinal medulla extend down to the level of the second sacral vertebra. Here they close down on the **filum terminale** [FIG. 187, and Vol. 3, p. 33] which receives a thin covering from them and continues on to the back of the coccyx.

2. The roots of five pairs of **sacral nerves** and one pair of **coccygeal nerves** pierce the arachnoid and dura and receive a sheath from each of them. The roots of the upper four sacral nerves unite at the ganglia in the lateral

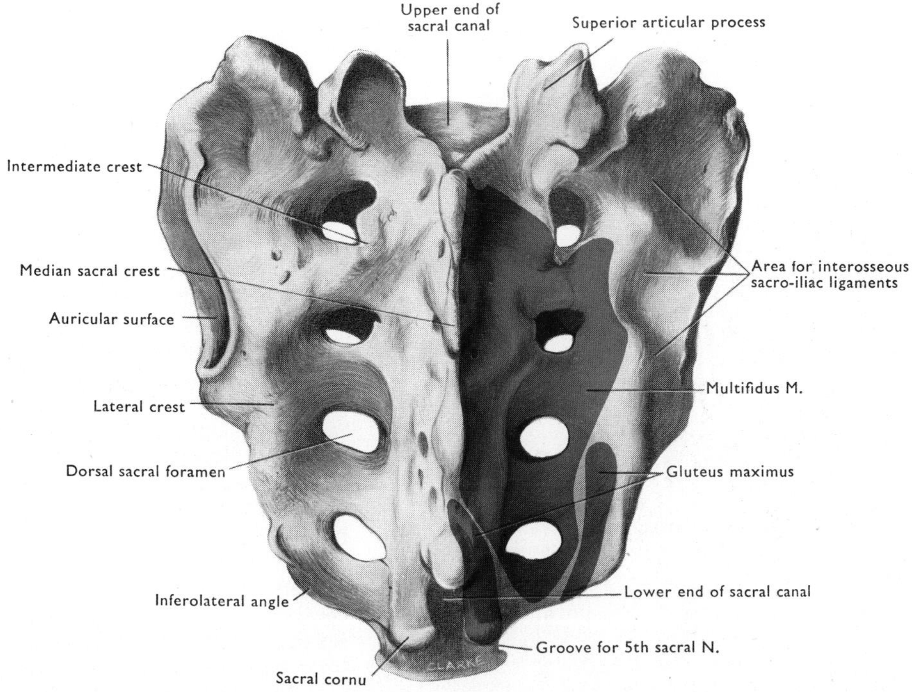

FIG. 186 The dorsal surface of the sacrum.

part of the sacral canal, and divide almost at once into dorsal and ventral rami. The small **dorsal rami** pass through the dorsal sacral foramina and supply the erector spinae and skin on the dorsum of the sacrum and adjacent gluteal region. The large **ventral rami** enter the pelvis through the pelvic sacral foramina to form the greater part of the **sacral plexus.**

The roots of the fifth pair of sacral nerves unite in the lower part of the sacral canal, and their rami escape through its inferior end. The roots of the coccygeal nerves unite within the dural sac, and piercing it, leave through the inferior end of the sacral canal. The dorsal rami of the fifth sacral and the coccygeal nerves unite, and communicating with the fourth sacral, supply the overlying skin. Their ventral rami run forwards through the sacrotuberous and sacrospinous ligaments, and entering the pelvis, form the coccygeal plexus. Around the dura and nerves is the inferior part of the internal vertebral venous plexus. It communicates with the pelvic veins through the pelvic sacral foramina [FIG. 230].

DISSECTION. Assuming that the gluteal region has been dissected, clean the iliolumbar ligaments and the ligaments on the posterior surface of the sacro-iliac joint by removing the overlying muscles and the posterior layer of the thoracolumbar fascia. Expose the dorsal sacral foramina and the dorsal rami of the sacral nerves passing through them together with small blood vessels. Clean the sacrotuberous ligament and define its attachments. Divide the ligament at its middle, and separate it from the sacrospinous ligament, noting any small nerves between them. Clean the sacrospinous ligament. On its lateral part and on the spine of the ischium, clean the pudendal nerve, the internal pudendal vessels, and the nerve to obturator internus.

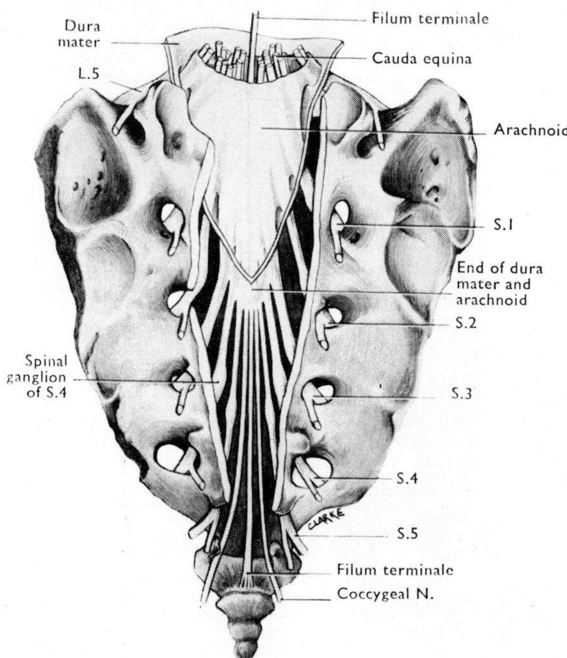

FIG. 187 A dissection to expose the sacral nerves and meninges within the sacral canal.

VERTEBROPELVIC LIGAMENTS
[FIGS. 192, 232, 233]

The **iliolumbar ligament** is a strong, triangular ligament that unites the thick transverse process of the fifth lumbar vertebra to the inner lip of the iliac crest posteriorly. It gives origin to part of the quadratus lumborum, and has the middle and anterior layers of the thoracolumbar fascia fused with it. Anteriorly it is covered by psoas, and posteriorly by erector spinae. It plays an important part in retaining the fifth lumbar vertebra in position, resisting the tendency of the weight of the body to force that vertebra antero-inferiorly on the sloping superior surface of the sacrum [FIGS. 91, 209].

The **sacrotuberous ligament** has a wide origin from the dorsal surfaces of the sacrum and coccyx and from both the posterior iliac spines. It passes downwards, forwards, and laterally, at first narrowing and then expanding again, to be attached to a curved, sharp ridge of bone along the medial margin of the ischial tuberosity. It is partly continuous with the tendon of biceps femoris, and the anterior margin curves forwards on the ischial ramus as the **falciform process.** The ligament forms part of the boundaries of both of the sciatic foramina and of the perineum [FIGS. 192, 233]. It gives origin superficially to gluteus maximus, and it crosses piriformis, the sacrospinous ligament, and the tendon of obturator internus. It is pierced by the perforating cutaneous nerve, the coccygeal and fifth sacral ventral rami, and by branches of the coccygeal plexus.

The **sacrospinous ligament** is the fibrous dorsal part of the coccygeus muscle. It extends as a thin, triangular sheet from the lateral margins of the last piece of the sacrum and the coccyx to the ischial spine, and thus separates the greater and lesser sciatic foramina. These foramina pass anteriorly into the pelvic cavity and the ischiorectal fossa respectively, for the one lies superior and the other inferior to the attachment of the levator ani to the pelvic surface of the **ischial spine.** Thus vessels and nerves passing from the pelvis to the ischiorectal fossa and perineum emerge through the greater foramen and enter the lesser, hooking over the sacrospinous ligament (pudendal nerve) or the **ischial spine** (internal pudendal vessels, and nerve to obturator internus). The medial part of the ligament is covered by the sacrotuberous ligament, and between them are parts of the perineal branch of the fourth sacral nerve and the perforating cutaneous nerve.

The **sacrotuberous** and **sacrospinous ligaments** bind the sacrum to the ischium, and holding down the posterior part of the sacrum, prevent the weight of the body depressing its anterior part around the sacro-iliac joints. Nevertheless they allow a small amount of movement which absorbs sudden increases in the loading.

SCIATIC FORAMINA

[FIGS. 232, 233]

The **greater sciatic foramen** is bounded by the greater sciatic notch of the hip bone and the sacrotuberous and sacrospinous ligaments. It is almost filled by piriformis, but it also transmits vessels and nerves to the buttock, posterior surface of the thigh, and perineum. The superior gluteal vessels and nerve emerge superior to the piriformis by hooking under the superior part of the greater sciatic notch. Inferior to piriformis is the large, sciatic nerve, deep to which is the nerve to quadratus femoris on the posterior surface of the acetabulum. The inferior gluteal vessels and nerve and the posterior cutaneous nerve of the thigh lie close to the medial side of the sciatic nerve. The vessels and nerves passing to the perineum have been seen already.

The **lesser sciatic foramen** is formed by the lesser sciatic notch and the two ligaments. The tendon of obturator internus emerges through it and turns laterally, often under cover of the gemelli. The nerve to obturator internus, the internal pudendal vessels, and the pudendal nerve enter the foramen.

THE POSITION OF THE PELVIC VISCERA

It is important that every student should study the pelvis of both sexes, and though for the purposes of dissection the two have to be treated separately, the features that are common to both should be noted.

In both sexes the **sigmoid colon** may be lifted out of the pelvis, but its inferior part is attached to the superior wall by the medial limb of the sigmoid mesocolon, and is continuous with the rectum on the third piece of the sacrum. The **rectum** follows the concavity of the sacrum and coccyx, and ends inferiorly in the anal canal.

The **urinary bladder** lies in the antero-inferior part of the cavity, posterosuperior to the pubic bones and symphysis. Between

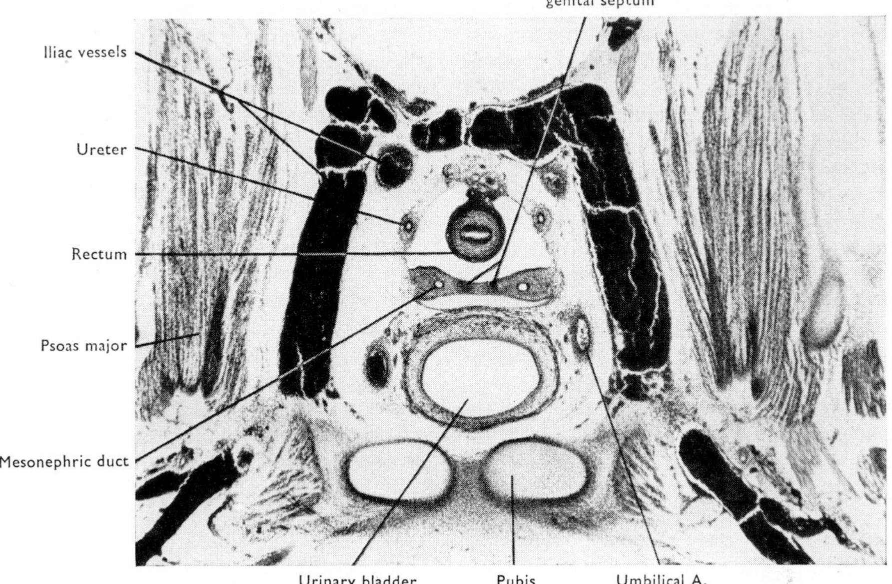

FIG. 188 A horizontal section through the lesser pelvis of an eight-week-old human foetus to show the subdivision of the pelvic cavity by the genital septum.

the bladder and the rectum there is a transverse connective tissue septum (*genital septum*) which is thin in the median plane, but thickens as it passes to the lateral wall of the pelvis. The ureters pass antero-inferiorly through this septum to the bladder. *In the male* the septum is small since it only contains a ductus deferens and a seminal vesicle on each side in addition to a ureter. Each **ductus deferens** sweeps postero-inferiorly from the deep inguinal ring across the anterolateral part of the pelvis, immediately inferior to the peritoneum. It hooks over the ureter and, running medially on the posterior surface (base) of the bladder in the septum, passes inferiorly along the medial side of the **seminal vesicle,** close to its fellow [FIG. 214]. It ends by uniting with the duct of the seminal vesicle to form the **ejaculatory duct,** posterior to the junction of the bladder and the prostate. This pierces the prostate to enter the prostatic part of the urethra, which traverses that gland from the neck of the bladder to the perineum.

In the female the septum is large and extends upwards into the lesser pelvis because it contains the uterus, uterine tubes, and ovaries in its superior part: the vagina is in the inferior part, posterior to the bladder and urethra. The **uterus** overhangs the bladder, and its rounded, free end (the fundus) is continuous through the adjoining two-thirds (body of the uterus) with the postero-inferior third, the cervix or neck. This is partly inserted into the anterior wall of the vagina.

The **vagina** extends antero-inferiorly between the rectum posteriorly and the bladder and urethra anteriorly (the latter almost incorporated in its anterior wall, FIG. 220), and opens with the urethra and rectum on the surface of the perineum.

On each side, from the junction of the fundus and body of the uterus, a **uterine tube** [FIG. 190] passes towards the lateral wall of the pelvis, and expanding (**ampulla**), recurves upon itself and forms a funnel-shaped end (**infundibulum**) which is directed medially towards the ovary. The infundibulum opens into the peritoneal cavity, and is surrounded by finger-like extensions of its walls (**fimbriae** of the tube), one or more of which is attached to the ovary (ovarian fimbria).

Also attached to the uterus at the junction of the fundus and body are two ligaments: (1) the **round ligament of the uterus** (antero-inferior to the tube) which curves anterolaterally to the deep inguinal ring in a position similar to that occupied by the ductus deferens in the male; and (2) the **ligament of the ovary** (posterosuperior to the tube) which joins the medial extremity of the ovary to the uterus. In addition, a ridge of fibrous tissue curves posterosuperiorly from the cervix of the uterus towards the lateral part of the sacrum, the **uterosacral ligament** [p. 207].

The **ureter** in the female follows the same course as in the male, but passes postero-medial to the ovary and lateral to the uppermost part of the vagina; its terminal part is therefore hidden by the genital septum.

PELVIC PERITONEUM
[FIGS. 189, 191]

The parietal abdominal peritoneum passes directly into the lesser pelvis over the margins of the superior aperture, and covers the surfaces of the pelvic organs, passing between them to produce peritoneal pouches and fossae. Anteriorly and posteriorly the arrangement of this peritoneum is virtually identical in the two sexes, but it differs in the intermediate region owing to the presence of the large genital septum and its contained structures in the female.

The posterosuperior surface of the pelvis is covered with peritoneum down to the second piece of the sacrum, except where the medial limb of the sigmoid mesocolon is attached [FIG. 124]. Inferior to this the rectum intervenes between the sacrum and the peritoneum. Superiorly the peritoneum covers the front and sides of the rectum, and then leaving it by turning forwards from the anterior surface of its middle third, runs upwards over the genital septum. Thus the peritoneum forms the **recto-uterine** (female) or **rectovesical** (male) pouch between the rectum and the contents of the genital septum, which are bent forwards over the superior surface of the bladder in the

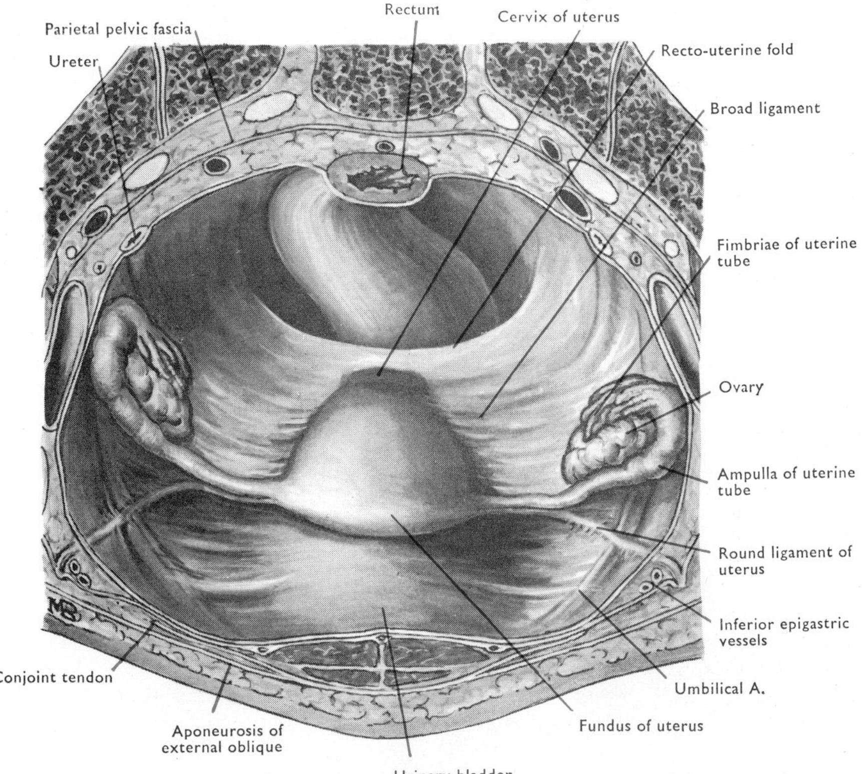

FIG. 189 The peritoneum of the lesser pelvis in the female.

female. *In the female*, the peritoneum in the median plane lies first on the superior part of the posterior vaginal wall, and passing over the posterosuperior surfaces of the cervix and body of the uterus, turns over the fundus to cover the antero-inferior surface of the body of the uterus [FIG. 209]. At the junction of the body and cervix, the peritoneum bends forwards over the superior surface of the bladder, thus forming the **uterovesical pouch of peritoneum.** It continues forwards over the bladder and passes directly on to the posterior surface of the anterior abdominal wall.

Lateral to the uterus, the peritoneum passes from the recto-uterine pouch to form a fold over the lateral part of the genital septum. It thus covers the uterosacral ligament (forming the **recto-uterine fold,** FIG. 189) and ovary (close to the lateral pelvic wall) on the posterosuperior surface of the fold, the uterine tube in the free margin, and the round ligament of the uterus on the antero-inferior wall. This fold of peritoneum and the connective tissue (**parametrium**) it contains form the **broad ligament** of the uterus, which widens laterally where the uterosacral ligaments pass posteriorly and the round ligaments curve anteriorly. Between these it is attached to the lateral pelvic wall across the external iliac vessels, the obliterated umbilical artery, and the obturator nerve and vessels. The part of the broad ligament beyond the end of the uterine tube is known as the **suspensory ligament of the ovary,** while the part between the ovary and

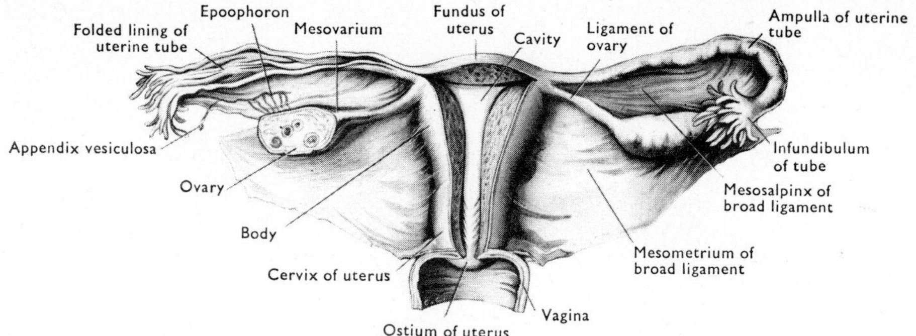

FIG. 190 The posterosuperior surface of the broad ligament and associated structures. The vagina, uterus, and left uterine tube have been opened, and the left ovary is sectioned parallel to the broad ligament.

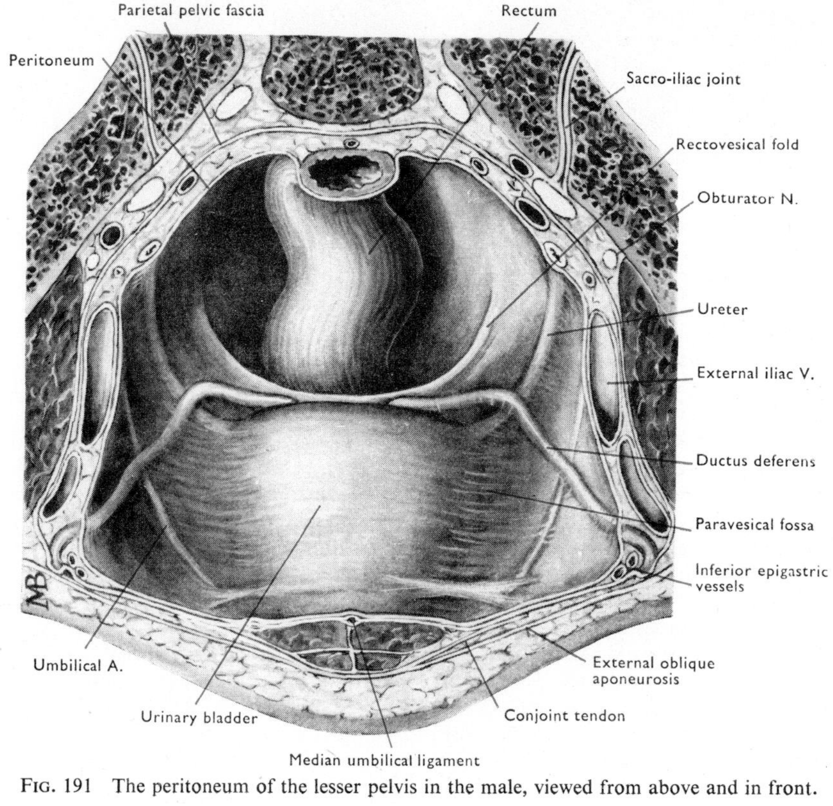

FIG. 191 The peritoneum of the lesser pelvis in the male, viewed from above and in front.

the uterine tube is the **mesosalpinx,** and the remainder is the **mesometrium** (mesentery of the uterus).

The uterus thus lies in a free, transverse fold which allows it to expand upwards into the abdominal cavity during pregnancy without disturbing its supporting structures. These, including the uterosacral ligaments, are composed of the connective tissue in the base of the broad ligament, which connects the cervix to the lateral walls of the pelvis, especially around the uterine arteries (sometimes known as the transverse ligaments).

Anterior to the broad ligament, and lateral to the bladder, the peritoneum passes forwards as the floor of a shallow **paravesical fossa** on each side [Fig. 191]. This is limited laterally by the ridge produced by the round ligament curving forwards to the deep inguinal ring. In the anterolateral part of the fossa is a slight ridge formed by the obliterated umbilical artery passing anteromedially towards the anterior abdominal wall.

In the male the peritoneum passes from the rectovesical fossa on to the superior part of the posterior surface of the bladder between the two deferent ducts. Occasionally it covers the superior surfaces of the seminal vesicles and the adjacent parts of the deferent ducts, which then raise a peritoneal fold that sweeps from the ducts posterolaterally towards the sacrum in the same position as the recto-uterine fold, the **rectovesical fold** [Fig. 191]. Anterior to this the peritoneum covers the entire superior surface of the bladder in the midline, but laterally it arches over the **ureter** which sweeps antero-inferiorly from the beginning of the external iliac artery to the superolateral angle of the base of the contracted bladder. The ureter forms the posterior limit of the **paravesical fossa** in the male, and is crossed by the ductus deferens [Fig. 191] where that duct turns medially on to the posterior surface of the bladder.

The greater part of the ductus deferens lies immediately inferior to the peritoneum. Anteriorly it is in the same position as the round ligament of the uterus in the female, but it extends further posteriorly [Figs. 189, 191] to reach the base of the bladder.

THE PERINEUM

The perineum consists of the structures that fill the inferior aperture of the pelvis. This diamond-shaped aperture lies between the upper parts of the thighs and the lower parts of the buttocks, and is almost completely hidden by them in the erect posture.

It extends from the inferior margin of the pubic symphysis to the coccyx, and its **lateral boundaries** are the inferior rami of the pubic bones, the rami and tuberosities of the ischium, and the sacrotuberous ligaments [Figs. 192, 193]. The perineum is considerably wider in the female than the male, and is divided into an anterior or urogenital region and a posterior or anal region by a transverse line passing through the ischial tuberosities immediately anterior to the anus.

The **urogenital region** contains: *in the male*, the urethra enclosed in the root of the penis, partly hidden anteriorly by the scrotum; *in the female*, the urethral and vaginal orifices, and the clitoris surrounded by the labia minora and majora. The **anal region** contains the terminal 3–4 cm. of the large intestine, the anal canal.

In the male, a median cutaneous ridge, the **raphe of the perineum,** extends from the anus over the inferior surfaces of the scrotum and penis. This marks the line of fusion of the structures that form the labia in the female, by which the floor of the urethra (labia minora) is completed and the two halves of the scrotum (labia majora) are brought together in the male.

THE FEMALE EXTERNAL GENITAL ORGANS

The pudendum femininum or vulva consists of the following structures [Fig. 194].

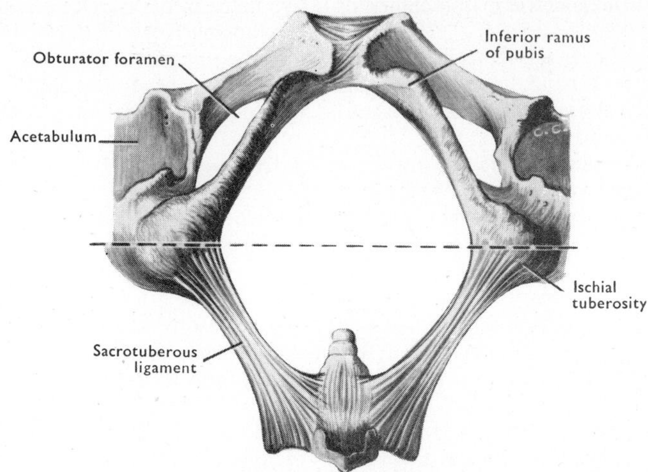

FIG. 192 The inferior aperture of the male pelvis.

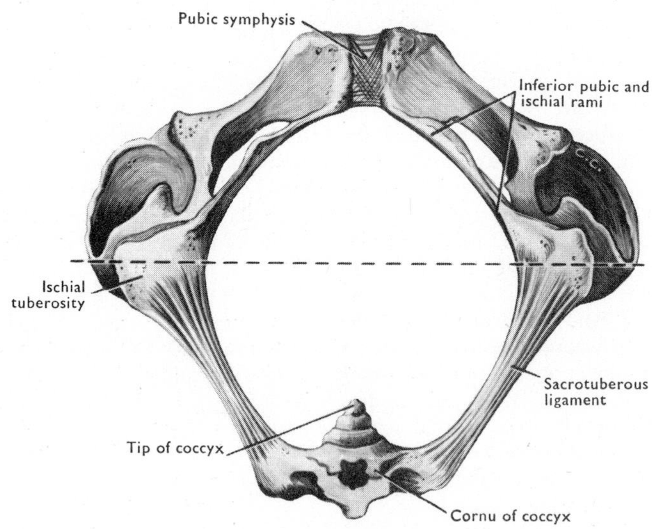

FIG. 193 The inferior aperture of the female pelvis.

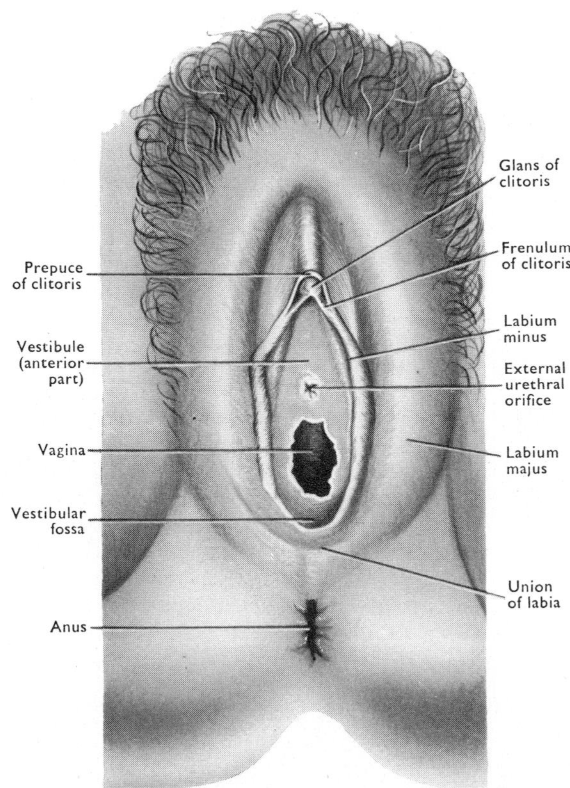

FIG. 194 The female external genital organs.

1. The **mons pubis** is produced by subcutaneous fat anterior to the pubic bones. It protrudes the overlying hairy skin, the hairs of which cease abruptly at a horizontal line where the mons meets the anterior abdominal wall.

2. The **labia majora,** which correspond to the halves of the scrotum, are a pair of rounded folds covered with skin which extend postero-inferiorly from the mons to surround the median pudendal cleft. They decrease in size posteriorly, and meet across the midline 2–3 cm. anterior to the anus. Laterally there are scattered hairs, particularly in the anterior parts, but their medial surfaces are smooth and lubricated by numerous sebaceous glands. The pudendal cleft contains the vaginal and urethral orifices and the remaining external genital organs.

3. The **labia minora** are a pair of smooth, pink folds, covered with stratified squamous epithelium, that lie between the labia majora. Anteriorly each splits into two as it approaches the clitoris [FIG. 194]. The smaller, posterior folds fuse and are attached to the inferior surface of the clitoris (**frenulum of the clitoris**). The anterior pair unite to form a hood over the clitoris, the **prepuce of the clitoris.** Posteriorly the labia minora are united by a transverse fold, the **frenulum of the labia,** which is separated from the vaginal orifice by the **vestibular fossa.** The frenulum labiorum is frequently absent owing to damage at childbirth.

4. The **clitoris** closely resembles the penis in appearance and structure, but is not traversed by the urethra. It lies in the anterior part of the pudendal cleft, and its downturned extremity ends in a sensitive tubercle, the **glans.** The clitoris can be made more obvious by pulling the glans out of the prepuce.

5. The **vestibule of the vagina** lies between the labia minora, and contains the orifices of the vagina, urethra, and of the ducts of a pair of greater vestibular glands which open between the labium minus and the margin of the vaginal orifice, one on each side.

6. The **vaginal orifice** lies in the posterior part of the vestibule, and is partly (or rarely completely) closed in the virgin by a thin membrane (**the hymen**) attached around the margins of the orifice. When the hymen has been ruptured, its position is marked by small, rounded tags, the **carunculae hymenales.**

7. The **orifice of the urethra** lies immediately anterior to the vaginal orifice, 2 cm. posterior to the clitoris. Its margins are raised, puckered, and palpable.

THE GENERAL ARRANGEMENT OF THE PERINEUM

The **urogenital region** has three layers of fascia separated by two layers of muscles and other structures. These layers are most obvious in the male, and consist of a superficial membranous layer that is attached laterally to the greater part of the inferior pubic rami and the ischial rami, close to the attachment of the fascia lata of the thighs. Anteriorly this layer continues its lateral attachments across the front of the pubic bones as far as the pubic tubercles, where it becomes continuous with the membranous layer of the superficial fascia of the anterior abdominal wall [FIG. 88]. Medial to these attachments it covers the scrotum as **dartos,** and forms the fascial sheath and suspensory ligament of the penis [p. 96]. Posteriorly the superficial membranous layer turns superiorly near the anterior margins of the ischial tuberosities, and becomes continuous with the posterior border of the middle fascial layer (the **inferior fascia of the urogenital diaphragm** or **perineal membrane**) which is also attached laterally to the pubic arch. The **superficial perineal space** is enclosed between these two layers of fascia. In the median plane where these two layers meet is the **central tendon of the perineum,** a fibrous body to which a number of perineal muscles are attached.

In the male, the **superficial perineal space** [FIG. 199] contains a number of nerves and blood vessels, and the root of the penis separated into its three elements [FIG. 201]: (1) the two crura attached to the everted edges of the ischiopubic rami, and each covered by an ischiocavernosus muscle; (2) the median bulb of the penis, which lies on the perineal membrane, is covered by the bulbospongiosus muscles, and contains the urethra which reaches it by piercing the perineal membrane. Lying transversely across the posterior margin of the space, and attached to the central tendon of the perineum and the ischium, are the superficial transverse perineal muscles.

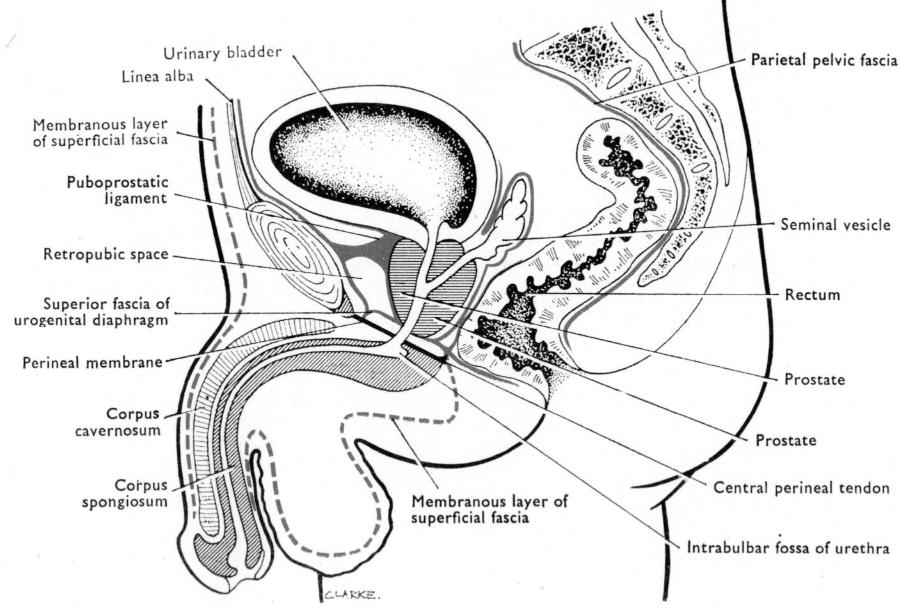

FIG. 195 A schematic median section through the male pelvis to show the parietal and visceral pelvic fascia (red).

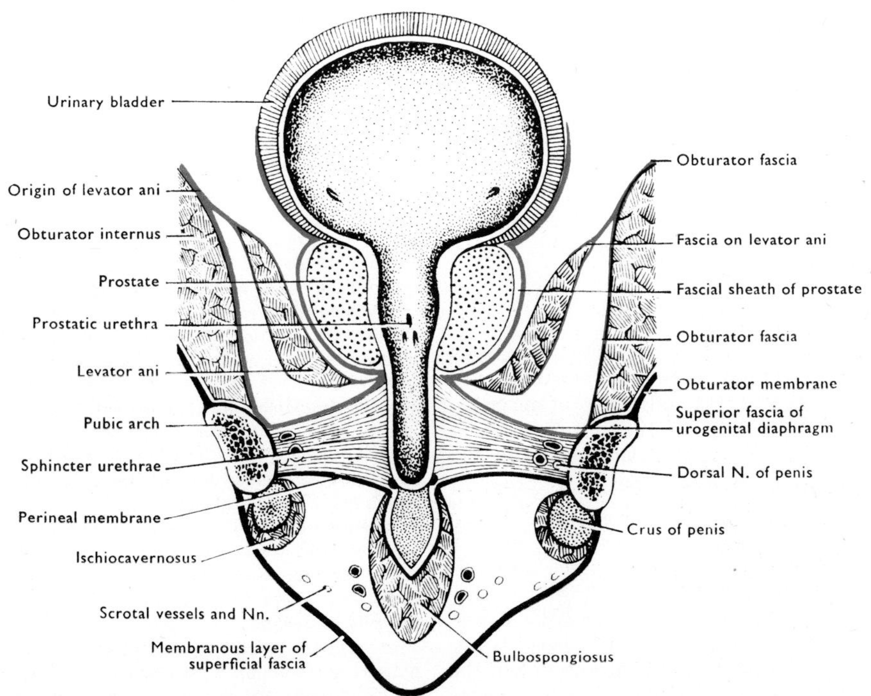

FIG. 196 A schematic coronal section through the male pelvis and perineum to show the arrangement of the pelvic (red) and perineal (black) fasciae.

Superior to the perineal membrane is a thin layer of muscle which stretches across the pubic arch [FIGS. 196, 203]. The main part of it surrounds the urethra **(sphincter urethrae),** while its posterior fibres pass more transversely, the **deep transverse perineal muscle.** This layer of muscle lies in the **deep perineal space,** which is limited superiorly by the third layer of fascia (**superior fascia of the urogenital diaphragm).** This is attached laterally to the pubic arch, and fuses posteriorly with the perineal membrane and the superficial membranous layer. Anteriorly, the superior and inferior fasciae of the urogenital diaphragm fuse, and are deficient immediately posterior to the pubic symphysis; the dorsal vein of the penis (or clitoris) enters the pelvis through the aperture so formed.

In the female, the same elements are present, but are split in the midline by the pudendal cleft and the vagina. Thus the superficial membranous fascia is a poorly defined layer confined to the labia majora. The perineal membrane, the sphincter urethrae, the bulb of the vestibule (which corresponds to the bulb of the penis, FIG. 202), and the bulbospongiosus [FIG. 200] are all split by the vagina. They are less well formed, and more difficult to define than in the male.

The **anal region** [FIGS. 199, 200]. In the midline this contains the lower part of the anal canal surrounded by the muscle, **sphincter ani externus,** and between this and the coccyx, a fibrous, fatty mass, the **anococcygeal ligament.** On each side, the fatty superficial fascia extends superiorly between the fascia covering the medial surface of obturator internus and that on the inferolateral surface of levator ani, to fill the **ischiorectal fossa** between them [FIG. 198].

THE PENIS AND URETHRA

The penis contains two **corpora cavernosa.** These are thick cylinders of spongy, fibro-elastic, erectile tissue bound together side by side [FIG. 197]. Each is enclosed in a thick layer of tough fibrous tissue (tunica albuginea) which only partly separates them. Their distal ends are embedded in the glans penis, the enlarged end of the third longitudinal body, the **corpus spongiosum.** Proximally the corpora cavernosa separate, and each tapering to a point is attached along the everted inferomedial surface of the ischiopubic ramus. The corpus spongiosum lies between and inferior to the corpora cavernosa in the body of the penis. It consists of delicate erectile tissue and a thin tunica albuginea, and is swollen proximally to form the bulb of the penis [FIG. 201]. It transmits the spongy part of the urethra.

The **urethra** *in the male* is approximately 20 cm. long, and extends from the most inferior part of the urinary bladder (**neck**) to the tip of the glans penis [FIGS. 195, 208]. It first traverses the prostate (**prostatic part,** 3 cm. long) from its base to a point anterior to the apex of the prostate [FIG. 195]; then pierces the superior and inferior fasciae of the urogenital diaphragm and the sphincter urethrae between them (**membranous part,** 1 cm. long). It then turns abruptly forwards, and sinking into the corpus spongiosum, dilates posteriorly to form the **intrabulbar fossa** [FIG. 195], and passes through the corpus spongiosum (**spongy part**) to expand in the glans (**navicular fossa**) and emerge from its apex.

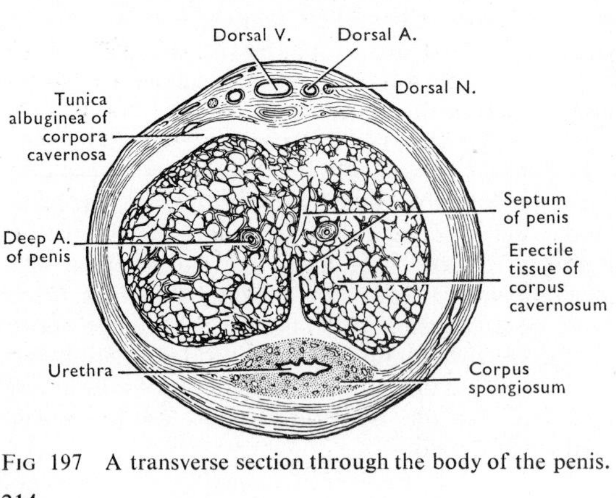

FIG 197 A transverse section through the body of the penis.

DISSECTION. Pass a greased bougie or blunt metal rod gently along the spongy part of the urethra in a plane parallel to the perineum. Direct the point towards the inferior surface of the penis to avoid recesses in the superior wall of the urethra, and palpate the point through the corpus spongiosum following its progress until it is arrested in the intrabulbar fossa, midway between the root of the scrotum and the anus. The point of the bougie should now be slipped through the membranous and prostatic parts by withdrawing it slightly, and carrying the handle in the median plane towards the thighs, while applying slight pressure on the point with a finger on the perineum. The point should enter the membranous part without force, and slip easily into the bladder. If this is not successful, do not try to force a passage, or the tissues will be damaged; try to guide the point into the membranous part of the urethra with a finger in the anal canal.

When the bougie is in position, note that it can be palpated easily as far as the bulb of the penis, and that it can be felt in the membranous part by a finger in the anal canal. It is scarcely palpable through the prostate by a finger in the rectum.

In the female, **identify the urethral orifice immediately anterior to the vagina. Pass a bougie along the urethra to the bladder, and note that it is readily palpable through the anterior vaginal wall. If possible, introduce a speculum into the vagina and examine the cervix uteri which protrudes through the anterior wall of the uppermost part of the vagina, with a sulcus (the fornices of the vagina) separating it from the vaginal walls. The aperture of the cervix (os uteri) is small, elongated transversely between the rounded lips of the cervix, and faces postero-inferiorly. In parous women the os is often enlarged and the lips are frequently cleft and scarred**

Make a transverse cut through the skin between the ischial tuberosities, immediately anterior to the anus. *In the male,* **make a median incision from the coccyx to the scrotum, encircling the anus.** *In the female,* **make the same incision to the mons pubis, but encircle the anus and the pudendal cleft. Reflect the flaps of skin produced by these two incisions, and note the radiating strands of involuntary muscle fibres passing outwards from the anus, the corrugator cutis ani. These fibres are the terminal parts of the longitudinal muscle layer of the intestine.**

Superficial Fascia

In the **anal region** this contains much lobulated fat and extends upwards into the ischiorectal fossa to form a movable pad on each side which allows for distension of the lower rectum and anal canal. In the **urogenital region** there is also a **membranous layer** which forms the floor of the superficial perineal space.

In the male, a **fibrous septum** passes superiorly from the membranous layer to the raphe between the bulbospongiosus muscles [FIG. 199]. This completely divides the space posteriorly, but is incomplete anteriorly. Towards the scrotum the fatty layer is progressively lost, and both fatty and membranous layers are replaced by smooth muscle (**dartos**).

In the female, both fatty and membranous layers are split by the pudendal cleft. The fatty layer is absent from the labium minus, and the membranous layer is continuous through the labia majora, and deep to the fat of the mons pubis, with the membranous layer of the superficial fascia on the anterior abdominal wall, as in the male.

DISSECTION. In the female, remove the fatty layer from the labium majus, and incising the membranous layer, explore the superficial perineal space with a finger. Note that the finger can readily be passed forwards on to the anterior abdominal wall, but is restricted posteriorly where the membranous layer turns upwards to fuse with the perineal membrane [p.212].

In the male, either explore one side of the space with a finger, or attempt to inflate it with air from a pump through a nozzle introduced through the membranous layer. In either case note the complete septum posteriorly, its incomplete nature anteriorly (which allows air to pass across the midline), and the continuity of the space anteriorly with the areolar tissue of the anterior abdominal wall deep to the membranous fascial layer. The introduction of air into the space mimics the effects of urine escaping from a ruptured urethra in the perineum.

Starting in the median plane at the root of the scrotum or frenulum of the labia, make two incisions through the membranous fascia, one to each ischial tuberosity Reflect the three flaps so formed and confirm their attachments, taking care not to damage the scrotal (labial) nerves and vessels which lie immediately deep to the fascia.

THE ANAL REGION

ANAL CANAL

This canal extends postero-inferiorly from the lower extremity of the rectum to the anus. It is 4 cm. long and its superior part lies in the pelvic cavity surrounded by the thickened inferior part of the circular muscle layer of the intestine, the involuntary **internal anal sphincter,** and with the lower parts of the levator ani muscles on each side of it. The inferior part of the anal canal lies in the perineum surrounded by the **external anal sphincter.**

Anococcygeal Ligament. This is a poorly defined, fibro-fatty mass permeated with muscle fibres from the levator ani muscles and the external anal sphincter. It extends from the anus to the tip of the coccyx, and lying inferior to the lower part of the rectum, helps to support it.

DISSECTION. Reflect the fascia from the external anal sphincter, and from the anococcygeal ligament, the margins of the anus, and the central perineal tendon. Clean the sphincter, and find the inferior rectal vessels and nerve in the ischiorectal fossa [Fig. 199], and the perineal branch of the fourth sacral nerve, which passes over the perineal surface of levator ani from the posterior angle of the ischiorectal fossa at the side of the coccyx, to supply the external sphincter and the overlying skin.

Sphincter Ani Externus

This muscle consists of: (1) a **subcutaneous part** that surrounds the anal orifice and has no bony attachments, but its fibres decussate anterior and posterior to the anus [FIGS. 199, 200]; (2) a **superficial part** which is oval in shape, with fibres that arise from the tip of the coccyx and anococcygeal ligament, and pass anteriorly around the anus to the central perineal tendon; and (3) a **deep part** which passes round the lower half of the anal canal from the central perineal tendon, and is fused with the inferior part of levator ani (**puborectalis**) which reinforces its action [FIG. 217].

Nerve supply: perineal branch of the fourth sacral and the inferior rectal nerves. Action: the subcutaneous and superficial parts close the anus, while the deep part, assisted by puborectalis, also draws the anal canal forwards, thus increasing the angle between it and the rectum [FIG. 208]. All parts of this sphincter are formed of striated muscle fibres, and it is under voluntary control.

ISCHIORECTAL FOSSA

This is the wedge-shaped space, filled with fat, lateral to the anus and levator ani. The *edge* lies superiorly where levator ani arises from the fascia covering obturator internus [FIG. 198]; the *base* is the perineal skin; the lateral and superomedial *walls* are formed by the fascia covering the perineal surfaces of obturator internus and levator ani respectively. The fossa is partly closed posteriorly by the sacrotuberous ligament, and anteriorly where the layers of perineal fascia fuse at the posterior border of the perineal membrane. Anterior to this, a narrow cleft filled with loose areolar tissue extends forwards from the ischiorectal fossa between levator ani and obturator internus, above the superior fascia of the urogenital diaphragm [FIG. 196].

The fossa is widest and deepest posteriorly, but becomes narrower and shallower anteriorly. Infections in the fat of the ischiorectal fossa are not uncommon either as a result of small tears of the anal mucous membrane or from disease of the perianal skin. If an abscess forms, it may either burst medially through the thin wall into the anal canal, or through the perianal skin, or both. In the latter case a track may lead from the skin to the anal canal, a *fistula in ano*.

The ischiorectal fossa contains the branches of the vessels and nerves that enter it through the lesser sciatic foramen (pudendal nerve, the internal pudendal vessels, and the nerve to obturator internus) and the perineal branch of the fourth sacral nerve.

DISSECTION. If the gluteal region has not been dissected, expose and clean the lower border of gluteus maximus by incising the superficial fascia from a point 2 cm. superior to the tip of the coccyx to the lateral side of the ischial tuberosity. Small gluteal branches of the posterior cutaneous nerve of the thigh may be seen curving round the inferior border of the muscle lateral to the ischial tuberosity. Identify the sacrotuberous ligament deep to this border of the gluteus maximus, and complete the cleaning of the inferior rectal vessels and nerve, following them to their origin on the lateral wall of the ischiorectal fossa. Expose the posterior scrotal (or labial) vessels and nerves in the angle between the posterior margin of the perineal membrane and the lateral wall, and follow them into the superficial perineal space. Clean the fat from the ischiorectal fossa, and identify and follow the pudendal nerve and vessels in the fascial pudendal canal on the lateral wall [Fig. 198].

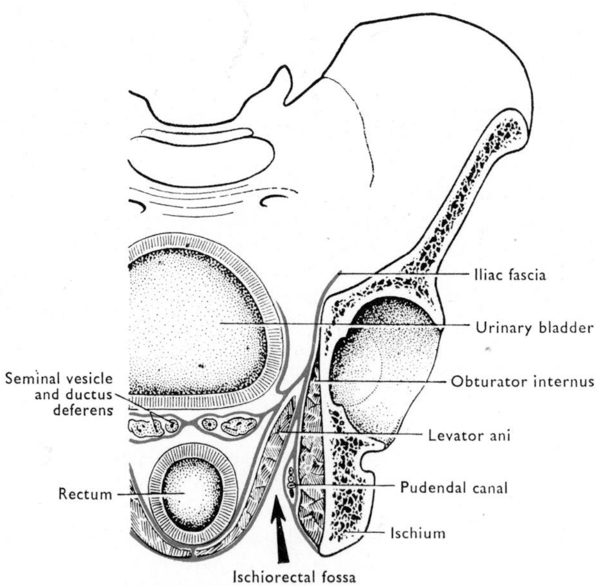

FIG. 198 A diagrammatic coronal section through the male pelvis to show the pelvic and perineal fasciae and levator ani.

Pudendal Nerve and Internal Pudendal Vessels

These give off the **inferior rectal branches** immediately on entering the pudendal canal (the inferior rectal nerve occasionally arises directly from the third and fourth sacral nerves in the pelvis). They pierce the medial wall of the canal, pass through the fat of the ischiorectal fossa, and supply levator ani, the external anal sphincter, and the overlying skin. The nerve communicates with the posterior scrotal (or labial) nerves, and with the perineal branch of the posterior cutaneous nerve of the thigh [FIG.

199], while the artery sends branches round the margin of gluteus maximus into the buttock.

As it gives off the inferior rectal nerve, the pudendal nerve divides into its terminal branches, the **perineal nerve** and the **dorsal nerve of the penis** or **clitoris,** which continue through the canal with the internal pudendal vessels. The **posterior scrotal** (or **labial**) **vessels and nerves** arise from the internal pudendal vessels and perineal nerve near the anterior part of the canal.

The **perineal branch of the fourth sacral nerve** enters the fossa at the side of the coccyx, and supplies the external anal sphincter and the skin posterior to the anus.

THE UROGENITAL REGION

DISSECTION. Follow the posterior scrotal (or labial) vessels and nerves through the superficial perineal space to the scrotum (or labium majus). Identify the perineal branch of the posterior cutaneous nerve of the thigh 2–3 cm. anterior to the ischial tuberosity, and follow its branches to the scrotum or labium majus.

Clean the structures in the superficial perineal space [Fig. 199]: (1) an ischiocavernosus muscle covers the inferior surface of each crus of the penis or clitoris

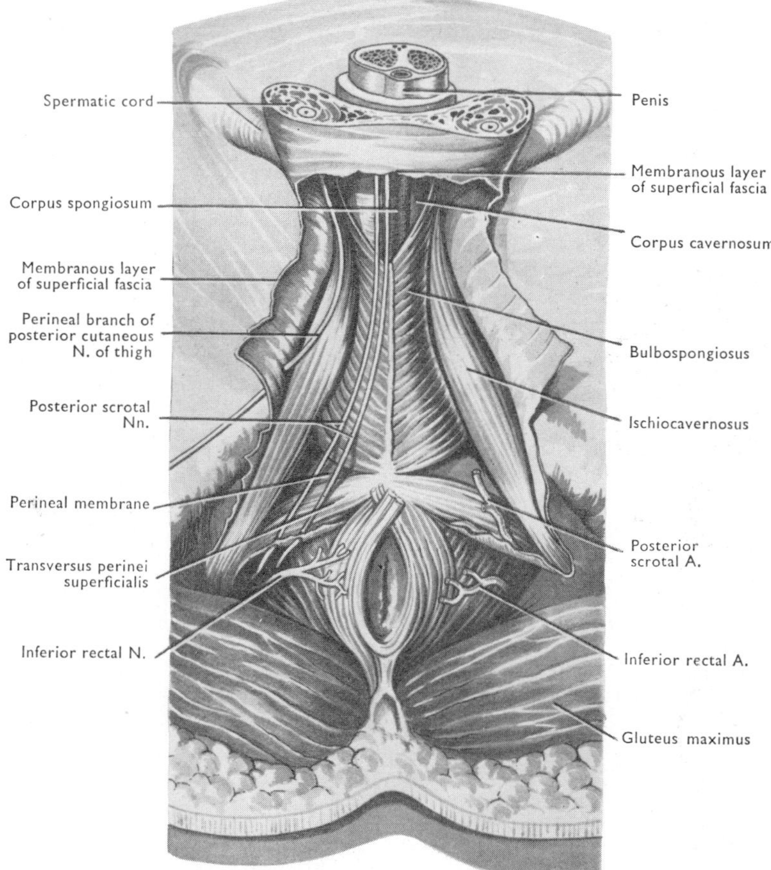

FIG. 199 A dissection of the male perineum. The penis and scrotum have been cut across and removed.

along the margin of the pubic arch; (2) the bulbospongiosus muscles in the male pass anterosuperiorly round each side of the bulb of the penis from a median, ventral raphe, which begins posteriorly in the central perineal tendon. They meet dorsal to the corpus spongiosum (in the female they are smaller and surround the sides of the vestibule from the central perineal tendon to the crura of the clitoris, Fig. 200); (3) the superficial transverse perineal muscles pass between the posterior ends of the other two in both sexes. Part of the perineal membrane can be seen in the triangular space between these three muscles.

NERVES AND VESSELS OF SUPERFICIAL PERINEAL SPACE

Two **posterior scrotal** or **labial nerves** (lateral and medial, S. 3, 4) arise from the perineal nerve in the anterior part of the pudendal canal. They cross the anterior part of the ischiorectal fossa, enter the superficial perineal space by piercing the membranous fascial layer, and passing deep or superficial to the transverse perineal muscle, supply the skin of the urogenital region, including the scrotum or labium majus.

Two **posterior scrotal** or **labial arteries** arise from the internal pudendal artery close to the nerves. They take the same course as the nerves, and one of them may give rise to a small **perineal artery** which runs on the superficial transverse perineal muscle to the central tendon of the perineum.

The **perineal branch** of the posterior cutaneous nerve of the thigh (S. 3) pierces the deep fascia anterolateral to the ischial tuberosity, and running anteromedially across the pubic arch, supplies the lateral and anterior parts of the scrotum or labium majus.

DISSECTION. Divide the posterior scrotal or labial arteries and nerves and turn them aside. Separate the superficial perineal muscles and expose the part of the perineal membrane between them. Cut the transverse perineal muscles from the central perineal tendon, and turning them aside, expose the terminal branches of the perineal nerve deep to the muscles [p. 223]. In the male, separate the two bulbospongiosus muscles along the raphe, and turn them away from the corpus spongiosum, following the fibres to their terminations. In the female, lift the bulbospongiosus muscles [Fig. 200] from the underlying masses of erectile tissue on each side of the vaginal orifice, the bulbs of the vestibule. In both sexes, strip the ischiocavernosus muscles from the crura of the penis or clitoris, and trace them to their termination.

SUPERFICIAL PERINEAL MUSCLES

The **superficial transverse perineal muscle** is a small slip that arises from the medial side of the ramus of the ischium close to the tuberosity, and joins its fellow in the central perineal tendon. In the female it is small, pale in colour, and difficult to define.

The **bulbospongiosus muscles** are understandably different in the two sexes. *In the male* [Fig. 199], they arise from the central perineal tendon and from the median raphe, and curve anterosuperiorly round the bulb and posterior part of the corpus spongiosum. The *posterior fibres* pass round the bulb to the perineal membrane, the *middle fibres* (the largest part) encircle the corpus spongiosum, uniting with their fellows in another raphe dorsal to it. The *anterior fibres* pass round the corpus spongiosum and the corpora cavernosa and unite dorsal to the penis **(bulbocavernosus).** *In the female* [Fig. 200], the fibres also arise from the central perineal tendon, but sweep round the sides of the vestibule over the inferior surfaces of the greater vestibular glands [Fig. 202] and the bulbs of the vestibule (the female equivalent of the corpus spongiosum), to be inserted into the sides and dorsum of the clitoris.

The **ischiocavernosus muscles** arise from the corresponding rami of the ischium close to the tuberosity. Each sweeps over the crus of the penis or clitoris and is inserted into the inferior and lateral surfaces of the anterior part of the crus. Nerve supply: the perineal nerve. Actions. The **transverse perineal muscles** help to fix the **central perineal tendon,** thus supporting the posterior part of the perineal membrane and the structures superior to it, *i.e.*, the prostate or vagina. The *ischiocavernosus* may assist with erection (which is due to the cavernous spaces of the penis or clitoris filling with blood) by compressing the deep vein which leaves the crus. The **bulbospongiosus** *in the male* compresses the bulb and corpus spongiosum, thus emptying the urethra of any residual urine or semen. Its anterior fibres can

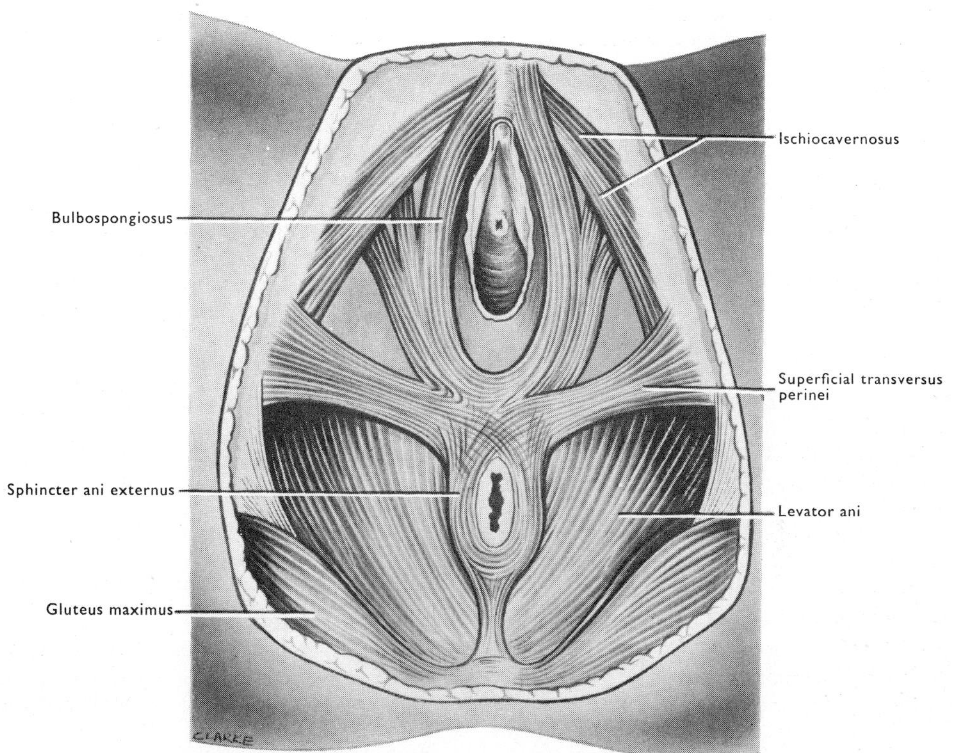

FIG. 200 The muscles of the female perineum.

compress the dorsal vein of the penis, and impeding the venous drainage from the cavernous tissue, assist with erection. *In the female*, it is a sphincter of the vagina, and is assisted by the underlying erectile tissue of the bulbs.

Central Tendon of Perineum. This indefinite mass of fibrous tissue lies between the anal canal and the bulb of the penis or the vagina. It gives attachment to the transverse perineal muscles, the bulbospongiosus, the superficial part of the external anal sphincter, some of the anterior fibres of levator ani, and longitudinal fibres of the rectal muscle. The tendon is an important structure, especially in the female, for if it is torn or stretched in childbirth it weakens the perineum which is no longer able to support the inferior part of the vagina, and thus facilitates the prolapse of a displaced uterus through the vaginal orifice.

CRURA OF PENIS AND CLITORIS

These are the divergent, posterior parts of the corpora cavernosa. Each is attached to the everted, medial surface of the pubic arch and the adjacent part of the perineal membrane, and is covered by, and gives attachment to the ischiocavernosus muscle. The **deep artery** and **vein** enter and leave its superior surface. At their distal ends the corpora cavernosa are inserted into the **glans** of the penis or clitoris; the former is the expanded end of the corpus spongiosum, while the latter is nearly a separate structure, but is united to the bulbs of the vestibule by connective tissue and a narrow strip of erectile tissue.

Bulb of Penis [FIGS. 195, 201]

This expanded proximal part of the corpus

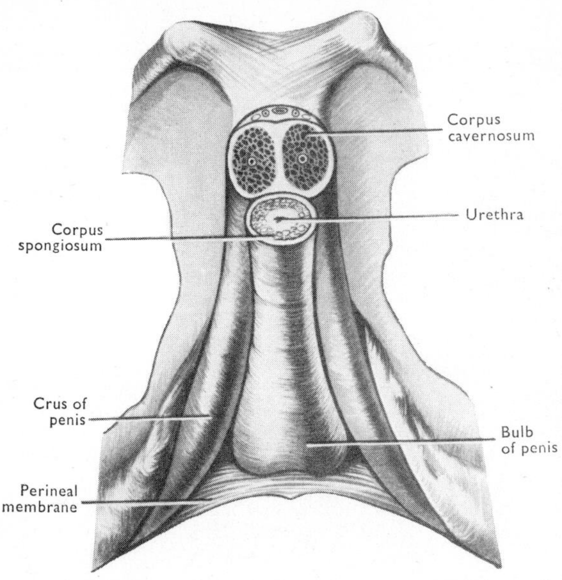

FIG. 201 The root of the penis. The corpora are shown in transverse section.

spongiosum is attached to the inferior surface of the perineal membrane by fibrous tissue, by the bulbospongiosus muscles, and by the **urethra** which pierces the perineal membrane to enter the corpus spongiosum immediately in front of its posterior end. The urethra is accompanied by the **ducts of the bulbo-urethral glands** and by the arteries of the bulb, both of which arise in the deep perineal space.

Bulbs of Vestibule

These oblong masses of erectile tissue lie one on each side of the vaginal orifice. Each, covered by a fibrous sheath and a bulbospongiosus muscle, is attached to the perineal membrane, and overlaps the corresponding greater vestibular gland posteriorly [FIG. 202]. The bulbs narrow anteriorly, and are united by a plexus of veins (the **commissure of the bulbs**) between the urethra and the clitoris. The commissure is attached to the glans of the clitoris by a thin strip of erectile tissue. The glans, the strip of erectile tissue, the commissure of the bulbs, and the bulbs together correspond to the corpus spongiosum and the glans penis.

Greater Vestibular Glands [FIG. 202]. These glands lie on the inferior surface of the perineal membrane beside the orifice of the vagina, covered by the bulbs of the vestibule. Each has a long duct that opens at the side of the vaginal orifice, between the hymen and the labium minus.

DISSECTION. Remove the superficial perineal muscles, and detach one crus of the penis or clitoris carefully, turning it forwards to expose the deep artery entering its superior surface. Find and clean the dorsal artery and nerve of the penis or clitoris close to the deep artery [Fig. 203]. Trace the dorsal artery and nerve to the penis or clitoris where they lie on the side of the median dorsal vein. Trace the vein proximally till it disappears into the pelvis between the pubic symphysis and the anterior margin of the perineal membrane [Fig. 204].

In the male, detach the posterior end of the bulb of

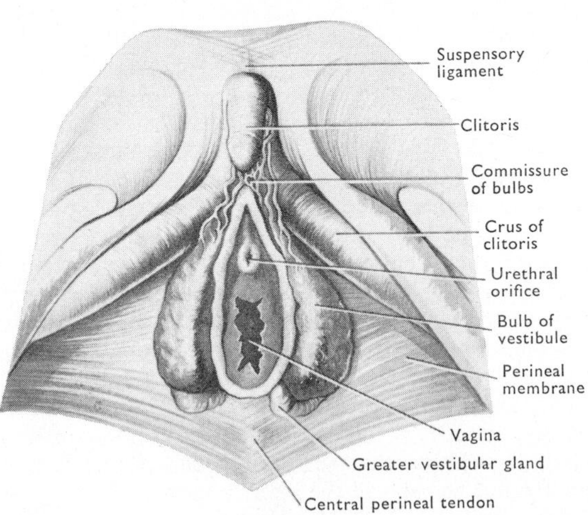

FIG. 202 A dissection of the superficial perineal space in the female.

the penis from the central perineal tendon, and turn it carefully forwards to expose the urethra and the artery of the bulb piercing the perineal membrane to enter the bulb. The ducts of the bulbo-urethral glands lie at the sides of the urethra but are difficult to identify. Clean as much of the perineal membrane as possible without damage to these structures.

In the female, gently raise the posterior part of the bulb of the vestibule and expose the greater vestibular gland. Follow it forwards to its duct, and expose the artery to the bulb. Divide the artery, and fold the bulb forwards. Clean as much of the perineal membrane as possible.

PERINEAL MEMBRANE (INFERIOR FASCIA OF UROGENITAL DIAPHRAGM)

The perineal membrane is a triangular fibrous sheet that extends from the central perineal tendon almost to the pubic symphysis, and is attached to the pubic arch laterally. Posteriorly it fuses with the membranous layer of the superficial perineal fascia and anteriorly and posteriorly with the fascia (superior fascia of the urogenital diaphragm) forming the roof of the deep perineal space; thus closing both perineal spaces posteriorly and the deep space anteriorly. At the latter fusion the anterior border of the perineal membrane is thickened to form the **transverse ligament of the perineum** immediately posterior to the **dorsal vein of the penis** or **clitoris** where it passes into the pelvis [FIG. 203].

The perineal membrane lies in a horizontal plane in the erect posture of the body. It is in contact inferiorly with the structures in the superficial perineal space, and superiorly with those in the deep space. It is pierced by: (1) the **urethra** (with the ducts of the bulbo-urethral glands in the male and the **vagina** in the female) in the median plane 2·5 cm. from the pubic symphysis in the male, but closer to it in the female; (2) the **arteries of the bulb** at the sides of the urethra in the male, or at the sides of the vagina in the female; and (3) the **internal pudendal vessels** with the **dorsal nerves of the penis** or **clitoris** at the sides of the perineal membrane anteriorly.

The urethral orifice in the perineal membrane is larger than the urethra, and its fascia is continued over the bulb of the penis as a fascial sheath for that structure.

DISSECTION. Carefully reflect the perineal membrane medially on the side from which the crus of the penis was removed, but leave the other half intact. This exposes a thin sheet of muscle which should be cleaned, but is difficult to dissect satisfactorily. It consists of the sphincter urethrae anteriorly and the deep transverse perineal muscles posteriorly.

Follow the internal pudendal artery forwards (with the dorsal nerve of the penis or clitoris) in this deep perineal space and through the perineal membrane to its division into the deep and dorsal arteries of the penis or clitoris. Find and trace the artery of the bulb.

In the male, look for the bulbo-urethral gland posterolateral to the urethra on the superior surface of the deep transverse perineal muscle.

DEEP PERINEAL SPACE

This space lies between the **perineal membrane** and the **superior fascia of the urogenital diaphragm.** It is pierced by the urethra (and the vagina in the female) and transmits the terminal parts of the internal pudendal vessels and the dorsal nerves of the penis or clitoris. It contains the sphincter urethrae and the deep transverse perineal muscles (and the bulbo-urethral glands in the male) which, with the enclosing fascial layers, form the **urogenital diaphragm.**

The sheet of muscle in the deep space consists of fibres which arise from the medial surface of the inferior pubic ramus. *In the male*, these pass to meet the corresponding fibres of the opposite side in a median raphe anterior and posterior to the urethra. The muscle fibres adjacent to the urethra pass circularly around it, and these together with the adjacent transverse fibres constitute the **sphincter urethrae,** while the most posterior transverse fibres form the **deep transverse perineal muscle.** *In the female*, the same arrangement exists, except that the posterior transverse fibres of sphincter urethrae are attached to the vaginal wall. Nerve supply: minute branches of the perineal nerve. Action: this is striated muscle which forms the *voluntary sphincter of the urethra.*

The **membranous part of the urethra** is only

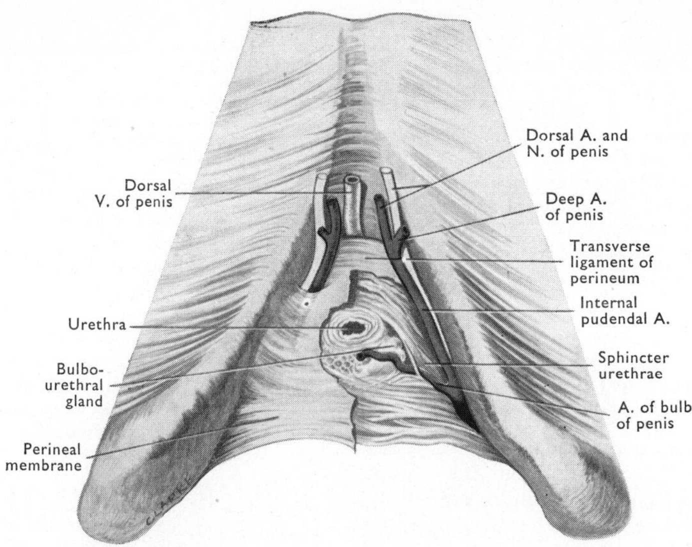

FIG. 203 A deep dissection of the male perineum. The penis has been removed, the urethra cut across, and the left half of the perineal membrane removed to expose sphincter urethrae and the artery to the bulb.

1 cm. long, and is the least distensible part. It extends for a short distance inferior to the perineal membrane to enter the spongy part, and is continuous with the prostatic part through the superior fascia of the urogenital diaphragm [FIG. 216]. It is lined with columnar epithelium.

Female Urethra

This tube is 4–5 cm. long and 6 mm. wide. It is very dilatable, and extends from the neck of the bladder, through the pelvic cavity and deep perineal space, to open immediately anterior to the vaginal orifice [FIG. 209]. Throughout its length it is attached to the anterior wall of the vagina, and a metal rod placed in it is readily felt through that wall. Most of the lining is stratified squamous or columnar epithelium, and a number of small mucous glands open into it.

Internal Pudendal Artery

This artery arises in the pelvis from the internal iliac artery. It passes through the gluteal region, and enters the ischiorectal fossa via the lesser sciatic foramen. Here it runs with the pudendal nerve and its terminal branches, in the fascia covering obturator internus, the **pudendal canal.** At the posterior border of the perineal membrane it enters the **deep perineal space,** and runs forwards with the dorsal nerve of the penis or clitoris. 1–2 cm. from the pubic symphysis it pierces the perineal membrane and divides into the dorsal and deep arteries of the penis or clitoris [FIG. 203]. It may divide while still in the deep perineal space.

Branches. The inferior rectal, perineal, and posterior scrotal or labial have been seen already [pp. 216, 218].

The **artery of the bulb** arises in the posterior part of the deep perineal space, and passing inferior to the sphincter urethrae, supplies it and the bulbo-urethral gland in the male. It then pierces the perineal membrane [p. 221] and entering the corpus spongiosum (or bulb of the vestibule in the female) runs through its whole length supplying it [FIG. 203].

The **deep artery of the penis** or **clitoris** enters

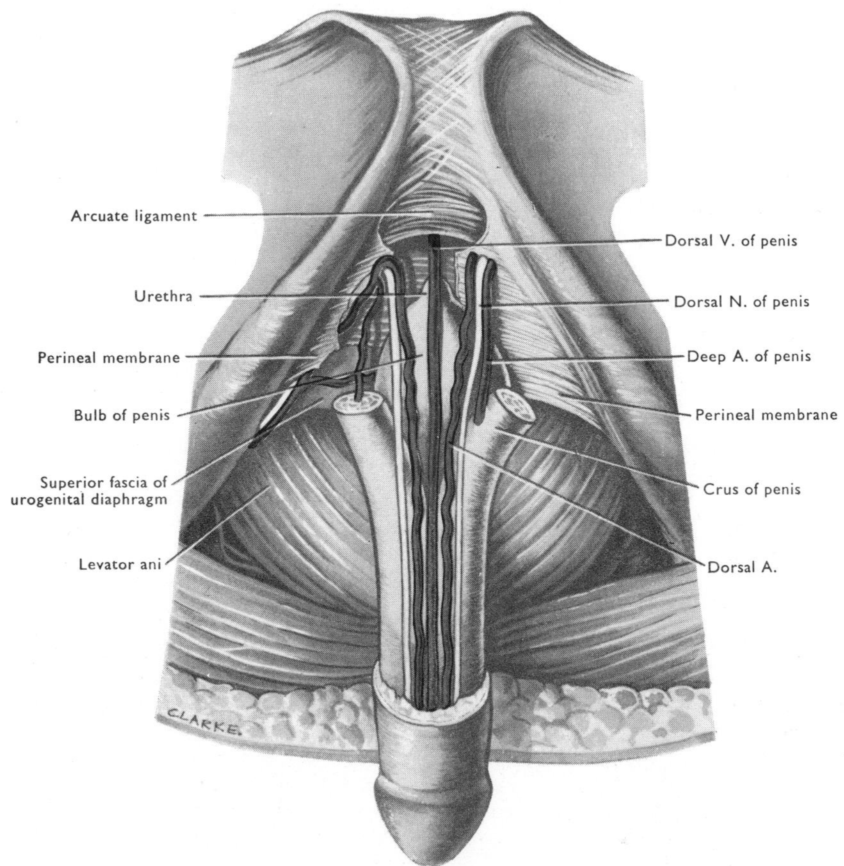

FIG. 204 A dissection to show the pubic symphysis and the dorsal vessels and nerves of the penis.

the crus, and passing forwards in the corpus cavernosum, supplies it [FIG. 108].

The **dorsal artery** passes anterosuperiorly between the crus and the bone to reach the dorsum of the penis or clitoris [FIG. 204].

Pudendal Nerve

This nerve arises from the sacral plexus (S.(1), 2, 3, 4) in the pelvis, leaves it through the lower part of the greater sciatic foramen, and passing over the sacrospinous ligament and through the lesser sciatic foramen, enters the pudendal canal in the perineum. It immediately gives off the inferior rectal nerve and divides into the perineal nerve and the dorsal nerve of the penis.

The **inferior rectal nerve** has been seen previously [p. 216].

The **perineal nerve** passes with the internal pudendal artery to the anterior end of the pudendal canal. Here it gives off two **posterior scrotal** or **labial nerves,** and divides into its terminal branches. These pass into the superficial and deep perineal spaces and supply the contained muscles and the bulb of the penis or of the vestibule.

The **dorsal nerve of the penis** or **clitoris** passes through the pudendal canal and deep perineal space close to the pubic arch. It gives a branch to the crus of the penis or clitoris, and piercing the perineal membrane 1–2 cm. from the pubic symphysis, passes with the dorsal artery to the penis or clitoris [FIG. 204], and sends branches round the side of that organ to its ventral surface. It supplies all the skin and the glans.

The pudendal nerve, in addition to its sensory fibres and the motor fibres to the perineal muscles, carries **autonomic fibres** to the erectile tissues supplied by its branches.

Bulbo-urethral Glands

These small glands lie posterolateral to the membranous urethra [FIG. 203] in the male. Their long ducts pierce the perineal membrane with the urethra. and running distally with it for a short distance, enter the spongy part of the urethra [FIGS. 218, 219].

LYMPH VESSELS OF PERINEUM

These important and numerous vessels are not demonstrable by ordinary dissection, but they drain anteriorly to the **medial superficial inguinal lymph nodes,** the enlargement of which may be the first sign of infection in this region. Lymph from all the perineal structures, including the inferior parts of the anal canal, vagina, and urethra, drain in this direction, but lymph vessels from the upper parts of the anal canal, vagina, and urethra drain superiorly into the pelvis [FIG. 228] together with some deep vessels which pass with the internal pudendal vessels and the dorsal vein of the penis or clitoris.

It is important to remember that the lymph vessels from the skin and fascial layers of the **scrotum** drain to the superficial inguinal nodes, but that the **testicular lymph vessels** drain via the spermatic cord to the *lumbar lymph nodes* on the abdominal aorta.

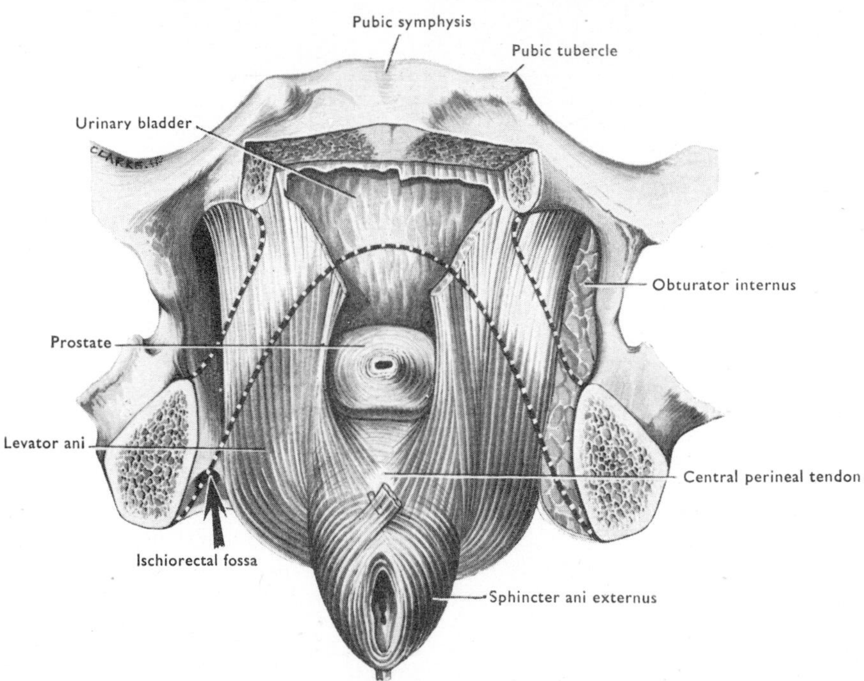

FIG. 205 A dissection of the levator ani muscles in the male. The perineum has been tilted forwards, the ischial rami and the inferior rami and parts of the bodies of the pubic bones (broken lines) have been removed together with the contents of the superficial and deep perineal spaces and of the ischiorectal fossae.

DISSECTION. **Remove the sphincter urethrae, the deep transverse perineal muscle, and the superior fascia of the urogenital diaphragm from the side on which the muscles are exposed. Clean as much as possible of the perineal surface of levator ani [Fig. 205]. Note that its anterior part has a free medial border which is separated from its fellow by a gap anterior to the central tendon of the perineum, into the superior surface of which these most medial fibres of levator ani are inserted. Confirm the fact that the gap transmits the urethra in the male, and the vagina and urethra in the female. Note that some of the fibres of levator ani, which pass to the central perineal tendon, turn round the posterior vaginal wall and form a partial sphincter for it. In the male, the inferior part of the prostate can be identified in the gap, the margins of the levator ani muscles passing inferior to its lateral parts and supporting it (levator prostatae).**

Trace the more posterior fibres of levator ani to the sides of the anal canal where they pass deep to the external sphincter. Some of the fibres join the longitudinal muscle layer, and extend inferiorly through the external sphincter to the perianal skin. Superiorly, confirm the attachment of levator ani to the fascia over obturator internus. Note that the posterior fibres of levator ani lie edge to edge with the coccygeus (which also arises from the ischial spine, and whose posterior part forms the sacrospinous ligament) which continues the plane of levator ani to the inferior margin of the greater sciatic foramen. Thus the levator ani muscles, together with the sacrospinous ligaments form a fibromuscular floor to the pelvic cavity, and this is deficient anteriorly between the medial margins of the levator ani muscles, where the gap is filled inferiorly by the urogenital diaphragm.

RETROPUBIC SPACE

This lies between the anterior surface of the bladder and the pelvic surfaces of the pubic bones. It is filled with loose, fatty connective tissue, the **retropubic pad of fat,** and it extends from the pubic symphysis posterolaterally around the sides of the bladder as far as the ureters. Posterior to the bodies of the pubic bones, the space is limited inferiorly by the strong **puboprostatic ligaments (pubovesical** or, more accurately, pubo-urethral in the female) which pass to the neck (lowest part) of the bladder and to the base (upper part) of the prostate (or urethra in the female). Superiorly the space is continuous with the loose extraperitoneal tissue which extends up the anterior abdominal wall to the level of the umbilicus, between the **lateral umbilical ligaments.** The bladder expands superiorly in this plane, and so may urine from a ruptured bladder.

DISSECTION. **Push a finger inferiorly between the bladder and the pubis till it reaches the resistance of the puboprostatic or pubovesical ligaments. Carry the finger posterolaterally to the side of the bladder, and note that the connective tissue here is also loose (as far posteriorly as the ureter or the base of the broad ligament) to allow for expansion of the bladder. Place a finger in the ischiorectal fossa, and note that the finger in the pelvic cavity is separated from it by the levator ani and the fascia covering it. As far as possible explore the relation of the finger in the pelvis to that in the perineum, passing both forwards to the puboprostatic ligaments.**

THE PELVIC VISCERA

OVARY

[Figs. 190, 206, 222]

The ovaries are pinkish white, ovoid structures, which are flattened supero-inferiorly. They measure approximately 3 cm. long, 1·5 cm. wide, and 1 cm. thick. Between them they usually produce one ripe ovum per menstrual cycle. This develops in a small cyst or **follicle** which ruptures approximately at the middle of the menstrual cycle, and releases the ovum into the peritoneal cavity. The remaining lining cells of the follicle then develop into a corpus luteum, which produces changes in the uterine lining (**endometrium**) that complete its preparation for implantation of the fertilized ovum. It the ovum is not fertilized, the corpus luteum degenerates towards the end of the menstrual cycle, and is gradually replaced by a fibrous scar (**corpus albicans).** Thus the originally smooth surface of the ovary becomes puckered with scars. In elderly women the entire ovary shrinks following its loss of stimulation by the pituitary gonadotrophic hormones after the menopause.

The ovary lies near the lateral wall of the pelvic cavity in a slight depression between the ureter posteromedially, the external iliac vein laterally, and the uterine tube in the free margin of the broad ligament anteriorly [FIG. 206]. The extremity of the uterine tube curves round the lateral end of the ovary and is attached to it by one of the fimbriae [FIG. 189]. The ovary is attached to the superior surface of the broad ligament by a very short peritoneal fold (the **mesovarium**) through which the ovarian vessels enter its **hilus.** The medial extremity of the ovary is attached to the uterus by the **ligament of the ovary.** The appendix vermiformis, if pelvic in position, may be very close to the right ovary.

In pregnancy the broad ligament and ovary are carried superiorly with the expanding uterus, and when this contracts, in the post-partum period, the ovary may return to a site other than that described above.

Vessels and Nerves. Each **ovarian artery** arises from the aorta below the renal artery, and descending over the posterior abdominal wall, crosses the external iliac artery, and enters the lateral part of the broad ligament (**suspensory ligament of the ovary**). It sends branches through the mesovarium to the ovary, and continuing medially in the broad ligament, gives twigs to the uterine tube, and anastomoses with the uterine artery.

The **veins** leave the hilus and form a **pampiniform plexus** on the artery. Near the superior aperture of the pelvis, a single ovarian vein is formed which ascends to the inferior vena cava (right vein) or the left renal vein (left vein).

The **lymph vessels** unite with those from the fundus of the uterus and the uterine tube, and ascend with the vein to end in the abdominal nodes from the bifurcation of the aorta to the level of the renal vessels.

Structure. Make a cut into the ovary and note its dense fibrous stroma. In a young individual this contains follicles in various stages of development and many large, scattered germ cells (oogonia) which can be seen under the microscope and which may develop into follicles. The surface of the ovary is covered by a cubical epithelium (**germinal epithelium**) which is continuous with the flattened mesothelium of the peritoneum at a white line which surrounds the margins of the mesovarium.

UTERINE TUBES
[FIGS. 189, 206, 221]

Each tube, approximately 10 cm. long, is narrow as it passes from its opening into the cavity of the uterus (at the junction of the fundus and body) through the wall of the uterus (**uterine part**) to join the narrow **isthmus** of the tube (2–3 cm. long) in the free edge of the broad ligament. The isthmus is continuous laterally with the expanded and slightly convoluted **ampulla** which forms most of the remainder of the tube, and passes towards the lateral pelvic wall. Here it rises out of the superior surface of the broad ligament on a short mesentery, and curving over the lateral extremity of the ovary, expands to form a funnel-shaped extremity (the **infundibulum**). This opens into the peritoneal cavity adjacent to the ovary, and has a fringe of finger-like processes (**fimbriae**) on its margin. One of these, the **ovarian fimbria,** is attached to the ovary. Near the time of ovulation, the tube becomes turgid and expands medially over the ovary. Thus the discharged ovum is easily carried into the tube by the action of cilia on the columnar epithelium covering the fimbriae and lining the mucous membrane of the tube, which is thrown into numerous longitudinal folds that virtually fill the muscular tube.

DISSECTION. Open one uterine tube longitudinally, and note the folds of its mucous membrane in the ampulla and infundibulum, and the variations in its internal diameter.

The ovum is fertilized in the ovarian end of the tube, and development begins as it slowly passes to the uterus. If this passage is delayed, the ovum may adhere to the tube and burrow into its wall. Unlike the uterus, the tube is too thin-walled to withstand the invading ovum, and rupture of the tube occurs with severe intraperitoneal bleeding: one cause of an acute abdominal emergency in women of child-bearing age. This is the commonest type of ectopic gestation; much more rarely a fertilized

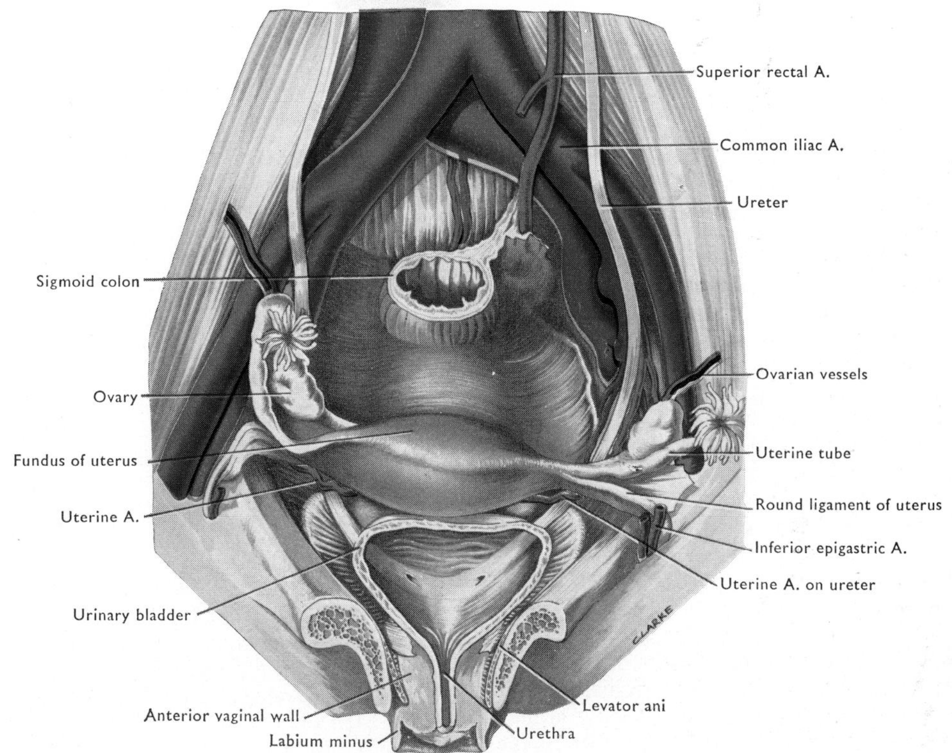

FIG. 206 A dissection of the female pelvis from the front after removal of the greater part of the bodies of the pubic bones and the anterior parts of the bladder and urethra.

ovum may fail to enter the tube and can then implant in the peritoneal surface of any of the pelvic viscera or walls.

Vessels. The blood vessels are branches of the ovarian and uterine vessels; the lymph vessels join those of the ovary and pass to the lumbar nodes.

Ligament of Ovary [FIG. 221]

This slender band of fibrous tissue and smooth muscle extends from the medial extremity of the ovary to the superior aspect of the junction of the uterine tube and uterus, and it forms a ridge on the superior surface of the broad ligament.

Round Ligament of Uterus [FIGS. 189, 206]

This slender band, composed of the same tissue as the ligament of the ovary, arises from the antero-inferior surface of the uterus opposite the attachment of the ligament of the ovary. The round ligament passes to the side wall of the pelvis, forming a ridge on the inferior surface of the broad ligament. It then sweeps forwards to the deep inguinal ring, crossing medial to the obturator vessels and nerve, the umbilical artery, and the external iliac vessels while immediately deep to the peritoneum. It then hooks round the lateral side of the inferior epigastric vessels, runs through the inguinal canal, and spreads out to its attachment in the labium majus.

The ligament of the ovary and the round ligament of the uterus together represent the remains of the **gubernaculum** in the embryo. This structure is partly responsible for the descent of the testis to the scrotum in the male. In the female, the persistence of the ducts forming the uterus and uterine tubes (which disappear in the male) interrupts the continuity of this structure and prevents it from drawing the ovary from its original position in the upper abdomen to the labium majus (the homologue of the scrotum). The ovary is drawn down to the greater pelvis, and later descends into the lesser pelvis when that structure enlarges to accommodate the bladder and uterus which are abdominal organs in the child [FIG. 211]. Very rarely the ovary may be drawn into the inguinal canal or even carried to the labium majus.

PELVIC PARTS OF URETERS

[FIGS. 189, 191, 222, 227]

Half of the 25 cm. long ureter lies in the pelvis and half in the abdomen.

The ureter crosses the origin of the external iliac artery, and runs postero-inferiorly along the front of the internal iliac artery, subjacent to the peritoneum of the lateral wall of the pelvis, and postero-inferior to the ovary in the female. At the level of the ischial spine, it curves anteromedially in the fat above levator ani. In the female, it passes inferior to the broad ligament and to the uterine artery which turns superiorly into that ligament. In the male it remains in contact with the peritoneum until it is separated from it by the ductus deferens a short distance before it reaches the posterosuperior angle of the bladder, the same point as in the female.

In both sexes the ureter passes obliquely through the bladder wall in an inferomedial direction, and opens at the superolateral angle of the trigone of the bladder [FIG. 207].

DISSECTION. Remove the peritoneum from the superior surface of the bladder, but do not carry this quite as far posteriorly as the depths of the uterovesical pouch in the female. Identify and clean the median umbilical ligament [Fig. 212] arising from the apex of the bladder. Clean the fat from the retropubic space and from the paravesical fossae, and displacing the apex of the bladder posteriorly, identify the puboprostatic or pubovesical ligaments.

In the male, clean the ductus deferens and ureter to the base of the bladder on both sides. In the female, clean the ligament of the ovary, the round ligament of the uterus, and the ureter on the side on which the uterine tube was opened. In following the ureter in the female, identify the uterine artery crossing superior to the ureter as it passes the side of the vagina.

Make an incision through the bladder wall along the junction of the superior and inferolateral surfaces [Fig. 212] from the apex as far as the lateral extremity of the base. Fold back the superior wall of the bladder and examine the internal surface [Figs. 206, 207].

INTERNAL SURFACE OF URINARY BLADDER

In the contracted bladder, the internal surface is ridged to a greater or lesser degree by folds of the mucous membrane, some of which cover protuberant bundles of the interlacing muscle especially in the hypertrophied bladder. On the posterior wall of the bladder is a smooth triangular area (the **trigone of the bladder**) the inferior angle of which lies at the median **internal urethral orifice,** while a small, obliquely placed **ureteric orifice** is present at each of the superolateral angles. The latter are joined by a well defined ridge which forms the superior side of the trigone, the **interureteric fold.**

Orifices of Ureters. Pass a fine seeker through each ureteric orifice, confirm that it passes into the corresponding ureter, and note the obliquity of its passage through the bladder wall. This oblique passage acts as a flap valve, thus any increase in intravesical pressure (due to contraction of the vesical musculature, *e.g.*, in urination) presses the walls of the intramural part of the ureter together and prevents the pressure in the bladder being transmitted to the ureter and kidney. This is an important feature, for raised pressure in the ureter and pelvis of the kidney, if continued, can cause irreversible damage to the kidney.

Internal Urethral Orifice. This is a Y-shaped slit at the inferior angle of the trigone. In the male the mucous membrane is bulged forwards (**uvula of the bladder**) between the limbs of the Y by the median lobe of the prostate which immediately underlies this part of the trigone.

PUBIC SYMPHYSIS

This is a secondary cartilaginous joint which is similar to an intervertebral disc, and unites

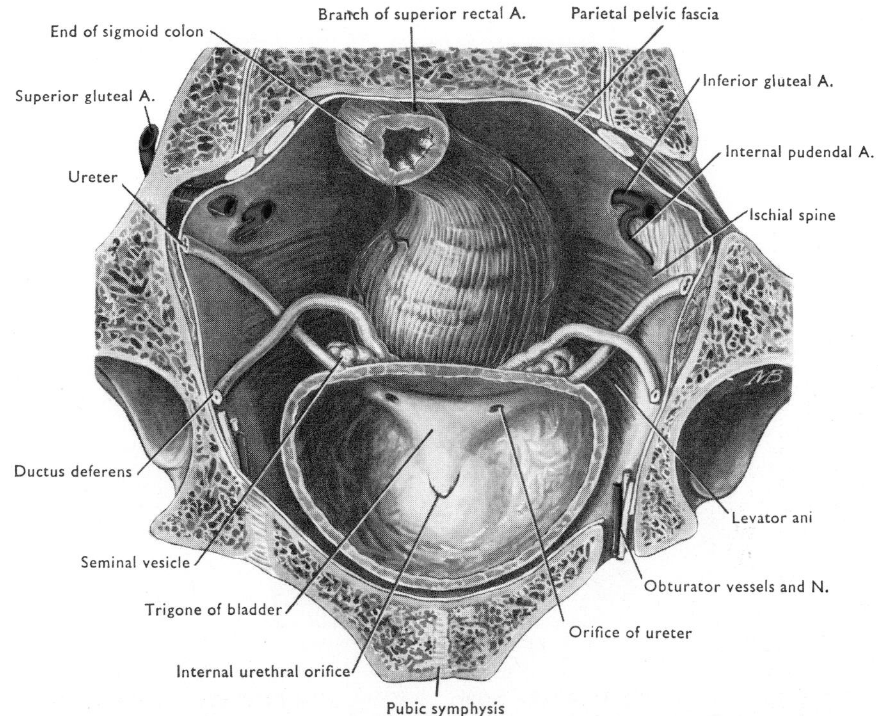

FIG. 207 Some of the contents of the male lesser pelvis seen from above and in front.

the two hip bones anteriorly. The articular surfaces of the pubic bones are covered with hyaline cartilage, and united by a disc of fibro-cartilage which has a central, slit-like cavity, and is surrounded by a ligamentous sheath. Posteriorly the ligament is thin; superiorly it unites the two pubic crests; anteriorly it is very strong and is composed of deep transverse, and superficial oblique fibres, bundles of the latter interdigitating with one another. The tendinous fibres of rectus abdominis and external oblique mingle with the superficial layer. The inferior or **arcuate ligament** is a strong, curved band which rounds off the apex of the pubic arch and extends along the inferior pubic rami. The **dorsal vein of the penis** or **clitoris** enters the pelvic cavity between the arcuate and transverse perineal ligaments [p. 221].

The pubic symphysis allows a small amount of movement between the hip bones, and tends to absorb shocks. In common with many other tissues, the disc contains more tissue fluid in the later stages of pregnancy, and may allow an increased range of movement during childbirth.

DISSECTION. Clean the surface of the pubic symphysis to expose the superior, anterior, and arcuate parts of its superficial ligament. Near the arcuate ligament, some ligamentous bundles arise from the antero-inferior surface of the pubic symphysis, and passing with the dorsal vein of the clitoris, are attached to the tissues around the urethra. This is the inferior part of the pubo-urethral ligament which stabilizes the urethra in the female.

In the male, make a median section through the penis and its corpus spongiosum to the bulb, opening the entire length of the spongy part of the urethra. Examine the internal surface of the urethra, and note any recesses or lacunae in its dorsal wall, especially at the proximal end of the fossa navicularis in the glans penis

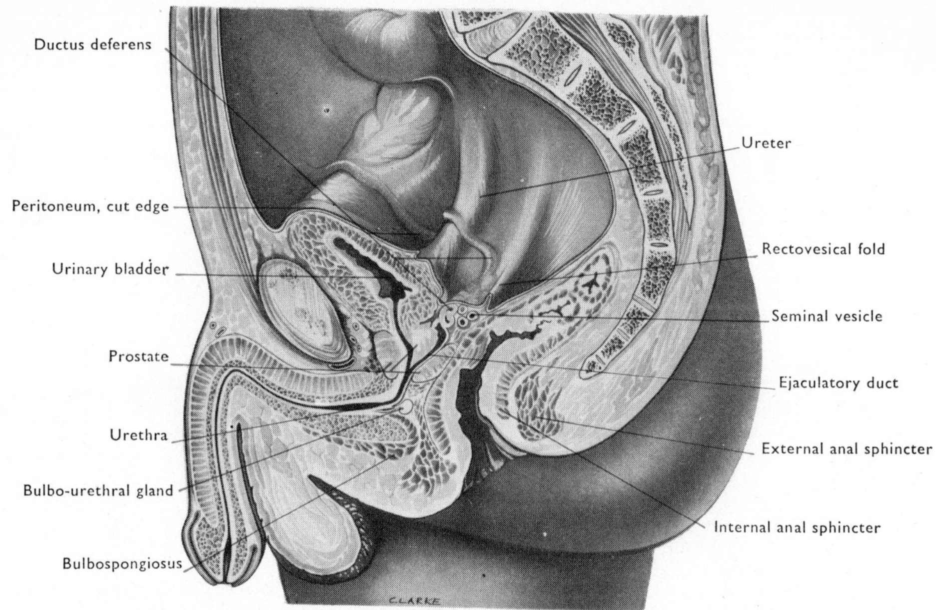

FIG. 208 A section through the male pelvis.

Identify the intrabulbar fossa and the opening of the membranous part into the spongy part. Pass a metal rod through the urethra to the bladder, from the external orifice in the female, or from the inferior extremity of the membranous part in the male.

Divide the pubic symphysis in the median plane, and cut down on to the metal rod, dividing the structures posterior to the pubic symphysis in the median plane, and opening the anterior wall of the urethra. Remove the metal rod and continue the median incision to the anterior surfaces of the sacrum and coccyx. In the perineum, this cut should pass through the middle of the central perineal tendon, anal canal, and anococcygeal ligament. In the pelvis it should divide the bladder through the internal urethral orifice and the middle of the interureteric fold, then pass either through the uterus and vagina or between the two deferent ducts, and divide the rectum longitudinally. Make a median, dorsal saw cut through the fourth and fifth lumbar vertebrae, the sacrum, coccyx, and the intervening intervertebral discs to meet the knife cut through the soft tissues, but avoid carrying the saw into the soft tissues of the pelvis.

Separate the two halves of the pelvis, clean out the rectum and vagina with a jet of water, and examine the cut surfaces of the pubic symphysis, the intervertebral discs, and the soft tissues [Figs. 208, 209].

URINARY BLADDER

[FIGS. 191, 207, 210, 212, 213, 214, 219, 222]

The interior of the urinary bladder has been seen already [p. 228]; its shape and position should now be studied.

This muscular urine store, when empty, lies in the antero-inferior part of the pelvis. Its superior surface is covered with peritoneum. This is reflected at the posterior border of the bladder on to the junction of the body and cervix of the uterus in the female (the utero-vesical pouch) and over the superior surfaces of the deferent ducts in the male. The bladder lies relatively free in the surrounding loose, extraperitoneal tissue except at its inferior part (**neck**) which is held firmly by the **pubo-prostatic** (male) or **pubovesical** (female) **ligaments.** Thus it is free to expand superiorly in the extraperitoneal tissue of the anterior abdominal wall, stripping the peritoneum from the transversalis fascia: a feature which allows the introduction of instruments into the distended bladder through the anterior

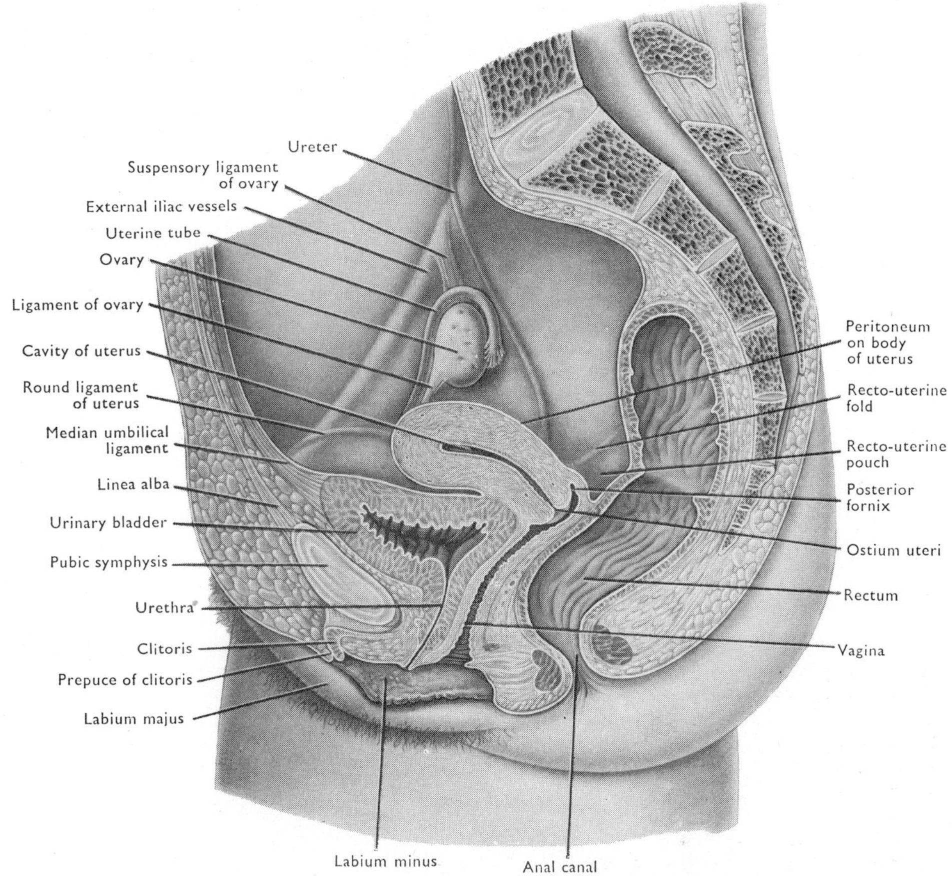

FIG. 209 A median section through the female pelvis.

abdominal wall without involvement of the peritoneal cavity.

In the child [FIG. 211] the bladder is an abdominal organ even when empty, and though the enlarging pelvis begins to accommodate it approximately at six years of age, it is not entirely a pelvic organ till after puberty.

Shape. The empty bladder has the shape of a three-sided pyramid with its apex anteriorly [FIG. 212], but becomes spherical when distended [FIG. 226]. The **apex** is directly continuous with the **median umbilical ligament** immediately posterior to the upper margin of the pubic symphysis. The median umbilical ligament is the fibrous remnant of the intra-abdominal part of the **allantois,** a tubular structure which extends from the bladder into the umbilical cord in the embryo. It may remain patent in part, or rarely throughout its length. In the latter case, urine may be discharged through the umbilicus when the umbilical cord is cut at birth.

The triangular **base** (or **fundus**) of the bladder faces postero-inferiorly, and is applied to the genital septum (and its contents) which separates it from the rectovesical (or recto-uterine) pouch and rectum.

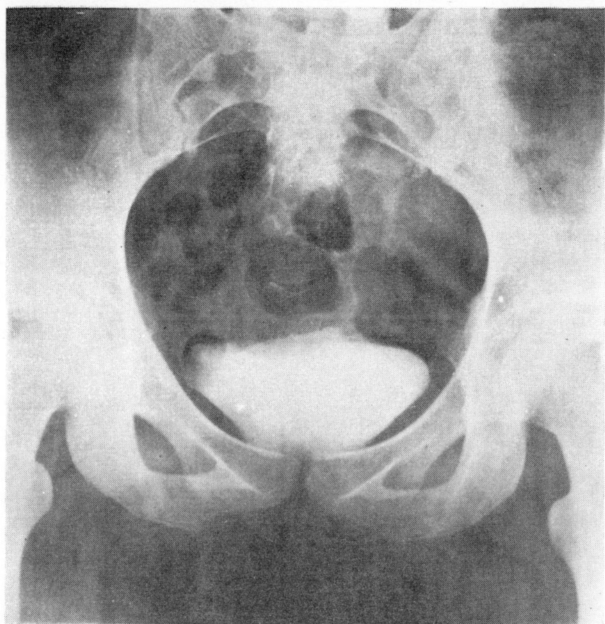

FIG. 210 A radiograph of the female pelvis to show the urinary bladder filled with contrast medium. Note the pyramidal shape of the partly distended bladder.

The sides of the pyramid consist of two **inferolateral surfaces** [FIG. 213] and one **superior surface,** all of which are slightly convex. The inferolateral surfaces lie parallel to the pelvic surfaces of the levator ani muscles on the retropubic pad of fat, and form the posterosuperior wall of the retropubic space. They meet at an edge (posterior to the pubic symphysis) which slopes postero-inferiorly from the apex to meet the inferior angle of the base at the most inferior part or **neck** of the bladder, where it is continuous with the urethra [FIGS. 208, 209].

The **base** (or fundus) and the superior surface are continuous at the posterior border, and the ureters join the bladder at the lateral ends of this border. *In the female*, the base is in contact with the cervix of the uterus and the upper part of the vagina. *In the male*, the two seminal vesicles, with the ampullae of the deferent ducts between them, cover all but a small, peritoneal covered, median part of the base, immediately below the posterior border [FIG. 214].

Structure of Bladder. The **muscle** layer is thick and strong, and consists of interlacing bundles of smooth muscle running in many directions (see gall-bladder, p. 173). Towards the neck, the bundles become finer, and are partly massed together to form a ring that surrounds the uppermost part of the urethra, the involuntary **sphincter of the bladder.** Other muscle fibres run radially in this region, and tend to pull open the internal urethral orifice when they contract on micturition. In the female, the muscle at the neck of the bladder is continuous with the urethral muscle inferiorly, while that in the male is continuous with the muscular stroma of the prostate gland.

The **mucous membrane** is lined with transitional epithelium which is urine proof and capable of considerable distension, but the underlying connective tissue is loose and inelastic, so that it becomes wrinkled on contraction except over the trigone where the epithelium is more firmly bound to the muscle and tends to remain smooth.

DISSECTION. Pull the half bladder medially and clean the structures on its lateral aspect, including the umbilical artery and its superior vesical branches passing to the bladder, the obturator nerve and vessels, and the superior part of levator ani.

In the male, follow the ductus deferens to the base of the bladder, clean it and the adjoining seminal vesicle down to the base of the prostate [Fig. 214]. Note the visceral pelvic fascia descending from these structures to form the fascial sheath over the posterior surface of the prostate (the rectovesical septum).

Follow the prostatic fascia inferiorly to the superior fascia of the urogenital diaphragm on the side where this fascia is intact.

Anteriorly, find the dorsal vein of the penis entering the pelvis to join the plexus of veins in the angle between the prostate and the bladder [Fig. 216]. Follow the

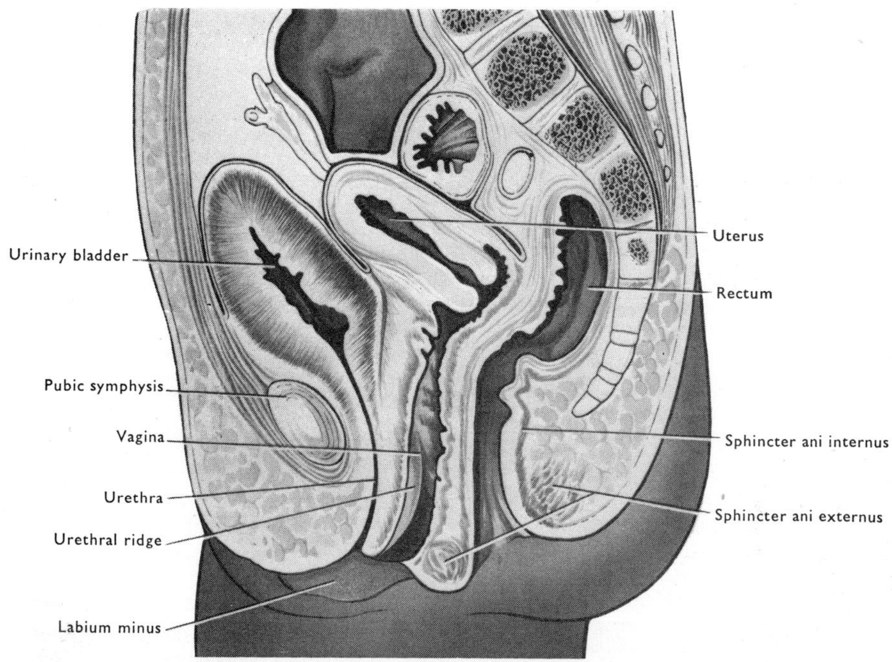

FIG. 211 A median section through the lower abdomen and pelvis of a new-born female child. Note that the urinary bladder and uterus lie in the abdomen.

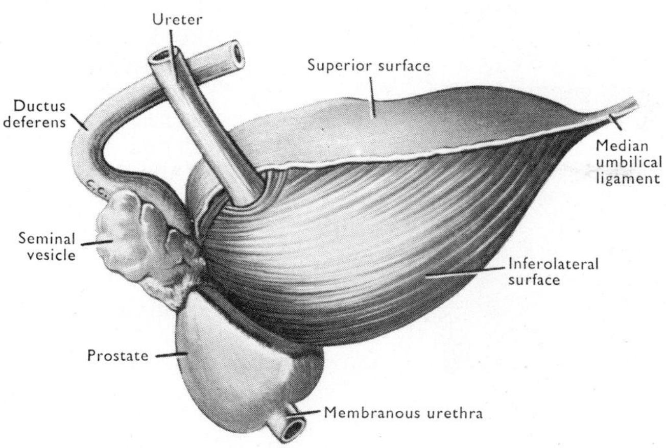

FIG. 212 A lateral view of the urinary bladder, prostate and seminal vesicle. The bladder is nearly empty.

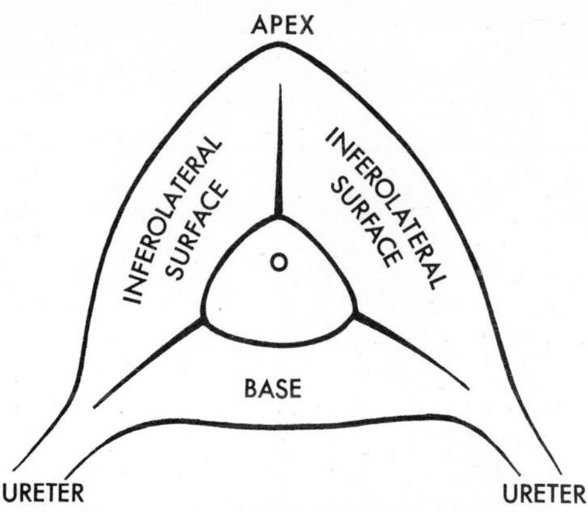

FIG. 213 A diagram of the urinary bladder as seen from below. The enclosed area marks the position of the prostate.

prostatic fascia on to the back of the pubic bone as the puboprostatic ligament.

Pull the bladder and prostate medially, and clean the medial margin of levator ani which lies immediately inferolateral to the prostate (levator prostatae muscle). Note that the urethra descends from the prostate into the deep perineal space through the gap between the medial margins of the two levator ani muscles, and that the apex of the prostate also protrudes through this gap on to the superior fascia of the urogenital diaphragm.

Note that the prostate is a firm structure which is traversed by the urethra and lies close to the anterior wall of the rectum with the rectovesical septum between.

Examine the prostatic urethra. Its upper and lower parts lie at an angle to each other, and immediately inferior to this, a small hillock (seminal colliculus) projects forwards from a median, posterior ridge (urethral crest, Fig. 219) which extends the length of the prostatic urethra with a groove on each side of it, the prostatic sinus. On the apex of the colliculus is the small opening of a blind, median pouch (prostatic utricle) which extends posterosuperiorly into the prostate, and is the remnant of the structure which forms the vagina in the female. On each side of the utricle is the smaller opening of an ejaculatory duct. Pass a fine seeker into the latter opening, and note that it enters either the ductus deferens or the seminal vesicle, which unite to form the ejaculatory duct near the base of the prostate [Fig. 218].

Find the beginning of the ejaculatory duct, and trace it antero-inferiorly through the posterior part of the prostate.

DUCTUS DEFERENS

[FIGS. 191, 208, 214, 227]

This thick-walled, muscular duct of the testis and epididymis has already been traced from the inferior pole of the testis through the spermatic cord and inguinal canal to the deep inguinal ring [pp. 108, 114]. At the deep inguinal ring it hooks round the lateral side of the inferior epigastric vessels, and runs posteriorly over the external iliac vessels on to the lateral wall of the lesser pelvis, immediately deep to the peritoneum. It then crosses [FIG. 207] the ureter near the posterolateral angle of the bladder, turns medially across the base of the bladder superior to the seminal vesicle, and bending inferiorly on the medial side of the seminal vesicle [FIG. 214], expands into a dilated and sacculated **ampulla.** This is enclosed with the seminal vesicle in the upper part of the fascial **rectovesical septum.** The ductus deferens then narrows rapidly and joins the duct of the seminal vesicle to form the **ejaculatory duct** immediately posterior to the neck of the bladder.

The thick **muscular wall** of the ductus deferens makes it readily palpable in the spermatic cord, and this smooth muscle is heavily innervated with atuonomic nerve

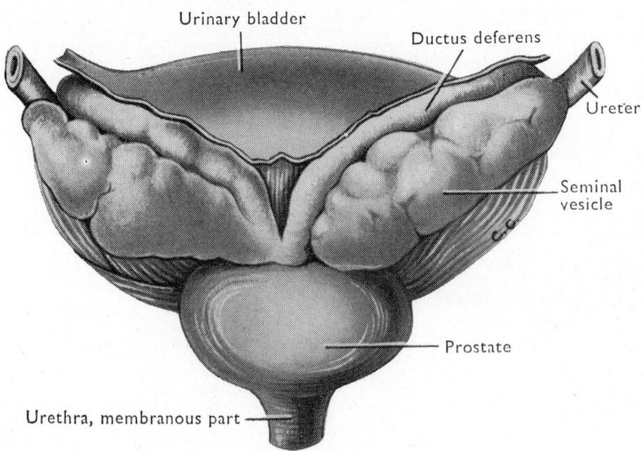

FIG. 214 The posterior surfaces of the urinary bladder, prostate. and seminal vesicles.

fibres to ensure rapid contraction and discharge of the contained spermatozoa and secretions.

SEMINAL VESICLE

[FIGS. 195, 212, 215]

This is a sacculated tube, approximately 15 cm. long, with short sacculated branches. It is coiled upon itself to form a piriform structure which is bound together and to the base of the bladder by the fascia of the upper part of the rectovesical septum. From its narrow, straight duct, which lies posterior to the neck of the bladder, the vesicle extends superolaterally to the entry of the ureter into the bladder, and lies lateral to the ampulla of the ductus deferens.

The seminal vesicle is not a store for spermatozoa. It produces a secretion which is mixed with the spermatozoa from the ductus deferens in the ejaculatory duct, when the muscular wall of the seminal vesicle contracts synchronously with that of the ductus deferens on ejaculation. The alkaline secretion contains fructose, mucus, and a coagulating enzyme. The vesicle has the same structure as the ampulla of the ductus deferens, is lined with columnar epithelium, and its thick secretion seems to be concerned with the nutrition of the spermatozoa.

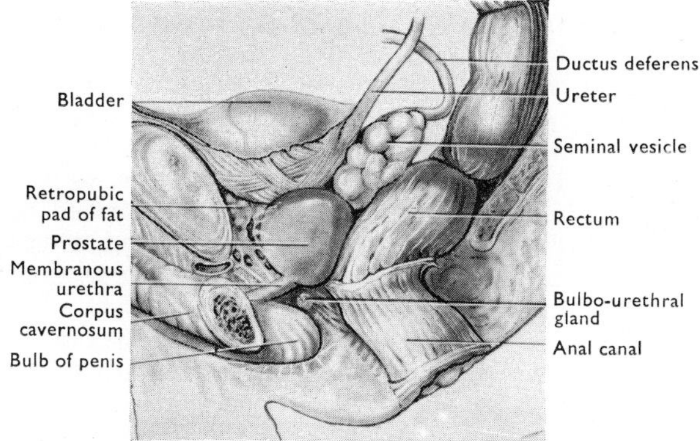

FIG. 215 Dissection of male pelvic organs from the left side.

Ejaculatory Duct [FIG. 218]

This slender duct is formed close to the median plane and posterior to the neck of the bladder by the union of the ductus deferens and the duct of the seminal vesicle. It is approximately 2 cm. long, and passes anteroinferiorly through the upper, posterior half of the prostate and along the side of the prostatic utricle, to open into the prostatic urethra on the seminal colliculus at the side of the utricle. The thin wall of the ejaculatory duct is formed by columnar epithelium and a thin layer of circular and longitudinal muscle.

PROSTATE

[FIGS. 205, 208, 212, 215, 217, 219]

This gland resembles an inverted, compressed cone, approximately 3 cm. from apex to base, and 3·5 cm. across the base. It is firm because of the dense fibromuscular stroma in which the complex glandular elements are buried, and which is directly continuous with the smooth muscle of the neck of the bladder at the **base** of the prostate. Peripherally, the base of the prostate is separated from the bladder by a groove which contains part of the **prostatic plexus of veins** and fat, and has the **ejaculatory ducts** entering it posteriorly.

The inferior end or **apex** of the prostate projects between the medial borders of the two levator ani muscles and rests on the superior fascia of the urogenital diaphragm which is continuous with the fascial sheath of the prostate. The urethra emerges from the prostate immediately anterosuperior to the apex.

The **inferolateral surfaces** are highly convex and lie on the medial margins of the levator ani muscles (**levator prostatae**) which clasp the lowest part of the prostate between them. The two inferolateral surfaces meet in a rounded anterior surface which is separated from the lower part of the pubic symphysis by some fatty areolar tissue.

The **posterior surface** of the

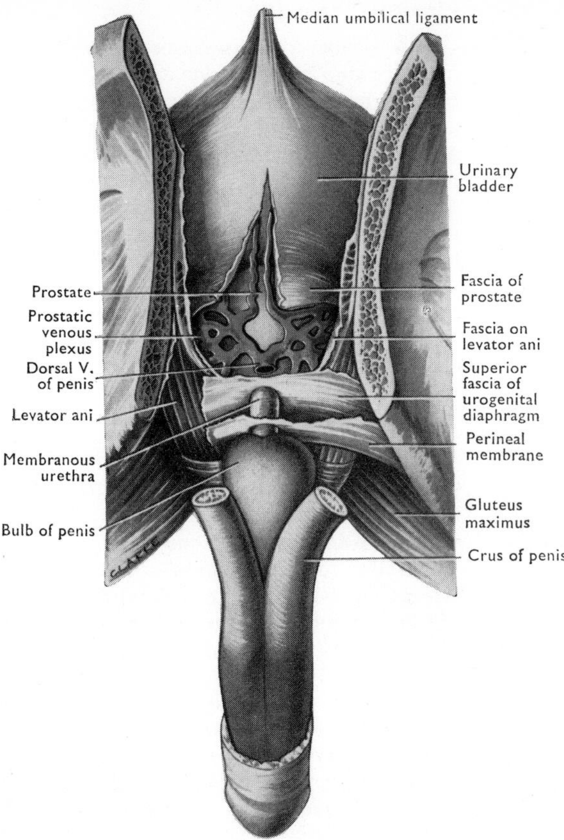

FIG. 216 A dissection of the retropubic space from the front.

prostate is nearly flat, and is separated from the lower part of the rectum only by the thickened part of its fascial sheath, the recto-vesical septum [FIG. 217]. It is, therefore, readily felt by a finger in the rectum.

The prostate has a thin **capsule** of fibro-muscular tissue, but is also enclosed in a loose **sheath** of visceral pelvic fascia which is separated from the capsule at the front and sides by the **prostatic venous plexus.** This drains the prostate and receives the dorsal vein of the penis anteriorly [FIG. 216].

Structure. The glandular part of the prostate develops as a considerable number of minute tubular outgrowths of the prostatic part of the urethra. These form the ducts of the numerous separate elements that make up the prostate but only those that arise from the posterior part of the urethra form glands of any size. Thus the major ducts enter the **prostatic sinuses,** and most of the glandular tissue lies in the posterior and lateral parts of the gland.

The median part of the prostate that lies superior to the prostatic utricle and the ejaculatory ducts, and posterior to the urethra, is the **median lobe.** It lies in direct contact with the inferior part of the trigone of the bladder, and bulges it upwards to produce the uvula of the bladder. Laterally, there is no clear separation of the median lobe from the remainder of the prostate, which is arbitrarily but incompletely divided into **right** and **left lobes** by the urethra.

The **prostatic secretion** is a watery, opalescent fluid which contains considerable quantities of acid phosphatase and protein. It is discharged into the urethra by the contraction of the muscular stroma at ejaculation, when the muscle of the ductus deferens and seminal vesicle also contracts. The size and activity both of the prostate and of the seminal vesicle is controlled by sex hormones. Thus both develop rapidly at puberty, and hypertrophy of the prostate is a common cause of obstruction of the urethra in elderly men.

Blood and Lymphatic Vessels of Bladder, Prostate, Seminal Vesicle, and Ductus Deferens. All these structures are supplied by three visceral branches of the internal iliac artery which are very variable in their arrangement.

The **superior vesical branches** of the umbilical artery supply the anterosuperior part of the bladder, and sometimes the superior parts of the seminal vesicle and ductus deferens.

The **inferior vesical artery** passes to the

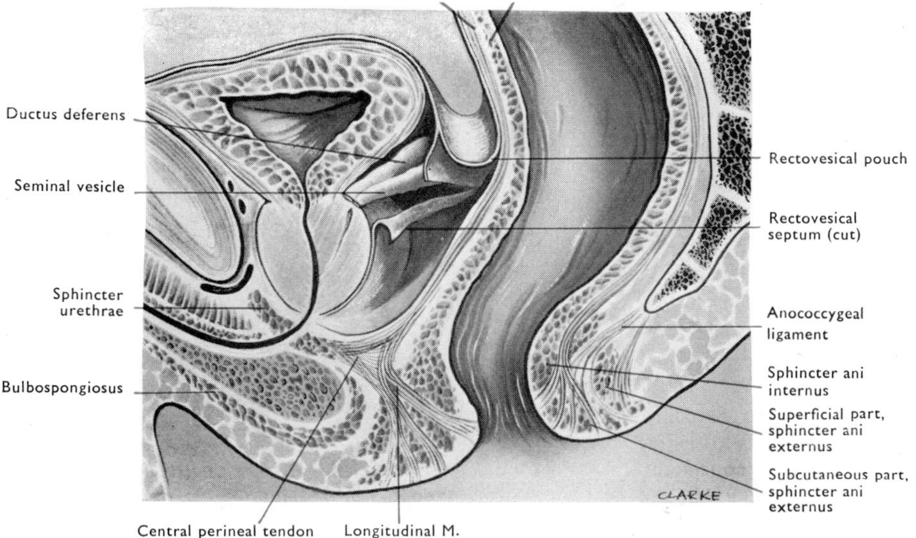

FIG. 217 A median section of the male pelvis.

posterior part of the bladder, and is joined by branches of the **middle rectal artery.** They supply this region, including the prostate (and its contained structures), the seminal vesicles, and the ampulla of the ductus deferens. A long slender branch (artery of the ductus deferens), usually from the inferior vesical artery, runs with the ductus to the inguinal canal.

The **veins** almost all correspond to the arteries, and drain to the internal iliac veins. The anterosuperior part of the bladder may drain to the external iliac vein, and the veins of the bladder and prostate, clustered around the neck of the bladder, also drain the dorsal vein of the penis and pass to the **inferior vesical veins.** These veins communicate through the anterior sacral foramina with the **internal vertebral venous plexuses** in the vertebral canal, and thus the blood from them may ascend either through the inferior vena cava or through the veins of the vertebral column.

The **lymph vessels** of the superior parts drain into the external iliac nodes, while those from the inferior parts pass to the internal iliac nodes. Some of the vessels from the region of the neck of the bladder pass to the sacral and common iliac nodes directly.

The **nerve supply** is by the **inferior hypogastric plexuses.** These contain sympathetic, parasympathetic, and sensory nerve fibres.

Puboprostatic and Pubovesical Ligaments

These ligaments are fibro-elastic condensations of the pelvic fascia which contain some smooth muscle. They pass from the back of the bodies of the pubic bones, close to the median plane, to be attached to the anterior surfaces of the fibrous sheath of the prostate and the neck of the bladder in the male, and to the neck of the bladder and the urethra in the female. They are united across the median plane by a thin fascial layer, and extend laterally to fuse with the fascia over the medial margins of the levator ani muscles. They are important structures in maintaining the position of the bladder, prostate, and urethra. *In the female*, the upper part of the S-shaped urethra is convex anteriorly because of the attachment of the pubo-urethral part of this ligament.

Inferiorly, the urethra curves forwards below the apex of the pubic arch to the external orifice, this inferior part being held by a pubo-urethral ligament that arises from the antero-inferior surface of the pubic symphysis.

MALE URETHRA
[Figs. 195, 208, 218, 219]

The parts of this tube have been described [p. 214], and the entire length has been opened. The urethra consists of a layer of fibro-elastic tissue and smooth muscle lined by a vascular submucous layer which contains many small mucous glands. The lining is predominantly of stratified columnar epithelium, except superior to the prostatic utricle where it is transitional in type, and at the navicular fossa which is lined by stratified squamous epithelium. The lining is pitted by a number of minute recesses (**urethral lacunae**) which face distally.

Prostatic Part. It is approximately 3 cm. long, and pierces the prostate from its base to a point immediately anterior to its apex. It is the widest and most dilatable part of the urethra, and is bent ventrally on itself in its superior half. A narrow, median ridge (**urethral crest**) with a groove (**prostatic sinus**) on each side, extends inferiorly on its posterior wall, from the internal urethral orifice to a rounded eminence (the **seminal colliculus**) on the crest about the middle of the prostatic urethra. The urethral crest then rapidly diminishes, disappearing inferiorly at the membranous part.

The seminal colliculus carries a small median opening (prostatic utricle) with a minute, slit-like aperture (**ejaculatory duct**) on each side, while most of the ducts of the prostate gland open into the prostatic sinuses.

The **prostatic utricle** (approximately 1 cm. long) is a blind sac which extends postero-superiorly into the prostate, and is wider than its aperture. It represents the remains of the parts of the fused paramesonephric ducts of the embryo which form the vagina in the female.

Membranous Part. This is the narrowest, shortest (1 cm.), and least dilatable part of the urethra. It pierces the superior and inferior fasciae of the urogenital diaphragm (which membranes give it its name) with the voluntary **sphincter urethrae** between. Immediately below the inferior fascia of the urogenital diaphragm (perineal membrane), the urethra inclines forwards and its posterior wall enters the bulb of the penis, but its anterior wall remains uncovered for a short distance. It is this part which is particularly liable to rupture if an attempt is made to pass a bougie into the membranous part before the point has reached the correct position.

Spongy Part. This is the longest part (16 cm.) of the urethra. It begins on the upper surface of the bulb of the penis, and extending downwards into it, forms the **intrabulbar fossa** [Figs. 195, 219], and then passes longitudinally through the centre of the corpus spongiosum. In the glans penis the urethra expands dorsoventrally to form the slit-like **fossa navicularis** which may be bounded posteriorly by a fold of mucous membrane in its roof. This forms a recess

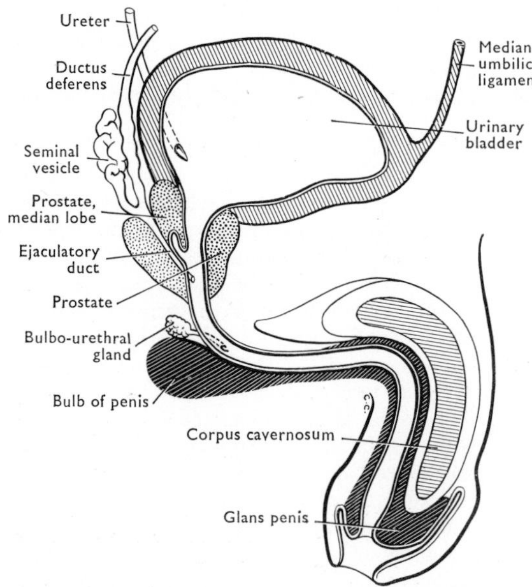

Fig. 218 A diagram of the bladder, urethra, and penis.

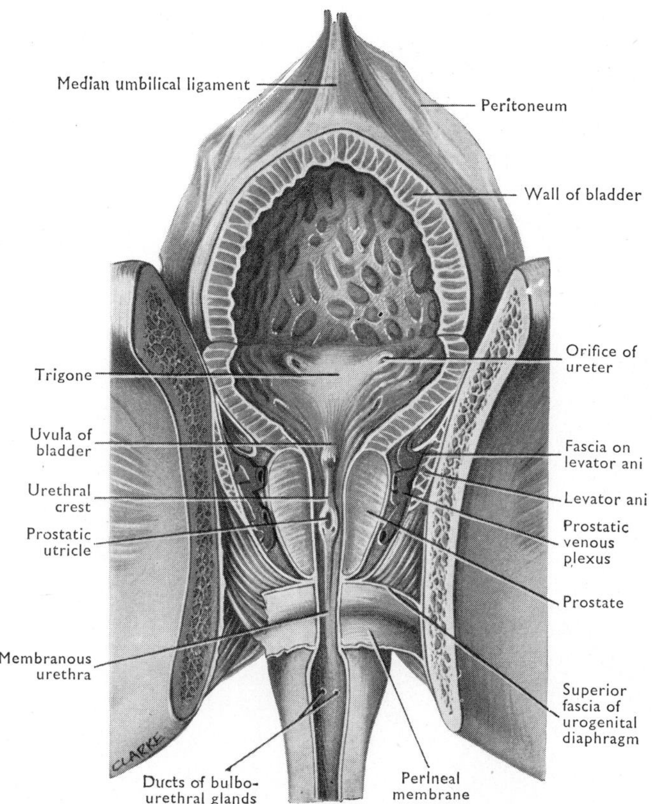

FIG. 219 A dissection of the urinary bladder and urethra from the front in the male. The contents of the deep perineal space have been removed except for the membranous urethra.

in which the tip of a catheter or bougie may catch [FIG. 107].

Vessels and Nerves. The urethra shares in the nerve, blood, and lymphatic supply of the prostate, urogenital diaphragm, and penis. Thus most of the lymph drains to the internal iliac lymph nodes, but some passes to the deep inguinal nodes (distal spongy part).

FEMALE URETHRA
[FIGS. 206, 209, 222]

In over-all length the female urethra is much shorter (4 cm.) than the male urethra, but is equal in length to its membranous and prostatic parts. It is also wider, more dilatable, and lined by stratified epithelium, squamous and columnar, becoming transitional epithelium in its uppermost part.

The mucous membrane contains **mucous glands** and is pitted by small **urethral lacunae** which face inferiorly. There are a number of small mucous **glands** (supposed to be homologous with the prostate in the male) on each side of the urethra, and these open at the margin of its external orifice by **para-urethral ducts.** There is a considerable layer of smooth muscle which is continuous superiorly with the muscle of the bladder. The female urethra is closely applied to the anterior vaginal wall, particularly in its inferior part, and may be bruised against the pubis in childbirth.

The female urethra is S-shaped when seen from the side. The superior part, corresponding to the prostatic urethra in position, is convex anteriorly, and is held by the **pubo-urethral** part of the **pubovesical ligament.** The inferior part curves forwards below the pubic symphysis, and is held in position by an **anterior pubo-urethral ligament** [p. 238].

Vessels. The blood supply is from the vaginal and internal pudendal vessels. The lymph vessels pass to the sacral and internal iliac nodes; a few from the inferior part pass to the inguinal nodes with the other lymphatics of the vestibule.

DISSECTION. Lift the divided uterus and confirm that the body is covered with peritoneum on its superior and inferior aspects, and is, therefore, freely mobile. Compare this with the fixity of the cervix, which is only covered with peritoneum on the posterosuperior surface

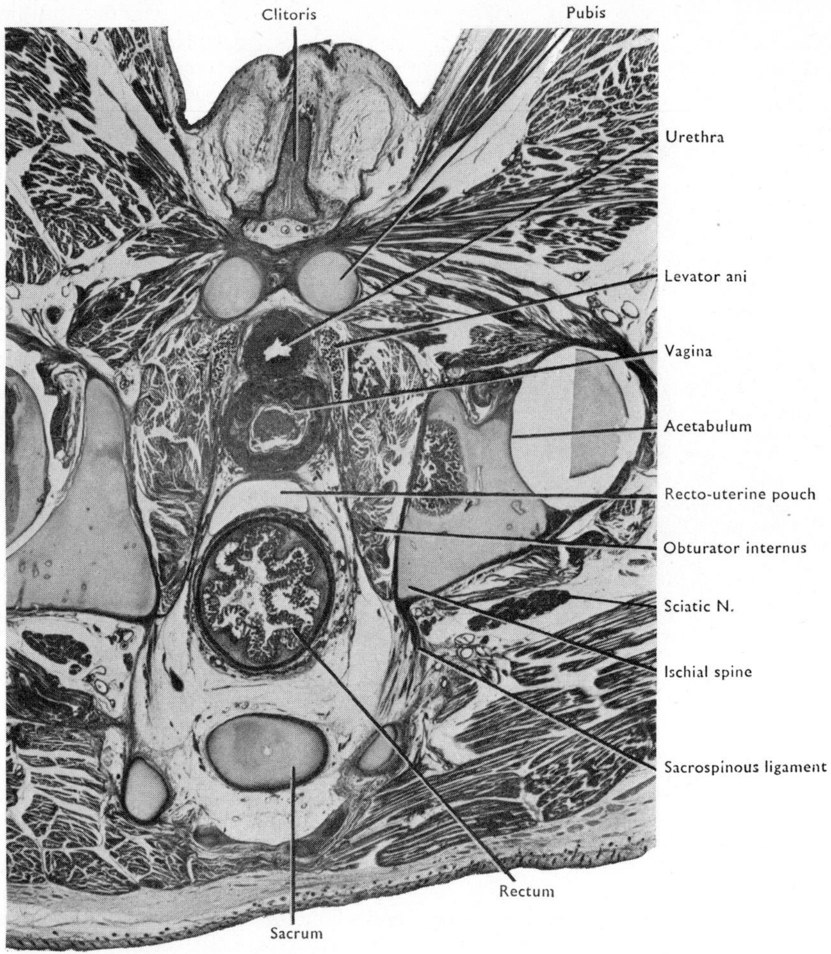

FIG. 220 A horizontal section through the lesser pelvis of a seven-month female human foetus.

of that part of it which lies outside the vagina (supravaginal part), and which is attached to the lateral pelvic wall by the thick base of the broad ligament and to the sacrum by its most posterior part, the uterosacral ligament. Examine the part of the cervix which projects into the vagina through the upper part of its anterior wall, and note that the cervix is surrounded on all sides by a narrow, slit-like part of the vaginal cavity, the fornices of the vagina.

If there is no fat in the broad ligament, transilluminate its thin superior part and attempt to see the remnants of the mesonephric tubules and duct (the epoophoron, Fig. 221) of the embryo. They are only rarely visible between the ovary and uterine tube, and they correspond to the efferent ductules of the testis and the epididymis in the male.

Note the position and examine the interior of the vagina. Compare the laxity of the tissue that separates it from the rectum with the dense tissue that binds it to the bladder and urethra. Confirm the attachment of the bladder and urethra to the pubis by the pubovesical ligaments.

UTERUS

[Figs. 206, 221–223]

This is a thick-walled, firm, muscular organ. It is lined with a mucous membrane (**endometrium**) that limits the narrow lumen and is firmly bound to the muscle (**myometrium**). The **endometrium** contains simple tubular glands that reach into the innermost layers of the muscle, and in the body of the uterus it undergoes cyclical changes induced by the changing ovarian hormones. The breakdown of all but the outermost layer of the endometrium produces the menstrual flow at the end of each cycle.

The uterus is 7–8 cm. long, and nearly half of the neck or **cervix** is inserted into the vagina through the uppermost part of its anterior wall. The **cervix** is approximately cylindrical, and has a diameter and length of 2·5 cm. The remainder of the uterus (the **body**) tapers from its widest part (the **fundus,** which is 5 cm. wide and 2·5 cm. thick) in the free edge of the broad ligament, to join the cervix at a slight constriction (the **isthmus**) which is only obvious prior to the first pregnancy. The uterine tubes pass laterally from the sides of the fundus (which usually lies slightly to the right of the median plane), and the ligaments of the ovaries and the round ligaments of the uterus are attached to the uterus respectively superior and inferior to the junction of uterus and tubes.

The uterus overlies the posterior part of the superior surface and the upper part of the base of the bladder. Thus when the bladder is empty, the uterus is tilted forwards at right angles to the vagina and to the pelvic brim [Fig. 222], and is therefore said to be *anteverted.* Also the body is slightly flexed at the isthmus on the firmer, more fibrous cervix [Fig. 209], and this curve is known as the *anteflexion* of the uterus. The body of the uterus, enclosed between the layers of the broad ligament, is freely mobile. Thus as the bladder fills, the uterus is raised, and may be forced back until it lies in line with the vagina when the bladder is fully distended: it is then said to be *retroverted.* In certain pathological conditions, the uterus may be permanently retroverted, and even extended on itself at the isthmus; a condition known as *retroflexion.*

Cervix

Nearly half of the cervix (the **vaginal part**) lies within the uppermost part of the vagina. This part is covered on its external surface by the mucous stratified squamous epithelium of the vagina. This epithelium is continuous with the simple columnar lining of the uterus just within the centrally placed **ostium uteri,** and peripherally, curves off the cervix on to the vaginal wall, thus surrounding an arch-like part of the vaginal cavity (the **fornix of the vagina**) which encircles the cervix. For descriptive purposes, the fornix is artificially divided into **anterior, posterior,** and right and

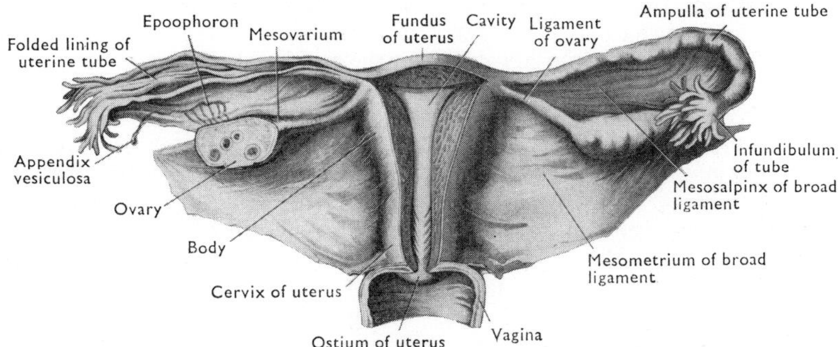

Fig. 221 The posterosuperior surface of the broad ligament and associated structures. The vagina, uterus, and left uterine tube have been opened, and the left ovary is sectioned parallel to the broad ligament.

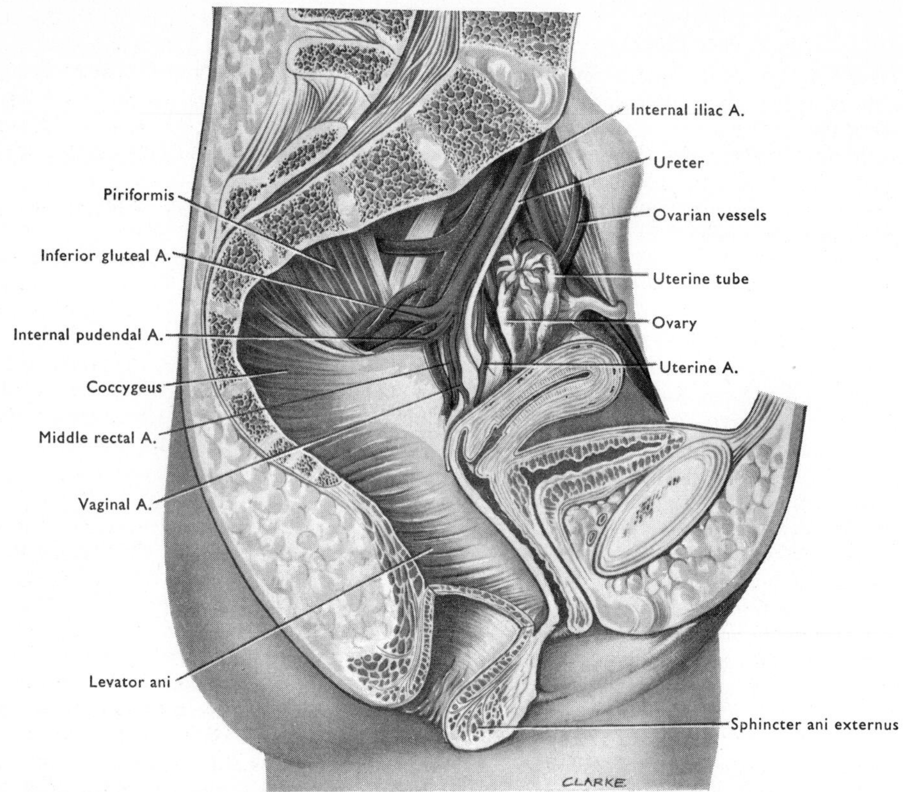

FIG. 222 A dissection of the structures in the left half of a female pelvis. The greater part of the rectum has been removed.

left **lateral fornices;** the anterior fornix being shallow because the cervix is inserted through the anterior vaginal wall [FIG. 222].

The posterosuperior surface of the supravaginal part of the cervix and the adjacent posterior vaginal fornix are the only parts of these structures covered with peritoneum. The antero-inferior surface of the cervix is directly in contact with the upper part of the base of the bladder [FIG. 222].

The **canal of the cervix** is spindle shaped. It is continuous superiorly with the cavity of the body of the uterus without any demarcation, except in the pregnant uterus where the cervix remains small and is not dilated until parturition. In the later stages of pregnancy the isthmus becomes the lower uterine segment. Inferiorly the canal of the cervix opens into the vagina through the **ostium uteri,** a narrow transverse slit with small anterior and large posterior lips. In nullipara, the endometrium of the cervix is thrown into folds arranged like the fronds of a palm leaf **(plicae palmatae).** It contains numerous tubular, branched glands, the ducts of which may be occluded so that the glands become distended with secretions and give rise to cysts in the cervix (Nabothian follicles). The endometrium of the cervix plays no part in the changes of menstruation.

The cervix, unlike the body of the uterus, is held in position by a number of structures which are principally condensations of fascia and some smooth muscle in the base of the broad ligament. The main mass surrounds the uterine artery (**transverse ligament of the cervix**), and passes from the cervix and lateral fornix on each side to the corresponding lateral wall of the pelvis. A similar condensation of connective tissue in each recto-uterine fold forms the **uterosacral ligament.** Thus the cervix tends to remain in position while the body of the uterus expands in pregnancy.

Body of Uterus

The **vesical surface** of the uterus is nearly flat. It is separated from the bladder by the **uterovesical pouch** of peritoneum which is empty unless the uterus is retroverted when a coil of intestine may lie in it. The pouch extends to the junction of the body and cervix where the peritoneum is reflected on to the posterior margin of the upper surface of the bladder.

The convex superior or **intestinal surface** of the uterus is covered with peritoneum which extends posteriorly over the supravaginal part of the cervix and the posterior fornix of the vagina. It is separated from the rectum by the **recto-uterine pouch** which contains loops of ileum and sigmoid colon.

The lateral surfaces of the uterus have the **broad ligament (parametrium)** attached to them, with the uterine vessels passing parallel to them between its layers.

The **cavity** of the body is a mere slit between the intestinal and vesical walls, but is triangular in outline. The uterine tubes enter it at the angles in the fundus, and the posterior angle is continuous with the cervical canal.

Vessels of Uterus. These are the uterine arteries and veins which enter the broad ligament beside the lateral fornices of the vagina, superior to the ureters [FIG. 223]. They pass along the lateral surfaces of the uterus, and turn laterally in the broad ligament to anastomose with the ovarian arteries. The large branches pass into the muscle of the uterus, and running within it, send smaller vessels into the endometrium to give a separate supply to the deepest and more superficial parts of that mucous lining. The arteries supplying the superficial layers of the endometrium (which are involved in menstruation) are **coiled arteries.** The presence of the large vessels within the muscle wall of the uterus ensures closure of these vessels when the uterus contracts at parturition. Thus when the placenta is discharged it leaves a large raw area from which severe haemorrhage can occur if the contraction is not maintained.

The **lymph vessels** pass by a number of routes [FIG. 228]: (1) from the cervix, fundus, and body they pass laterally through the broad ligament (occasionally interrupted by small para-uterine nodes in the broad ligament) to the external iliac nodes; (2) from the fundus they pass with the ovarian lymph vessels to the lumbar nodes and along the round ligament of the uterus to the superficial inguinal nodes; and (3) from the cervix to the internal iliac and sacral nodes.

The **nerves** of the uterus come from the inferior hypogastric plexus, many of the postganglionic parasympathetic nerve fibres arising in large pelvic ganglia close to the cervix.

VAGINA

[FIGS. 209, 222, 223]

This tube extends antero-inferiorly from its posterior fornix to pass between the medial borders of the two levator ani muscles. It then pierces the superior and inferior fasciae of the urogenital diaphragm with the sphincter urethrae between them, and opens into the vestibule between the labia minora. The anterior wall is 7·5 cm. long, while the posterior wall, which reaches the posterior fornix, is 9 cm. long. The anterior and posterior walls are in contact except where the vaginal part of the cervix intervenes and the cavity is slightly larger.

The **anterior wall** is in contact with the base of the bladder and the terminal parts of the ureters, and is tightly bound to the neck of the bladder and to the urethra, and thus to the pubis through the pubovesical ligaments.

The **posterior fornix** is covered with peritoneum, and injuries to this part of the vagina may involve the peritoneal cavity. Below this, loose areolar tissue separates the **posterior wall** from the lowest part of the rectum; a feature which allows the vaginal wall to separate from

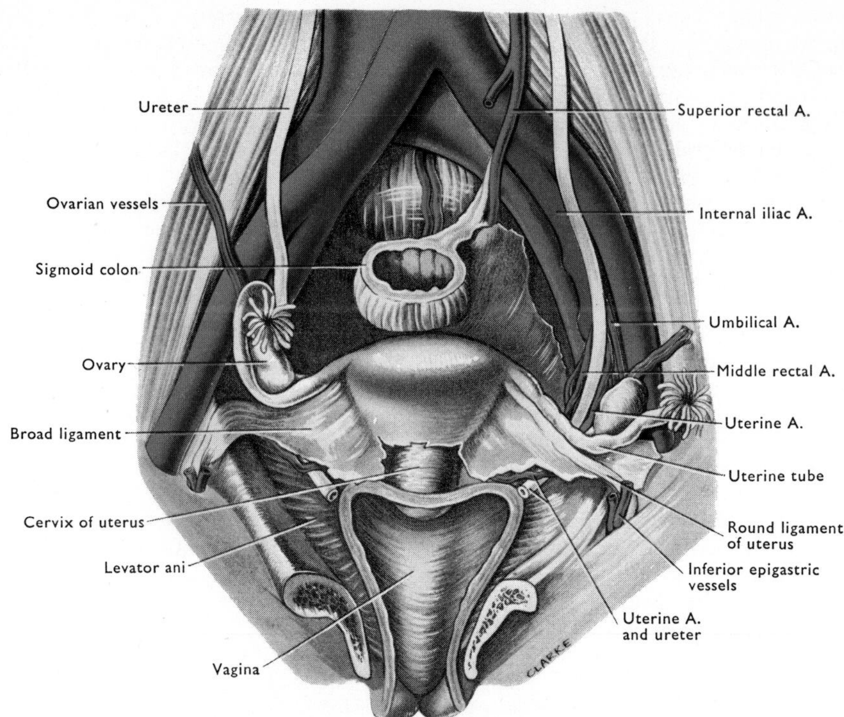

FIG. 223 A dissection of the female pelvis from the front. The uterus has been displaced backwards, and the bladder, urethra, and anterior wall of the vagina removed.

the rectum and protrude through the vaginal orifice when the cervix descends from its normal position in prolapse of the uterus. This can only occur when the **central perineal tendon,** which supports the lowest part of the posterior wall, is weakened or torn, and the cervical ligaments are stretched, as may happen in childbirth.

In the region of the lateral fornices, the **lateral walls** give attachment to the base of the broad ligament which here contains the uterine vessels and ureters. Pulsations of the uterine arteries may be felt through the lateral fornices in the living. Inferiorly the lateral walls are in contact with the levator ani and sphincter urethrae muscles, and the greater vestibular glands and the bulb of the vestibule inferior to the perineal membrane.

Vessels of Vagina. The vaginal artery supplies it on each side, and is supplemented by twigs from the uterine, middle rectal, and arteries of the bulbs of the vestibule. The veins form submucous and adventitial plexuses. The former are so thin walled and numerous as to resemble erectile tissue, and are liable to be distended and varicose. The veins drain along the arteries.

The **lymph vessels** of the upper part drain with the uterine vessels to the external and internal iliac nodes. The middle part drains with the vaginal blood vessels to the internal iliac nodes. The inferior part drains either to the sacral and common iliac nodes, or with the vessels of the vulva to the superficial inguinal nodes [FIG. 228].

Structure. This highly distensible tube is lined with mucous stratified squamous epithelium, with an elastic areolar submucous layer that contains many veins, a few lymphatic follicles, but no glands. The muscle layer contains bundles of longitudinal and circular smooth muscle, but without definite layers. At the margin of the orifice of the vagina, the mucous membrane may extend inwards in the form of a circular fold, the **hymen.** Rarely this may be a complete membrane which prevents the discharge of the menstrual flow after puberty. More usually an incomplete ring, the hymen is torn at childbirth, and remains as the **caruncluae hymenales** [p. 211].

DISSECTION. Confirm the relation of the peritoneum to the upper two thirds of the rectum [p. 206]. Examine the mucous membrane of the rectum. Identify its transverse folds, and then strip some of it from the upper part of the rectum. Note the relative laxity of the submucosa (less obvious in fixed than in fresh tissue), and look for evidence of the submucous venous plexus. Clean part of the circular muscle layer.

Find the superior rectal artery. Trace it on to the posterior surface of the upper part of the rectum, and follow its branches downwards on the posterolateral surfaces of the rectum to its lower part [Fig. 225]. Strip the remainder of the peritoneum and fascia from the external surface of the rectum, and identify the outer, longitudinal layer of muscle.

RECTUM

[FIGS. 207–209, 224, 225]

The rectum begins as the continuation of the sigmoid colon on the pelvic surface of the third piece of the sacrum. It is approximately 12 cm. long, and first follows the curve of the sacrum and coccyx. It then runs antero-inferiorly to the central perineal tendon, lying above the anococcygeal ligament in the groove between the parts of the levator ani muscles passing to the anococcygeal ligament. It ends by turning postero-inferiorly as the **anal canal,** 2–3 cm. beyond the tip of the coccyx, and

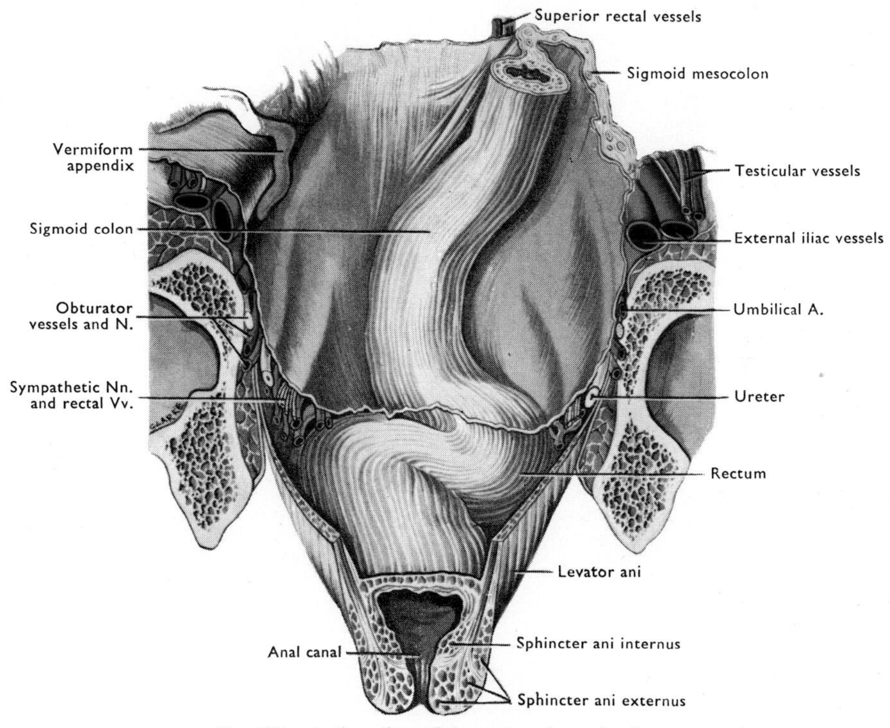

FIG. 224 A dissection of the rectum from the front.

immediately posterior to the **central perineal tendon** and to the apex of the prostate in the male. The lower part, frequently more distended than the remainder, is known as the **ampulla.**

In spite of its name, the rectum is not straight, but follows the curve of the sacrum and coccyx in the sagittal plane [FIG. 195]. In the coronal plane [FIG. 224] it follows a triple sinuous curve, the angularity of which increases inferiorly.

Peritoneum covers the front and sides of the upper third of the rectum, and gradually passing forwards, turns off the front of the rectum, at the junction of its middle and lower thirds, on to the back of the bladder (male) or the posterior fornix of the vagina (female), to form the floor of the **rectovesical** or **recto-uterine pouch.** Thus the upper two-thirds of the rectum are in contact anteriorly with coils of the pelvic colon and ileum. The lower third is *either* separated from the base of the bladder by the seminal vesicles and deferent ducts and from the prostate by the rectovesical septum *in the male*, *or* from the vagina by loose areolar tissue *in the female*.

The **recto-urethralis muscle** consists of some weak bundles of longitudinal rectal muscle which pass forwards to the apex of the prostate and the adjacent urethra *in the male*, or to the back of the vagina *in the female* [FIG. 217].

Posterolaterally, the branches of the superior rectal artery lie on the wall of the rectum, which

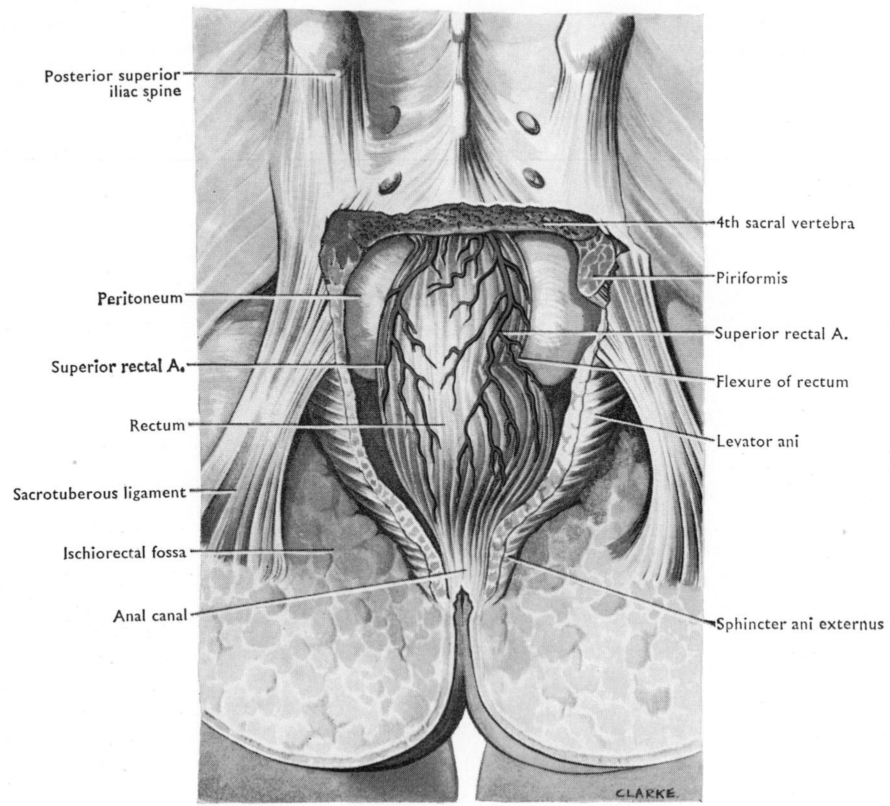

FIG. 225 A dissection of the rectum from behind.

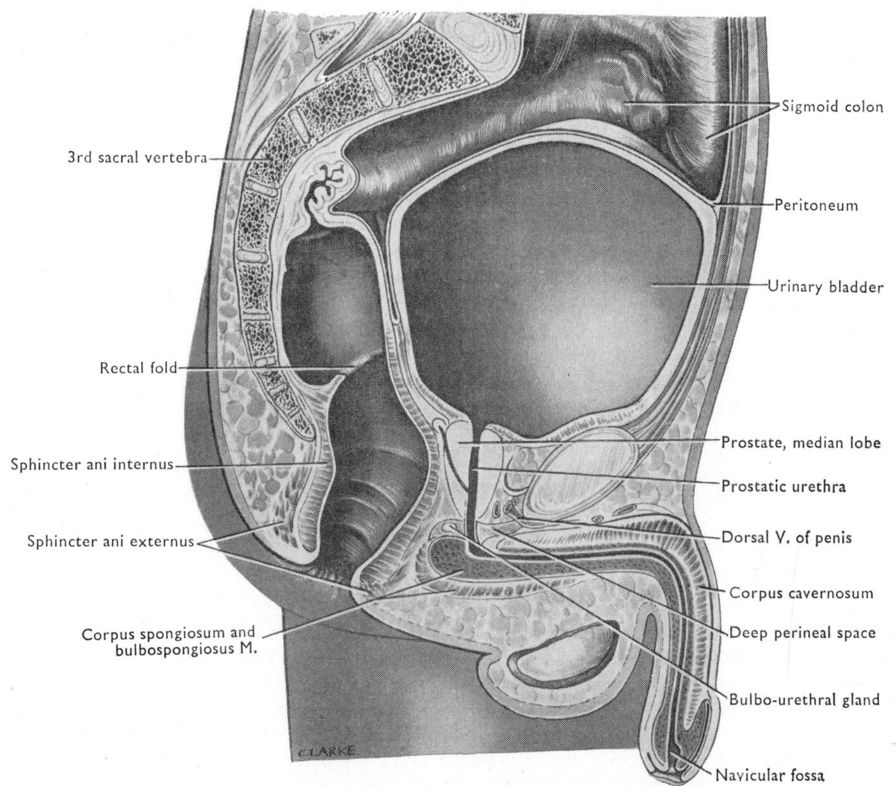

FIG. 226 A section through the male pelvis. The urinary bladder and rectum are distended. Note that the peritoneum is removed from the lower part of the anterior abdominal wall by the distended bladder.

is applied in the median plane to the sacrum, coccyx, and anococcygeal ligament, and on each side to the muscles attached to these (piriformis, coccygeus, and levator ani). Between these structures and the layer of pelvic fascia which separates them from the rectum, are the median sacral vessels, a sympathetic trunk on each side, and the ganglion impar on the coccyx, and lateral to these, the lateral sacral vessels and the lower sacral and coccygeal nerves.

Laterally, the rectum is in contact with the peritoneum superiorly, and inferiorly with the fat and fascia over coccygeus and the levator ani muscles. Some of this fascia is condensed around the middle rectal artery and attached to the fascial sheath of the rectum, thus helping to hold the rectum in position.

Rectal and Vaginal Examinations

In the male, a finger in the rectum may be used to palpate the posterior surface of the prostate, or the seminal vesicles and terminal parts of the deferent ducts superior to the prostate. *In the female*, the firm cervix may also be palpated through the rectal and vaginal walls, and it is possible to examine the cervix and body of the uterus by bimanual palpation with two fingers in the vagina and a hand on the anterior abdominal wall. This method also allows palpation of the ovaries through the lateral fornices, particularly when they are enlarged by any pathological process.

DISSECTION. Examine the lining of the anal canal. Identify, if possible, the junction between the mucous membrane and skin, which is usually below the middle of the canal. The mucous membrane is thrown into a number of vertical folds (anal columns) which are united inferiorly by small, horizontal, semilunar folds (anal valves). These enclose small pockets of the mucous membrane (anal sinuses), and all are covered with columnar epithelium. Inferior to this the epithelium becomes transitional in type, and joins the skin at a bluish-white line.

When these structures have been identified, strip the mucous membrane and skin from a sector of the anal canal. Identify the internal anal sphincter, and note that the anal valves lie approximately opposite the middle of that structure. Follow the circular muscle of the sphincter superiorly into continuity with the corresponding layer in the rectum.

ANAL CANAL

This terminal part of the large intestine is approximately 4 cm. long. It descends postero-inferiorly between the levator ani muscles and through the internal and external sphincters of the anus, to end at the anus.

The **internal sphincter** consists of a thickening of the circular smooth muscle of the intestine, and it surrounds the upper two-thirds of the anal canal. The **external sphincter** [p. 215] surrounds the lower two-thirds of the anal canal. It thus overlaps the internal sphincter and the fibres of **levator ani** which pass to the wall of the anal canal between them. Of the latter, the **puborectales** (see below) sweep round the sides and posterior aspect of the anorectal junction, and pulling this anteriorly, increase the angle between the rectum and anal canal and act as a sphincter. Some of the more **vertical fibres** of the levator ani muscles pass in to join the longitudinal muscle of the intestine and run with it through the bundles of the external sphincter to the perineal skin, thus anchoring the longitudinal muscle and levator ani inferiorly. Longitudinal muscle bundles of the rectum pass forwards into the central perineal tendon, and help to maintain the ano-rectal flexure [FIG. 217].

The anal canal lies between the anococcygeal ligament and the central perineal tendon in the median plane. Laterally it is in contact with the levator ani muscles and the ischiorectal fat inferior to that.

Structure of Rectum and Anal Canal

The **rectum** is surrounded by a fascial layer and separated from the sacrum and coccyx by a layer of pelvic fascia. The smooth **muscle** layers are of outer longitudinal and inner circular fibres. The longitudinal layer is of more uniform thickness than in the colon, for the taeniae coli thicken and spread out as they reach the rectum to form a continuous layer which is especially thickened anteriorly and posteriorly. These longitudinal thickenings tend to maintain the flexures of the rectum.

The **submucous layer** is formed of loose areolar tissue which allows the mucous membrane to slide freely on the muscle. It contains an extensive plexus of veins which link the superior (inferior mesenteric) and inferior (internal pudendal) rectal veins. When distended, this plexus forms haemorrhoids (piles).

The **mucous layer** is thick. It consists of numerous simple tubular glands which extend into a connective tissue layer rich in lymphocytes and plasma cells, and the simple columnar epithelium contains large numbers of goblet cells. In the ampulla, some **deep glands** extend into the submucosa, and some may penetrate the muscle. The mucosa is so loosely connected to the muscle layer that it may prolapse through the anus with the dilated submucous veins. The mucosa is raised into three **transverse folds,** one opposite the concavity of each rectal flexure, and these folds include the mucous, submucous, and some of the muscle layers of the rectal wall. The right fold is the largest and lies at the level of the floor of the rectovesical (or recto-uterine) pouch, the other two are approximately 4 cm. above and below it.

The **anal canal** has the same layers as the rectum in its upper two-thirds, but the lower third is lined by skin. It is surrounded by the sphincter layers described above. The mucous layer forms a series of longitudinal ridges

(anal columns) which are united to each other inferiorly by small, horizontal, semilunar folds **(anal valves)** near the mucocutaneous junction, thus forming a series of small pockets (**anal sinuses**) each at the inferior end of a groove between two ridges. The anal valves are liable to be torn by the passage of a hard mass of faeces, and this may allow infection to spread into the wall of the anal canal (fissure *in ano*).

The anal valves lie at the level formerly occupied by the anal part of the cloacal membrane. In the embryo this temporarily closes the anal end of the alimentary canal, and if it persists, leads to the condition known as imperforate anus.

Vessels

There are five **rectal arteries:** one superior rectal (from the inferior mesenteric); two middle rectal (from the internal iliac); two inferior rectal (from the internal pudendal in the ischiorectal fossa). The **veins** form submucous and adventitial plexuses, and drain along the arteries to the internal iliac and portal veins.

Lymph vessels [FIG. 228] drain by a number of routes: (1) From the lower part of the anal canal and surrounding perineal skin they run forwards to the medial **superficial inguinal lymph nodes.** (2) From the upper part of the anal canal, lymph vessels either drain across the ischiorectal fossa to the internal pudendal vessels, or ascend with vessels from the lower part of the rectum to the **internal iliac nodes.** (3) Other rectal lymph vessels pass to the **sacral** and **common iliac lymph nodes.** (4) Some ascend with the inferior mesenteric vessels to the inferior mesenteric and **lumbar nodes.**

THE VESSELS OF THE LESSER PELVIS

DISSECTION. Clean the internal iliac vessels and their branches and tributaries [Figs. 222, 227]. Pull the pelvic viscera away from the pelvic walls so as to follow the vessels to the viscera. If necessary remove the veins to get a clear exposure of the arteries. Note any parts of the hypogastric plexus and the lymph nodes that are exposed as the vessels are cleaned.

Superior Rectal Artery. This is the continuation of the inferior mesenteric artery. It begins on the middle of the left common iliac artery, and descending in the medial limb of the sigmoid mesocolon, divides into two branches on the third piece of the sacrum. These branches descend first on the back and then on the sides of the rectum. They divide into circumferential branches which pierce the muscle layers near the middle of the rectum, and descend in the submucosa to the anal canal where they anastomose with the branches of the inferior rectal artery.

The **superior rectal vein** accompanies the artery to become the inferior mesenteric vein. It drains the rectal venous plexuses directly, but may also drain other visceral pelvic plexuses which anastomose with the rectal plexuses (see below).

INTERNAL ILIAC ARTERY
[FIGS. 222, 227]

In the adult this is the smaller of the two branches of the common iliac artery, though it is the larger in the foetus when it transmits blood to the placenta through the **umbilical artery.** At birth the umbilical arteries are tied, and rapidly degenerate into a fibrous cord to the level of their last persistent branch, the superior vesical artery.

The internal iliac artery supplies the contents of the lesser pelvis (except those parts supplied by the superior rectal, ovarian, and median sacral arteries), the perineum, the greater part of the gluteal region, and the iliac fossa. The arrangement of its branches, particularly the visceral branches, is subject to wide variation.

The artery begins medial to psoas major and anterior to the sacro-iliac joint, at the level of the lumbosacral disc. It passes posteriorly into the lesser pelvis over the medial aspect of the external iliac vein, the brim and upper part of the lateral wall of the lesser pelvis and the obturator nerve. The artery is immediately lateral to the pelvic peritoneum, and lies between the ureter inferiorly and the internal iliac vein superiorly.

Posterior Branches

1. The **superior gluteal artery** is the direct continuation of the artery. It pierces the pelvic fascia, and passing between the lumbosacral trunk and the ventral ramus of the first sacral nerve, leaves the lesser pelvis through the uppermost part of the greater sciatic foramen, above piriformis, in company with the corresponding vein and the superior gluteal nerve.

2. The **iliolumbar artery** ascends deep to psoas where it divides into iliac and lumbar branches. The **iliac branch** passes laterally and appears on the abdominal surface of iliacus. The lumbar branch ascends posterior to psoas, supplies quadratus lumborum, and may form the fifth lumbar artery. The corresponding **vein** does not enter the pelvis, but joins the common iliac vein.

3. The **lateral sacral arteries** (two in number on each side) pass medially and descend in front of the sacral ventral rami. Each artery divides into two, one of which passes through each pelvic sacral foramen to supply the structures in the sacral canal [p. 202] and continue through the corresponding dorsal sacral foramen to supply the overlying muscles and skin.

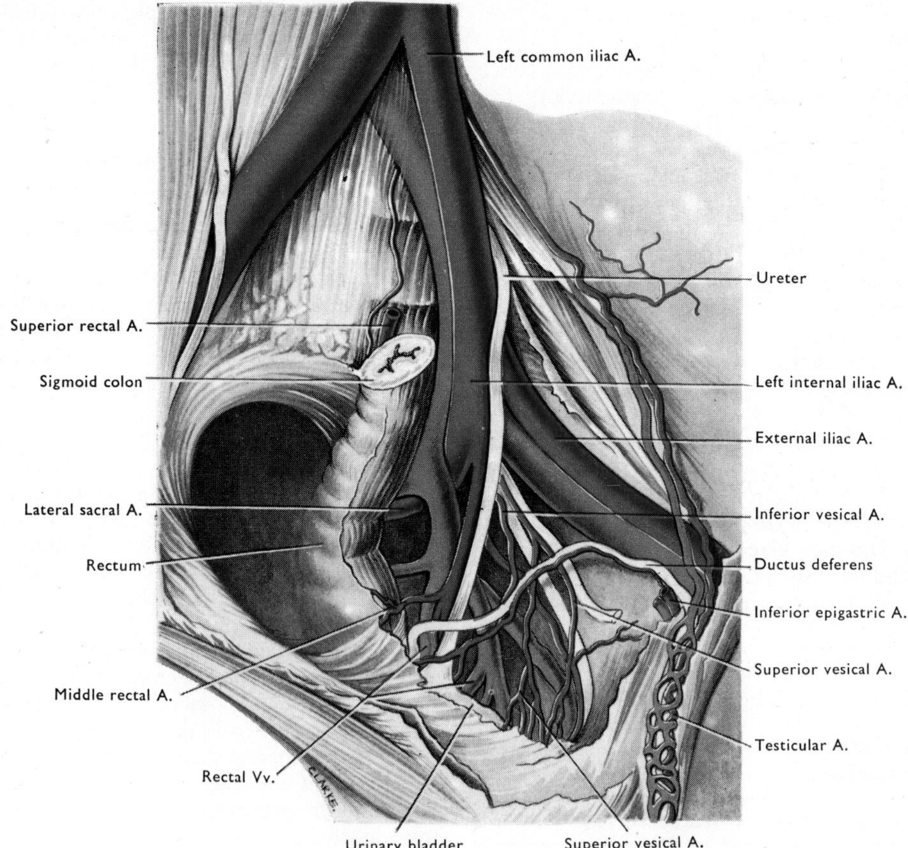

FIG. 227 The structures on the lateral wall of the male pelvis. These are exposed by retracting the bladder and rectum and removing the peritoneum and extraperitoneal fat.

Anterior Branches

These are usually divided into visceral and parietal branches, but are listed here in the order in which they frequently arise.

1. The **umbilical artery** runs antero-inferiorly between the side of the bladder and the lateral wall of the pelvis, giving two or three **superior vesical** branches to the bladder. It then loses its lumen, and leaving the anterior part of the pelvis, passes superomedially through the extraperitoneal tissue of the anterior abdominal wall to the umbilicus as the **lateral umbilical ligament.** The **umbilical vein** does not run with the artery, but passes directly to the liver from the umbilical cord in the foetus, and persists as the ligamentum teres after birth.

2. The **obturator artery** arises close to the umbilical. It passes with the obturator nerve and vein to the obturator canal, through which it escapes into the adductor compartment of the thigh. It gives some small branches to the surrounding structures. One of these, the **pubic branch,** passes on to the pelvic surface of the pubis to anastomose with the pubic branch of the inferior epigastric artery [p. 111]. This anastomosis may supply part or all of the obturator artery (**accessory obturator artery**), and may or may not be accompanied by an abnormal obturator vein.

3. The **inferior vesical artery** is only found in the male. It runs forwards to the base of the bladder where it supplies the seminal vesicle, prostate, postero-inferior part of the bladder, and the ductus deferens through a long, slender branch which runs on that structure to the testis. The latter is variable in its origin and may arise from the superior vesical or umbilical arteries.

3a. The **vaginal artery** in the female corresponds to the inferior vesical artery in the male. The vaginal artery passes forwards to supply the vagina, the postero-inferior parts of the bladder, and the pelvic part of the urethra.

4. The **uterine artery** [FIG. 223] is either separate or may arise with the vaginal, umbilical, or middle rectal arteries. It passes along the root of the broad ligament, and crossing medially above the ureter at the side of the lateral vaginal fornix, runs tortuously along the lateral margin of the uterus between the layers of the broad ligament. It supplies the superior part of the vagina, the uterus, and part of the uterine tube, and it ends by anastomosing with the corresponding ovarian artery in the broad ligament.

In its course to the side of the cervix, the uterine artery lies in the condensed connective tissue which helps to hold the cervix in position by attaching it to the lateral pelvic wall.

5. The **middle rectal artery** is a small branch which passes medially to the rectum. It supplies branches to the rectum and to the vagina or seminal vesicle and prostate. It is surrounded by a condensation of connective tissue which helps to hold the rectum in position.

6. The **internal pudendal artery** descends anterior to the piriformis and the nerves of the sacral plexus, and piercing the pelvic fascia, leaves the pelvis through the inferior part of the greater sciatic foramen, between piriformis and coccygeus. It then crosses the gluteal aspect of the ischial spine, and entering the lesser sciatic foramen, is distributed to the perineum [p. 222].

7. The **inferior gluteal artery** pierces the pelvic fascia, and passing between the ventral rami of the first and second sacral nerves, emerges into the gluteal region inferior to piriformis and either medial or posterior to the sciatic nerve. It has no branches of consequence in the pelvis.

Pelvic Hernia. The branches of the internal iliac artery that leave the pelvis pierce the pelvic fascia, and these may be sites for pelvic herniae. Such herniae can therefore occur along the superior gluteal, inferior gluteal, or obturator arteries.

The Median Sacral Artery. This small vessel, originally the caudal part of the aorta, arises from the posterior surface of the aorta immediately above the bifurcation. It descends in the median plane, on the vertebral column, to the coccyx where it ends in a cellular body, the **glomus coccygeum.** It gives off: (1) the fifth lumbar arteries; (2) small branches to the back of the rectum; and (3) anastomotic twigs to the lateral sacral arteries.

VEINS OF PELVIS
[FIGS. 222, 227]

The venous drainage of the pelvis is through the internal iliac veins, except for the blood which passes by the superior rectal, median sacral, and ovarian veins, and the veins which pass through the pelvic sacral foramina to communicate with the internal vertebral venous plexus in the vertebral canal.

The **internal iliac vein** lies superior to the artery and receives veins that correspond to branches of the artery, except for the umbilical which goes to the liver and the iliolumbar which drains into the common iliac. The largest tributary is the superior gluteal vein.

Pelvic Venous Plexuses

The veins of the pelvis form a number of complicated intercommunicating plexuses. These are extremely difficult to dissect, but are of considerable importance.

The **rectal venous plexuses** lie on the surface of the rectum and in its submucosa. They drain by way of the superior, middle, and inferior rectal veins, and hence form a route of communication between the portal and systemic venous systems. Thus blockage of the portal vein leads to distension of this plexus, though this most commonly occurs without portal obstruction. When distended to form haemorrhoids, the submucous plexus may even cause prolapse of the rectal mucosa through the anus. Since the rectal plexuses communicate with the other pelvic plexuses, distension of these plexuses (see below) may also occur in portal obstruction, but is most obvious in association with the increased blood flow through the pelvis which occurs in pregnancy, and to a much lesser degree, at menstruation.

The **vesical venous plexus,** *in the male*, is principally found on the base of the bladder around the seminal vesicles, deferent ducts, and the ends of the ureters. It drains through the inferior vesical veins to the internal iliac veins, and also along the rectovesical fold to the anterior surface of the sacrum. Thence it may drain either through the pelvic sacral foramina to the internal vertebral venous plexus with some tributaries from the rectum, or through the lateral sacral veins to the internal iliac vein. The size of the **internal vertebral venous plexus** is such that it can form an alternative route for all the blood in the inferior vena cava when this vein is obstructed.

The **prostatic venous plexus** lies on the front and sides of the prostate within its fascial sheath. It receives the dorsal vein of the penis, and drains into the vesical venous plexus.

In the female, the vesical venous plexus surrounds the pelvic part of the urethra and the neck of the bladder. It receives the dorsal vein of the clitoris, and drains into the **vaginal plexuses.** These lie on the sides of the vagina and in its submucosa. They communicate with the rectal and uterine plexuses, and drain mainly through the vaginal veins.

The **uterine plexuses** lie principally at the sides of the uterus between the layers of the broad ligament. They drain into the uterine veins that pass along the uterine arteries, but they also communicate through the broad ligament with the pampiniform plexus, and thus drain partly with the ovarian veins.

LYMPH NODES AND VESSELS OF PELVIS
[FIGS. 176, 228]

These are numerous and difficult to demonstrate.

The **external iliac nodes** [p. 190] not only drain lymph from the lower limb and abdomen, but also receive direct vessels from the bladder, prostate, and uterus.

The **internal iliac nodes** lie along the artery and its branches. They receive lymph from all the pelvic contents, from the perineum (internal pudendal), from the deeper parts of the gluteal region (superior and inferior gluteal vessels) and from the back of the thigh. Like the external iliac nodes, they drain to the common iliac nodes.

The **sacral nodes** lie along the median and lateral sacral arteries. They drain the dorsal wall of the pelvis, and also the rectum, neck of

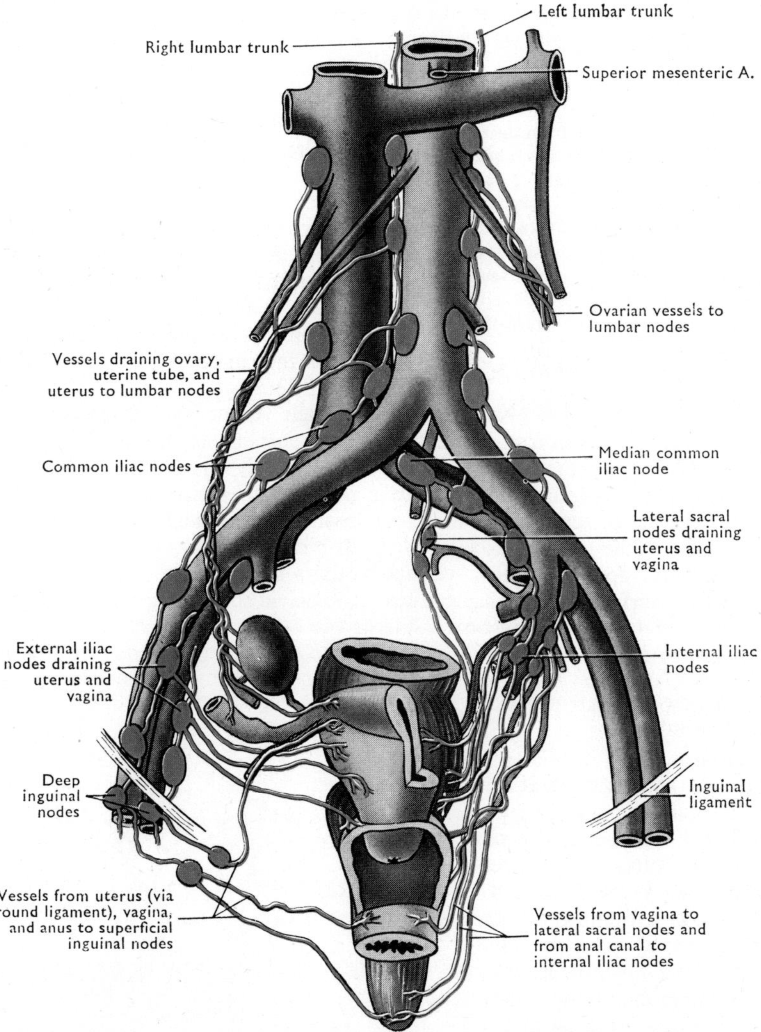

FIG. 228 A diagram of the lymph vessels and nodes of the female pelvis and abdomen.

the bladder and prostate, or cervix of the uterus. They drain to the common iliac nodes.

In addition to these groups, small, intermediate nodes lie in the broad ligament and in the fascial sheaths of the bladder and rectum.

DISSECTION. Find the sympathetic trunk as it enters the pelvis, and trace it to its termination on the coccyx. Take care not to damage its delicate branches but identify the grey ramus communicans that it sends to the ventral ramus of each sacral nerve as the ramus emerges from the pelvic sacral foramen. If the superior hypogastric plexus can be identified anterior to the common iliac vessels, follow it to the inferior hypogastric plexus in the pelvis, and note any branches of the second to fourth sacral ventral rami (pelvic splanchnic nerves) passing to that plexus.

Clean the umbosacral trunk and each of the five sacral ventral rami in turn. Follow them inferolaterally on the piriformis muscle where they unite to form the sacral plexus.

Find and clean the two nerves (to quadratus femoris and obturator internus) that arise from the front of the sacral plexus, and follow them till they leave the pelvis through the greater sciatic foramen. Lift the sacral plexus forwards and clean it to its terminal branches (the sciatic and pudendal nerves). Then find and clean the branches that arise from the dorsal surface of the plexus. Trace part of the fourth sacral ventral ramus inferiorly to join the fifth and the coccygeal nerve and form the coccygeal plexus on the pelvic surface of coccygeus.

THE NERVES OF THE LESSER PELVIS

LUMBOSACRAL TRUNK

This is a thick cord formed from the entire ventral ramus of the fifth lumbar nerve and the descending part of the fourth. It descends obliquely over the ala of the sacrum into the pelvis (posterior to the pelvic fascia), and passing above the superior gluteal vessels across the pelvic surface of the sacro-iliac joint, joins the sacral ventral rami on the front of piriformis.

SACRAL AND COCCYGEAL VENTRAL RAMI

The upper four sacral ventral rami emerge through the pelvic sacral foramina; the fifth and coccygeal pierce the sacrospinous ligament and coccygeus, above and below the transverse process of the coccyx respectively. The first and second sacral ventral rami are large, the remainder diminish rapidly in size from above downwards.

The lumbosacral trunk and the **first sacral ventral ramus** are separated by the superior gluteal vessels, but both cross the pelvic surface of the sacro-iliac joint before passing on to the surface of piriformis to unite. Thus both may be involved in pathological changes in this joint. The first sacral ventral ramus is separated from the **second** by the inferior gluteal vessels, and the second, third, and part of the fourth lie between the anterior surface of piriformis and the pelvic fascia. They converge with the other nerves towards the lower part of the greater sciatic foramen, and form a solid triangular mass of nerve fibres and connective tissue (**the sacral plexus**), which splits into a smaller, medial, **pudendal nerve** and a larger, lateral, **sciatic nerve.** The other branches arise from the dorsal and pelvic surfaces of the plexus. The internal pudendal vessels descend across the front of the nerves, and the rectum (separated by pelvic fascia) overlaps these nerves from the third downwards. The remaining part of the fourth sacral ventral ramus turns inferiorly to join the coccygeal plexus on the surface of coccygeus.

Each ventral ramus receives a **grey ramus communicans** from the sympathetic trunk immediately on entering the pelvis, and before they unite in the plexus they give rise to certain branches: (1) twigs from the first and second to piriformis; (2) irregular branches from the others to coccygeus and levator ani; and (3) the pelvic splanchnic nerves.

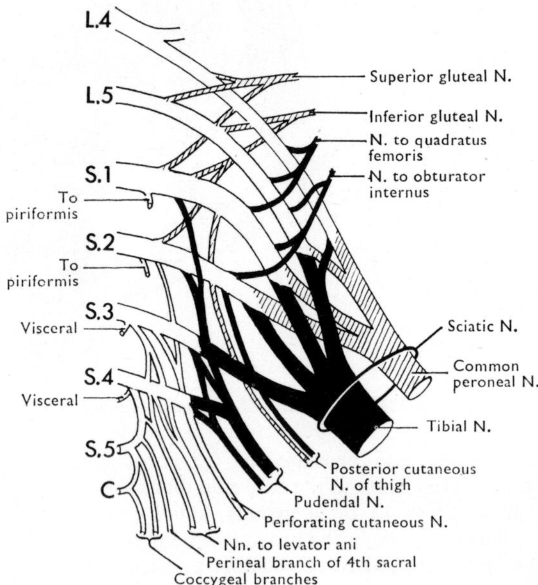

FIG. 229 A diagram of the sacral and coccygeal plexuses. Ventral divisions of the ventral rami, black; dorsal divisions, cross hatched. See also FIG. 178.

The **pelvic splanchnic nerves** are slender branches that pass from the third and fourth or second and third sacral ventral rami to the inferior hypogastric plexus. They consist of preganglionic parasympathetic fibres that are distributed through the peripheral parasympathetic ganglia to the pelvic viscera and to the descending and sigmoid parts of the colon.

Terminal Branches of Sacral Plexus

The **sciatic nerve** (L. 4, 5; S. 1, 2, 3) forms on the front of piriformis, and leaves the pelvis through the lower part of the greater sciatic foramen. In the back of the thigh it divides into **tibial** and **common peroneal nerves.** Occasionally this division occurs in the pelvis, in which case the common peroneal nerve usually pierces the piriformis as it leaves the pelvis. It may then be possible to demonstrate the origin of the tibial nerve from the ventral divisions of the ventral rami, and the common peroneal nerve from their dorsal divisions (c.f., femoral and obturator nerves).

The **pudendal nerve** (S. (1), 2, 3, 4) arises by separate branches from these ventral rami, and leaves the pelvis between piriformis and coccygeus; hooking round the sacrospinous ligament to pass into the perineum.

Nerves arising from the Pelvic Surface of the Plexus

The **nerve to quadratus femoris** (L. 4, 5; S. 1) passes out of the pelvis on the anterior surface of the sciatic nerve.

The **nerve to obturator internus** (L. 5; S. 1, 2) leaves the pelvis between the sciatic and pudendal nerves, and follows the latter into the ischiorectal fossa.

Nerves arising from Dorsal Surface of Plexus

The **superior gluteal nerve** (L. 4, 5; S. 1) arises above piriformis and accompanies the superior gluteal vessels.

The **inferior gluteal nerve** (L. 5; S. 1, 2) and the **posterior cutaneous nerve of the thigh** (S. 1, 2, 3) arise partly by the same roots. They leave the pelvis either immediately posterior or medial to the sciatic nerve.

The **perforating cutaneous nerve** (S. 2, 3) descends on piriformis and coccygeus. It then either pierces coccygeus or passes between it and levator ani to reach and pierce the sacrotuberous ligament and the overlying gluteus maximus. It supplies skin in the gluteal region.

The **perineal branch of the fourth sacral nerve** descends on coccygeus, pierces it, and passing deep to the sacrospinous and sacrotuberous ligaments, appears in the posterior angle of the ischiorectal fossa at the side of the coccyx. It passes forwards over the perineal surface of levator ani to supply the external anal sphincter and the surrounding skin.

Coccygeal Plexus (S. 4, 5; Co.)

This minute plexus lies on the pelvic surface of coccygeus. It supplies that muscle and part of levator ani, and piercing coccygeus and the ligaments, supplies the skin on the dorsum of the coccyx and between it and the anus.

OBTURATOR NERVE

[FIGS. 179, 227]

This nerve is formed from the ventral divisions of the ventral rami of the second, third, and fourth lumbar nerves in the substance of psoas. It descends behind psoas, and emerging from its medial aspect deep to the common iliac vessels, crosses the margin of the superior aperture of the pelvis, lateral to the ureter and the internal iliac vessels. It then runs antero-inferiorly over obturator internus, in front of the obturator artery and vein, and leaves the pelvis through the obturator canal. In the last part of its course it lies postero-lateral to the ovary (and may be involved in pathological changes in that organ), and is crossed either by the attachment of the broad ligament and the round ligament of the uterus or by the ductus deferens.

AUTONOMIC NERVES OF THE PELVIS

The Sympathetic Trunk

This descends into the pelvis over the medial part of the ala of the sacrum, and then crosses the medial margins of the pelvic sacral foramina to join its fellow in the median **ganglion impar** on the coccyx. At first posterior to the pelvic peritoneum and pelvic fascia, the rectum lies anterior to it below the third piece of the sacrum.

There are four sacral ganglia on each trunk and the common ganglion impar.

Branches. (1) Grey rami communicantes to all the sacral and coccygeal ventral rami. (2) Small filaments to the median sacral artery. (3) Branches to the inferior hypogastric plexuses from the upper ganglia. (4) Branches to the rectum from the lower ganglia. (5) Twigs to the glomus coccygeum from the ganglion impar.

Inferior Hypogastric Plexuses

The superior hypogastric plexus descends into the pelvis, and divides into two inferior hypogastric (pelvic) plexuses. Each of these surrounds the corresponding internal iliac artery, and receives branches from the upper sacral ganglia of the sympathetic trunk. The main plexus separates into subsidiary plexuses along the branches of the internal iliac artery (principally the visceral branches). These plexuses communicate with each other and receive branches from the **pelvic splanchnic nerves.** Small **ganglia** are found on these plexuses and their extensions on to the viscera.

Visceral Plexuses. These are extensions of the inferior hypogastric plexuses on to the walls of the pelvic viscera: (1) The **rectal plexus** receives a contribution from the inferior mesenteric plexus, and sends ascending parasympathetic fibres for distribution along the branches of the inferior mesenteric artery. (2) The **vesical plexus** is continuous with that over the ductus deferens and seminal vesicle, and inferiorly with the **prostatic plexus** which sends cavernous nerves (greater and lesser) along the membranous urethra to the penis. (3) The **uterine** and **vaginal plexuses** accompany the corresponding arteries, and the vaginal plexus also supplies the urethra, bulbs of the vestibule, and the clitoris.

DISSECTION. Clean the piriformis, define its attachment to the sacrum, and follow it till it disappears through the greater sciatic foramen. If the gluteal region is already dissected, follow piriformis to the greater trochanter of the femur on the posterior surface of the specimen. Identify the ischial spine [Fig. 184] and the fibres of coccygeus and levator ani that are attached to it [Fig. 231]. Turn the bladder, prostate (or uterus and vagina), and rectum medially, and complete the cleaning of the superior surface of levator ani. Take particular care posteriorly where the muscle is thin. Trace its fibres inferomedially to their insertion. With a finger in the ischiorectal fossa, determine the origin of the muscle from the ischial spine to the pelvic surface of the body of the pubis, across the fascia covering obturator internus. Clean the free medial border of the muscle, removing the attachment of the lateral part of the puboprostatic (pubovesical) ligament from the fascia covering levator ani.

THE MUSCLES OF THE LESSER PELVIS

Piriformis

This muscle arises from the pelvic surface of the second, third, and fourth pieces of the sacrum, lateral to and between the pelvic sacral foramina. Its fibres converge inferolaterally, to pass inferior to the sacro-iliac joint and through the greater sciatic foramen. In the gluteal region it crosses the posterior surface of the hip joint, and is inserted into the tip of the greater trochanter of the femur by a narrow tendon. Nerve supply: twigs from the ventral rami of the first and second sacral nerves. Action: it is one of the short muscles around the hip joint which help to stabilize that joint. It can act as a lateral rotator of the extended femur, or an abductor of the flexed femur.

Coccygeus Muscle

This is the muscular anterior part of the sacrospinous ligament. It passes from the ischial spine to the lateral margins of the last piece of the sacrum and the first piece of the coccyx. It lies along the inferior margin of piriformis (but is separated from it by the structures that leave the pelvis inferior to that muscle), and is edge to edge with the posterior border of levator ani. It thus forms the lowest part of the posterior wall of the pelvis, and together with levator ani, produces the muscular **pelvic diaphragm.** In many mammals, coccygeus and levator ani are both concerned with

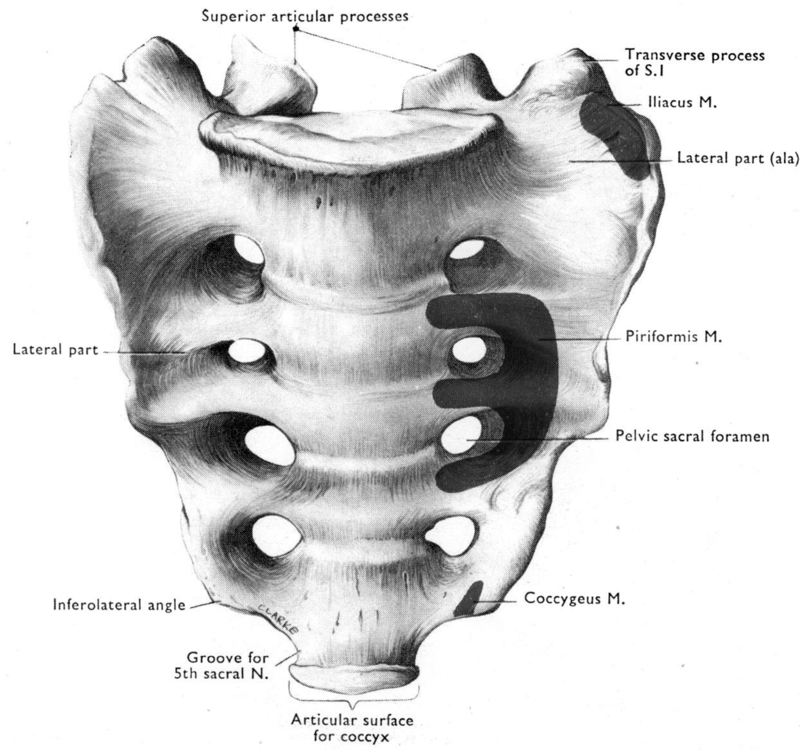

FIG. 230 The pelvic surface of the sacrum.

movements of the tail. With the loss of this organ in Man, coccygeus is virtually replaced by ligamentous tissue, and levator ani takes on an important role in supporting the pelvic floor in the erect posture. Nerve supply: coccygeus is supplied by the lower sacral ventral rami. Action: it may assist the sacrospinous ligament in supporting the pelvic contents, but it can only produce minor movements of the coccyx.

Levator Ani Muscle [FIGS. 204, 205, 219, 222, 225]

This is a wide, thin, curved sheet of muscle, which forms the floor of the pelvic cavity, and separates it from the ischiorectal fossa.

It has a long origin from the pelvic surface of the body of the pubic bone to the ischial spine, arising from the tendinous arch of the obturator fascia between these two bony points. The muscle fibres converge, and are inserted with the opposite muscle into the central perineal tendon, the anal canal, the anococcygeal ligament, and the coccyx. The anterior fibres, therefore, pass nearly horizontally backwards below the prostate (**levator prostatae**) and bladder or beside the vagina (**pubovaginalis**) to the central perineal tendon, and are separated from the muscle of the opposite side by a gap which transmits the urethra (and vagina). The posterior fibres run inferomedially; those that join the anal canal pass between the internal and external anal sphincters to join the longitudinal smooth muscle layer, and are inserted with it into the perianal skin. Those that pass to the anococcygeal ligament run inferior to the terminal part of the rectum and support it.

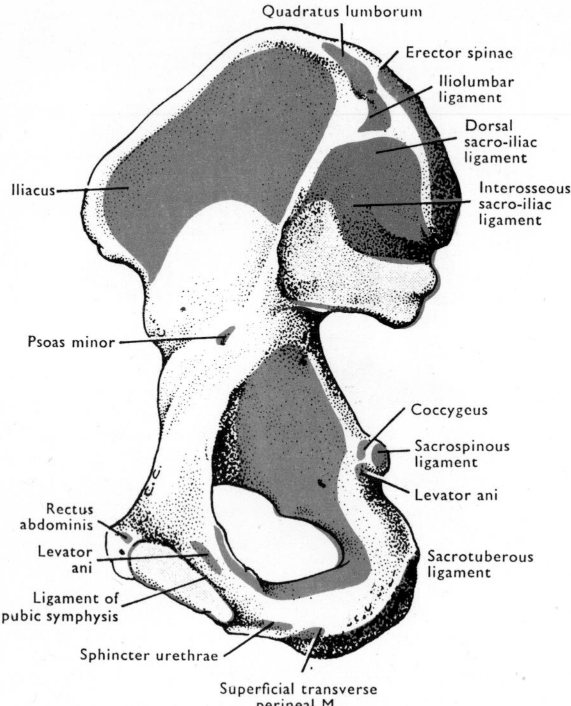

FIG. 231 The medial aspect of the right hip bone. Muscle attachments, red; ligamentous attachments, blue. The lower of the two large red areas indicates the attachment of obturator internus.

Part of the muscle that arises from the pubic bone forms a separate bundle which passes posteriorly on the upper surface of the other fibres of levator ani. It loops round the side and posterior surface of the anorectal junction to meet the corresponding fibres of the opposite muscle, and together they form a U-shaped sling, the **puborectalis muscle.**

Nerve supply: nerve fibres from the inferior rectal nerve enter the perineal surface, while the pelvic surface receives branches from the ventral rami of the coccygeal and lower sacral nerves.

Action: the two levator ani muscles act together to raise the pelvic diaphragm. This assists the muscles of the abdominal wall to compress the abdominal contents, *e.g.*, in forced expiration, vomiting, defaecation, and in fixing the trunk for strong movements of the upper limbs. The fibres that are inserted into the central perineal tendon support the prostate and the posterior wall of the vagina, and together with the bulbospongiosus muscles act as an incomplete sphincter of the vagina. The fibres that are inserted into the anal canal and central perineal tendon pull the canal over the descending mass of faeces. The **puborectalis** pulls the anorectal junction forwards, increases the angle between the rectum and the anal canal, and prevents the passage of faeces from the rectum into the anal canal. In childbirth, the whole muscle supports the head of the foetus during the dilatation of the cervix, and the anterior part may be torn as the head passes through the vagina.

DISSECTION. When the levator ani has been fully dissected, separate it from its origin and expose the full extent of the obturator fascia. Note the arrangement of this fascia, and cleaning it from the obturator internus, identify the pudendal canal with its contents and the attachment of the sacrotuberous ligament at its inferior margin. Clean the surface of obturator internus and trace its fibres to the lesser sciatic notch. Lift its tendon from the notch and identify the bursa between it and the bone.

Obturator Internus

This is a thick, fan-shaped muscle that covers most of the side wall of the lesser pelvis. It arises from the obturator membrane, the margins of the obturator foramen (except at the obturator sulcus), and a wide area between the obturator foramen and the greater sciatic notch, medial to the acetabulum. The fibres converge postero-inferiorly on a strong tendon that hooks round the bone of the lesser sciatic notch, and runs laterally over the posterior surface of the hip joint to the medial aspect of the greater trochanter. In this last part of its course, it is accompanied by the gemelli.

Nerve supply: a special nerve from the sacral plexus [p. 255]. Action: it helps to stabilize the hip joint, and acts as a lateral rotator of the femur in the erect posture, but abducts it when the hip joint is flexed.

Obturator Fascia. This dense layer of fascia covers the pelvic surface of obturator internus. It fuses with the periosteum at the margins of the muscle except: (1) at the obturator sulcus where it turns over the anterosuperior surface of the muscle to fuse with the obturator membrane and form the floor of the obturator canal which transmits the obturator vessels and nerve; and (2) postero-inferiorly where it joins the falciform process of the sacrotuberous ligament [Fig. 233].

It gives origin to most of the levator ani from the thickened **tendinous arch** between the ischial spine and the body of the pubis. Inferior to this it forms the lateral wall of the ischiorectal fossa, and splits to form the pudendal canal medial to the ischial tuberosity.

THE JOINTS OF THE PELVIS

The sacrum, coccyx, and hip bones make up the pelvis. The five pieces of the sacrum are fused together and are joined to the coccyx by the sacrococcygeal joint [p. 260]. The sacrum lies posterosuperiorly between the two hip bones, articulating with each at a sacro-iliac joint formed by the ilium and the lateral part of the sacrum. These joints are principally maintained by strong interosseous and dorsal sacro-iliac ligaments, but the sacrum and coccyx are also held in position relative to the hip bones by the sacrotuberous [p. 204] and sacrospinous [p. 204] ligaments [Fig. 232]. Anteriorly the hip bones are united in the pubic symphysis [p. 228]. Superiorly the sacrum is joined to the remainder of the vertebral column by the lumbosacral joints, which are further supported by the iliolumbar ligaments.

DISSECTION. The iliolumbar and dorsal sacro-iliac ligaments have already been partly cleaned [p. 203]. Complete the cleaning of these structures by removing all of erector spinae and the thoracolumbar fascia from the dorsal surface of the sacrum and fifth lumbar vertebra. Identify the ventral sacro-iliac ligament on the pelvic surface of the sacro-iliac joint, and if fusion between the ala of the sacrum and the ilium has not occurred, divide the ligament and open the joint by bending the sacrum backwards against the ilium. Identify the cartilage on the joint surfaces, and note the thinness of the ventral sacro-iliac ligament and the manner in which the apposed surfaces of the sacrum and ilium fit together so as to leave only the smallest room for movement.

Clean and then strip off the dorsal sacro-iliac ligaments to expose the interosseous sacro-iliac ligaments which lie deep to them. Divide the interosseous ligaments and separate the sacrum and ilium. Examine the joint surfaces again.

LUMBOSACRAL JOINTS

These joints are similar to those between the lumbar vertebrae [p. 87], but the lumbosacral intervertebral disc is more wedge-shaped than the others to take up the considerable angulation between the adjacent surfaces of the fifth lumbar vertebra and the sacrum [Fig. 209]. The stability of this articulation is increased by: (1) the widely spaced articular processes; and (2) the strong **iliolumbar ligament,** which extends from the stout transverse process of the fifth lumbar vertebra to the iliac crest, and fans inferiorly to the lateral part of the ala of the sacrum as the **lateral lumbosacral ligament** [Fig. 91].

This articulation is subject to a number of variations which can give rise to symptoms. The fifth lumbar vertebra or its transverse process may be fused on one or both sides with the sacrum, or the transverse process may articulate with the ala of the sacrum. The first sacral vertebra may be partly separated from the remainder of the sacrum. The normal sacral hiatus may extend superiorly into the lumbar region (spina bifida), thus weakening the neural arch of the fifth lumbar vertebra. Rarely the spine, laminae, and inferior articular processes of the fifth lumbar vertebra are separate from the remainder of the vertebra. This is a condition which allows the remainder of the fifth lumbar vertebra to slide forwards on the sloping superior surface of the sacrum (spondylolisthesis).

The **sacrococcygeal joint** has a narrow intervertebral disc and ligaments corresponding to the anterior and posterior longitudinal ligaments of the other intervertebral joints. The sacral and coccygeal cornua and transverse processes are also linked by ligaments, which may be ossified. The coccygeal joints are found in young subjects. They consist of intervertebral discs and ligaments, but they ossify early.

SACRO-ILIAC JOINT

The sacro-iliac joint is very strong, and is responsible for transmitting the weight of the body to the hip bones. It is a synovial joint of considerable complexity and little movement. The sacrum is wedged between the iliac bones so that the articular cartilage on the irregular auricular surfaces of both bones are tightly apposed and held in position by strong interosseous and dorsal sacro-iliac ligaments.

The weight of the body tends to drive the base of the sacrum downwards between the hip bones, thus tightening the sacro-iliac ligaments and drawing the articular surfaces closer together. The same force tends to tilt the apex of the sacrum upwards, but this is prevented by the **sacrotuberous** and **sacrospinous ligaments** [p. 204].

The **ventral sacro-iliac ligament** is a thin ribbon of transverse fibres between the convex margins of the articular surfaces. It does little more than close the abdominopelvic surface of the joint.

The **interosseous sacro-iliac ligaments** are very strong, and unite the wide, rough areas that adjoin the concave margins of the articular surfaces [FIGS. 184, 186]. They close the sacro-iliac joint dorsally.

The **dorsal sacro-iliac ligaments** are immediately superficial to the interosseous ligaments and fused with them. They consist of: (1) short transverse fibres that pass from the ilium to the first and second transverse tubercles of the sacrum; and (2) a longer, more vertical band from the posterior superior iliac spine to the third and fourth sacral transverse tubercles.

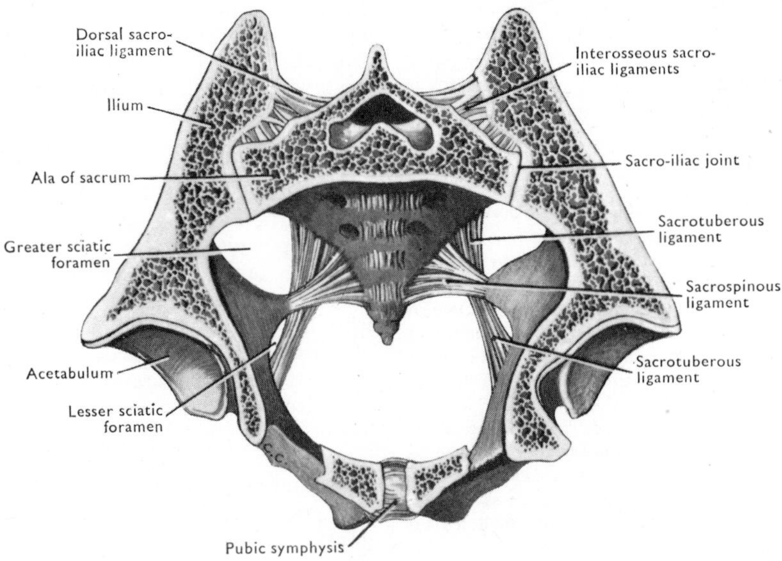

FIG. 232 An oblique section through the lesser pelvis to show the ligaments and sacro-iliac joints.

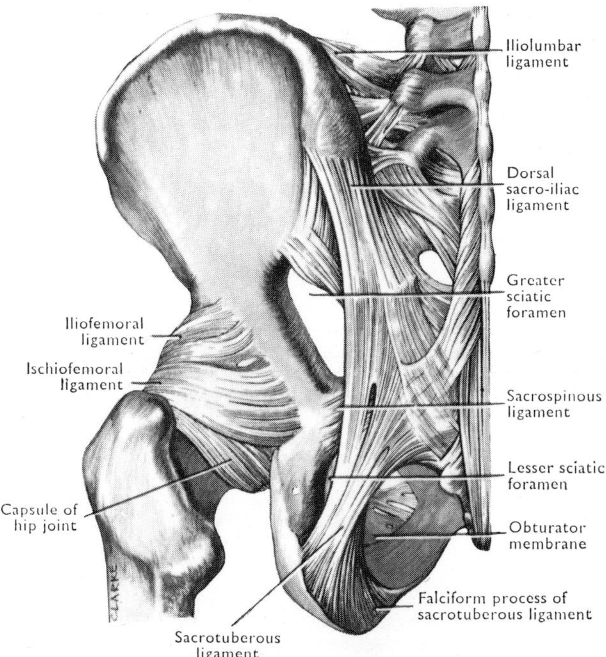

FIG. 233 Dorsal view of the pelvic ligaments and the hip joint.

The latter blends with the medial edge of the sacrotuberous ligament.

Posteriorly the joint is covered by the erector spinae and gluteus maximus muscles. The skin dimple marking the posterior superior iliac spine lies opposite the middle of the joint, while the posterior inferior spine marks the posterior and most superficial part of the joint.

The abdominal surface of the joint is covered by iliacus and psoas, with the obturator and femoral nerves close to it. The pelvic surface is crossed by the lumbosacral trunk and the first sacral ventral ramus. Both of these may be involved in disease of the joint and give rise to pain which is felt in the distribution of these nerves, *i.e.*, below the knee. The internal iliac vein and the superior gluteal vessels are also in contact with the pelvic surface of the joint.

Movement at the joint is limited to a slight rotation towards the end of full flexion of the trunk and the hip joints, as in touching the toes, but the main function is to prevent the direct transmission to the vertebral column of forces applied to the feet, and thus to cushion the shock. The joint may become ossified with increasing age, especially in males.

In some animals, and possibly also in Man, the sacro-iliac ligaments become softer and more yielding in the later stages of pregnancy. They share this property with the pubic symphysis and sacrococcygeal ligaments, and the combined effect facilitates the passage of the foetus through the pelvis at term.

INDEX

Entries in bold refer to the pages on which the major descriptions are given; those followed by an asterisk indicate the pages on which the bones are illustrated.